Perceptions of Health and Illness

Perceptions of Health and Illness

Current Research and Applications

Edited by

Keith J. Petrie
The Faculty of Medicine and Health Science,
The University of Auckland, Auckland, New Zealand

and

John A. Weinman
United Medical and Dental Schools, London, United Kingdom

harwood academic publishers
Australia • Canada • China • France • Germany • India • Japan
Luxembourg • Malaysia • The Netherlands • Russia • Singapore
Switzerland • Thailand • United Kingdom

Copyright © 1997 OPA (Overseas Publishers Association) Amsterdam B.V. Published in The Netherlands by Harwood Academic Publishers.

Amsteldijk 166
1st Floor
1079 LH Amsterdam
The Netherlands

British Library Cataloguing in Publication Data

Perceptions of health and illness : current research and
    applications
    1. Medicine and psychology   2. Sick — Psychology
    I. Petrie, Keith J.   II. Weinman, John A.
    610.1'9

    ISBN 90-5702-102-1 (Hardcover)

Contents

List of Contributors

Charles Abraham
School of Social Science, University of Sussex, Brighton, UK

Yael Benyamini
Department of Psychology and Institute for Health, Rutgers University, New Jersey, USA

Susan Brownlee
Department of Psychology and Institute for Health, Rutgers University, New Jersey, USA

Deanna L. Buick
Department of Psychiatry and Behavioural Science, The University of Auckland, New Zealand

Linda D. Cameron
Department of Psychology, Saint Joseph's University, Pennsylvania, USA

Melissa Crouch
Department of Psychology and Institute for Health, Rutgers University, New Jersey, USA

Robert T. Croyle
Department of Psychology, University of Utah, Utah, USA

Kathryn P. Davison
Psychology Department, Southern Methodist University, Dallas, Texas, USA

Michael Diefenbach
Department of Psychology and Institute for Health, Rutgers University, New Jersey, USA

Christine Eiser
Department of Psychology, University of Exeter, UK

Sarah E. Hampson
Department of Psychology, University of Surrey, Guildford, UK

Marybeth Hart
Department of Psychology, University of Utah, Utah, USA

Robert Horne
John Harris Clinical Pharmacy Unit, University of Brighton, UK

Marie Johnston
Department of Psychology, University of St Andrews, Fife, Scotland UK

Adrian Kaptein
Department of Psychiatry, University of Leiden, The Netherlands

Sheryl J. Kopel
Department of Psychology, University of Exeter, UK

Elaine A. Leventhal
Department of Medicine, University of Medicine and Dentistry of New Jersey, New Jersey, USA

Howard Leventhal
Centre for Research on Health and Behavior, Institute for Health, Rutgers University, New Jersey, USA

Theresa M. Marteau
Psychology and Genetics Research Group, United Medical and Dental Schools, Guy's Campus, London, UK

Rona Moss-Morris
Department of Psychiatry and Behavioural Science, The University of Auckland, New Zealand

Linda Patrick-Miller
Department of Psychology and Institute for Health, Rutgers University, New Jersey, USA

James W. Pennebaker
Psychology Department, Southern Methodist University, Dallas, Texas, USA

Keith J. Petrie
Department of Psychiatry and Behavioural Science, The University of Auckland, New Zealand

Theo J. Pimm
Principal Clinical Psychologist, Community Physical Rehabilitation Services, Aylesbury, UK

Chantal Robitaille
Department of Psychology and Institute for Health, Rutgers University, New Jersey, USA

Margreet Scharloo
Department of Psychiatry, University of Leiden, The Netherlands

Vicky Senior
Psychology and Genetics Research Group, United Medical and Dental Schools, Guy's Campus, London, UK

Paschal Sheeran
Department of Psychology, University of Sheffield, UK

Yi-Chun Sun
Department of Psychology, University of Utah, Utah, USA

John A. Weinman
Unit of Psychology, United Medical and Dental Schools, Guy's Campus, London, UK

Acknowledgements

In this book we have endeavoured to draw together a field that has developed rapidly over the preceding few years and to provide a comprehensive and up-to-date overview of psychological research on illness perceptions. All the invited authors have made a significant recent contribution in this area and we are indebted to them for providing such excellent chapters within the tight time limit which we set. We are particularly grateful for the effort and expertise of Denise Reynolds who assisted tremendously in bringing the book to completion and also to Max Wong for her cover illustration. Finally we wish to thank our close colleagues and collaborators Roger Booth, Rob Horne, Rob Kydd, Rona Moss-Morris and Jamie Pennebaker for their continued good humour and support.

Perceptions of Health and Illness

John A. Weinman & Keith J. Petrie*

Changes in the landscape of health care over the past 20 years have been of great significance for research in the field of illness perceptions. The importance of psychological factors in the management of chronic illnesses has received increasing attention in the health field. There has been a greater emphasis on prevention of disease in healthy populations and on understanding and improving rates of adherence to treatment programmes in those with chronic conditions. Advances in the field of·genetics are offering patients and their health care providers greater options in the areas of screening and prevention. These changes have increasingly challenged the established view of the patient as a passive and obliging participant in the health care process. Patients now have higher expectations of health care providers to be informed about diagnosis and treatments as well as having their views taken into account in medical interactions.

These changes are compatible with the illness perceptions approach which sees the patient as an active participant in the health care process. The field has been well served by Leventhal's seminal theoretical work examining how patients evaluate health threats by constructing their own representations or perceptions

*The authors wish to express warm thanks to Denise Reynolds for her expert assistance in preparing the manuscripts for this book.

which influence their patterns of coping. A book by Skelton and Croyle (1991) gathered together much of the available research in the field at that time. Since then the area has expanded rapidly and we believe it is timely to gather these major threads of research together. In particular, there is now sufficient research in specific areas to merit separate coverage of these. For example a number of diseases have been investigated from an illness perception perspective and good examples of this can be seen in the final section of this book. Similarly there is now a growing and influential body of work on the importance of cognitive processes in determining the response to health screening and preventive initiatives in health care, and this area forms the focus of the second section of this book. The opening section sets the scene for the whole book by reviewing a number of basic conceptual, theoretical, and methodological issues.

ILLNESS PERCEPTION THEORY AND MEASUREMENT

The papers in the first section of the book provide a background to the more applied contributions in the following two sections. Quite appropriately the opening chapter is from Howard Leventhal and his colleagues. This begins by examining the origins of the illness perceptions approach arising from early research on the rather minimal impact of fear messages in relation to responses to health threats. This early work quickly raised the possibility that there was parallel processing of health information, since it indicated that the cognitive representations of the threat and the emotional representation (e.g. fear arousal) could be processed independently. It also identified the need to distinguish the cognitive representations of the threat from the actions or action plans necessary for dealing with it. This distinction between cognitive representations, emotional responses, and action plans underpins a great deal of current work in this area and is a theme which runs through a number of other chapters in the book, particularly in the second section. Further early work led to the notion that illness representations contained a number of discrete attributes (i.e. identity; cause; time-line; consequences; controllability) which provided the basis for the coping responses or procedures for dealing with the health threat. Thus, in being faced with a situation such as the experience of an unusual symptom, or the provision of a diagnosis from a doctor, individuals will construct their own representation which, in turn, will determine their behaviour and other responses, including help-seeking and medicine-taking. In addition to representations of the threat, the individual will also draw upon their expectations and beliefs about the different behavioural choices, including adherence to prescribed medicines. In a later chapter, Robert Horne provides further evidence about the role of medicines beliefs in influencing people's willingness to adhere to recommended treatment.

These cognitive, emotional, and behavioural responses are self-regulatory in that they both impinge upon and are influenced by the individual's self concept. Thus health threats can have major effects on self-perception but also appraisals of health threat can be moderated by such factors as personality (e.g. optimism) and age. Although the main focus of this work has been on the individual, taking a psychological perspective, it is clear that social and cultural factors shape both the appraisal processes and the behaviours chosen for controlling or dealing with the situation. In the final section of their paper, Leventhal and colleagues stress the importance of understanding self-regulatory processes within the social and cultural contexts in which they occur. This is identified as a key area for future work and is consistent with the need for health psychology to move more strongly in this direction (Landrine & Klonoff, 1992).

From this opening chapter it becomes clear that representations of health threats are a function of an individual's semantic knowledge (e.g. relation of symptoms to diseases; understanding of disease and treatment options etc.), and specific contextual factors such as the nature of somatic changes and the situations in which these occur. This semantic knowledge accumulates across the lifespan and the symptoms and contexts will vary as a function of the age and social circumstances of individuals. These developing and cumulative aspects of health and illness related cognitions are addressed directly in the next two chapters.

The chapter by Christine Eiser and Sheryl Kopel is concerned with the way children gain an understanding of the concepts of health and illness. While much of the earlier work on this used a

Piagetian framework for describing different developmental stages in this understanding, more recent studies encourage a move away from a purely cognitive, stage-based approach. There is an increasing awareness of the importance of the child's own experience and the realisation that children develop accurate, functional accounts of illness-related events. Rather than seeing a child's developmental stage as the key determinant of their thinking about health and illness it is becoming clear that at any age or stage children can differ in these beliefs about health and illness. They provide examples of this in their discussion of children's perceptions of control, risk, and personal vulnerability. These insights into children's understanding can be used in various ways for developing health education campaigns and in the delivery of effective health care. From their chapter it becomes clear that children's experiences and social circumstances are of great importance in determining how they make sense of and respond to health and illness information. Knowledge and understanding do evolve but in a less orderly and stage-based approach than previously proposed and parents can play a crucial role in providing information and support, as well as behavioural models. Rather than regarding children as emerging but imperfect versions of adults, we need to understand them as self-regulating individuals who are capable of making decisions and choices on the basis of their own representations of health threats and illness. As with any self-regulatory process, there is also a need to understand the role of immediate (e.g. family circumstances; parental behaviour) and broader social and cultural contexts for understanding children's health and illness behaviour.

The following chapter by Elaine Leventhal and Melissa Crouch examines changes in self-regulatory processes in relation to health and illness across the lifespan, with a particular focus on older people. They provide evidence of a complex set of interacting cognitive, biological, and contextual factors which can be used to explain changing patterns of help-seeking and health care utilisation in older people. This evidence indicates that these changing patterns are not a direct effect of ageing per se but a reflection of age-related modifications in the way symptoms are perceived and evaluated, resulting in more benign attributions and possible delays in help-seeking. However, compensatory behaviours, based around an increased sense of vulnerability combined with the need to reduce health risks and conserve personal resources, ensure that older people show higher levels of most preventive behaviours and better adherence to treatment. With a marked increase in the proportion of older people in many countries, there is an urgent need to optimise the planning and organisation of preventive services and health care delivery. A good awareness of the understanding and self-regulatory processes of older people will be vital in this respect, and this chapter provides some important insights.

One of the problems confronting researchers investigating illness perceptions is the task of eliciting and measuring people's cognitions. The original work used semi-structured interviews to identify the different dimension of illness perception and some studies still use this approach. Recently a theoretically-based questionnaire has become available and this can provide a convenient and valid measure of all five dimensions (Weinman, Petrie, Moss-Morris & Horne, 1996). However, the question of what to measure and the choice of method is an important one which is examined critically in the chapter by Margareet Scharloo and colleagues. They have conducted a systematic review of recent studies on the assessment of illness perceptions in chronic illness, using appropriate databases from 1985 to 1995. Their search has unearthed a large number of studies and provides clear indications about the focus and methods of existing research. Of the five dimensions of illness perception, perceived control is the mostly widely studied and chronic pain patients were the most frequently investigated group. Most studies are restricted to the assessment of one or two dimensions and very little work has examined the relations between dimensions. However, there do appear to be some consistent relations between different illness perception dimensions and different health outcomes. These are explored in much more detail in the chapters in Section 3, each of which focuses on a specific health problem, including cancer, chronic fatigue syndrome, diabetes, arthritis and heart disease.

The survey of methodologies for assessing illness cognitions highlights the range of methods and approaches which have been developed. Since this area of research is still very much in a developing phase it is not surprising that no 'gold standard' measure has emerged yet. Moreover there is a need for studies which compare the reliability and validity of different approaches, in order to provide researchers with a basis for choosing an appropriate method for a particular study. In the same way that Jensen *et al.* (1986)

have provided a critical comparison of methods for assessing pain, there is now a need for evaluative and comparison studies of illness perception assessment methods. There is also a need to determine what other cognitions and related processes need to be incorporated into adequate models of health and illness behaviour. From the pioneering work of Howard Leventhal and his colleagues, there is clearly a consensus about the five dimensions of illness perception but there is a growing awareness of other processes which need to be incorporated into explanatory models. For example, in addition to assessing illness perceptions, there is a need to understand people's views about the treatment or advice they are given.

A particular need to understand patient's beliefs about their treatment arises from the relatively high rates of non-adherence which have been reported widely (Meichenbaum & Turk, 1987). This forms the starting point for Robert Horne's chapter which reviews older work on people's beliefs about medicines and reports the development of new measures to assess these beliefs. The majority of previous work is qualitative and, although it has been based on diverse clinical groups in a wide range of contexts, it has provided consistent evidence that there are widespread beliefs about the positive therapeutic gains as well as the potentially harmful effects of medicine taking. Robert Horne has developed new scales which measure these positive and negative beliefs not only about medicines in general, but also about specific prescribed medicines. Using these scales, he has been able to demonstrate their predictive value in explaining treatment adherence and has developed an augmented version of Leventhal's self-regulatory model, in which medicines beliefs combine with illness representations as determinants of medicine taking. His data are consistent with those of Leventhal, in that the concrete experiences of different illnesses and their treatments are instrumental in generating different illness and medicines representations which, in turn, are associated with particular patterns of coping and medication adherence.

In the final chapter of the first section, Marie Johnston explores the role of patients' cognitions as determinants of disability. Starting with dissatisfaction with the World Health Organisation (WHO) model of disability, which postulates a direct relationship between impairment and disability, she develops a psychological model. This is built on the premise that since the WHO model defines disability in behavioural terms, then it is necessary to search for psychological determinants (i.e. cognitions; emotions). She begins by examining the role of cognitions and coping as predictors of behavioural impairment, using the self-regulatory model as a basis, but only finds partial success with this. In common with a number of other recent studies (e.g. Moss-Morris, Petrie & Weinman, 1996), cognitions, particularly control cognitions, are found to predict level of disability but they do not appear to do this by their effects on coping, as would be predicted by the Self-Regulatory Model. An alternative model (The Theory of Planned Behaviour — Ajzen, 1988) is proposed for linking the cognitive predictors and behavioural concomitants of disability. In doing this she recognises the lack of attention in existing cognitive models to what Schwarzer (1992) calls "the action phase" of health behaviour which focuses directly on the factors which determine whether a specific behaviour is engaged in. This focus on behaviour is obviously a key issue in understanding disability and in developing successful rehabilitation programmes. A model of disability based on cognitions, emotions, and the organisation and planning of behaviour will not only provide a more complete understanding of how impairments create disability but will also provide pointers for new ways of intervening to improve functioning.

ILLNESS PERCEPTIONS IN PREVENTION AND HEALTH SCREENING

Research on health and illness perception has two distinct origins. Work on illness perception has developed from studies examining the sense that people make of health threats and symptoms and how these act as a guide for coping responses, such as help-seeking and treatment adherence (see the opening chapter in the book by Leventhal and colleagues). Studies of health related behaviour in healthy populations have examined the role of different cognitions in explaining the wide variations which have been reported in the adoption of preventive health behaviour (Connor & Norman, 1996). Health screening lies somewhere between these two areas of work since people may enter screening as healthy but emerge with a possible or actual threat to their health. Health screening is therefore of particular interest in research on health and illness cognitions since it offers the chance to examine changes in cognition at a clearly defined point in time that lies somewhere between the perception of health and of illness or health threat.

The four chapters in this section of the book examine cognitive processes in health screening and preventive contexts. The first chapter in this section by Charles Abraham and Paschal Sheeran and final one by Linda Cameron have a common starting point in that they both begin by evaluating the contribution of traditional social cognition models to the explanation of health-related behaviour. Whereas Linda Cameron recognises their limitations in taking account of emotional responses, Charles Abraham and Paschal Sheeran perceive the limitations of these models in failing to explain how actions are initiated and carried out.

They begin by examining the contribution social cognition models have made to our understanding of preventive behaviour. They note that widely used models such as the Health Belief Model, focus on the salience of a health threat together with some general evaluations of the associated behaviour change but provide little or no direct insight into the cognitive precursors of the action process. Some insights into these precursors can be gained from considering cognitions such as specific self-efficacy beliefs (Bandura, 1986) which can influence intentions to engage in a behaviour as well as the likelihood of the behaviour itself. Their chapter reveals the move from a concern with the processes involved in the appraisal of health threats and the appropriateness of a particular action toward an understanding of the cognitive underpinnings of action regulation. They emphasize the importance of planning specific actions in relation to particular anticipated contexts but question the utility of stage models of action generation. Finally, they highlight a core set of cognitive measures which are likely to distinguish between those who do and those who do not adopt preventive health behaviours.

In the second chapter, Theresa Marteau and Vicky Senior focus on one specific cognitive process, namely, the adoption of causal explanations for a real or potential threat to health arising from a screening test. Earlier studies (e.g. Turnquist *et al.*, 1988) have reported that a greater number of attributions are reported by more distressed individuals, but the nature of this relationship is still unclear. Theresa Marteau and Vicky Senior concentrate more on the nature of attributions which are chosen and their psychological impact on those who are affected. They also consider attributional processes and their effects in significant others, such as spouses and health care professionals. Their exploration of attributional processes emphasizes the direct links between the beliefs about the cause of an event and the subsequent perception of control over that event or future ones, as well as the role of these perceptions as determinants of future health behaviour. However, the primary emphasis of their chapter is on what happens to attributions and subsequent behaviour in genetic screening tests, where one specific attribution, namely a genetic cause, is provided for those who are screened positive. Their focus on this is extremely timely, given the rapid recent developments in molecular biology and screening tests for diseases with a known genetic basis. Their studies show that, although genetic explanations are commonly adopted by individuals to explain the onset of illness, causal attributions for genetically-based conditions are more complex than would be expected. Even when a condition has been identified as having been genetically transmitted, other possible causal attributions (e.g. stress; past behaviour etc.) may still continue to be held. At the same time, potentially protective health behaviours may be evaluated as less viable or worthwhile since a genetic condition is seen as less controllable or preventable.

In the following chapter Robert Croyle and colleagues describe ways in which individual representations of health threats can become distorted or less accessible following the receipt of positive information from health screening tests, such as a cholesterol check. They have investigated detection behaviour and responses to real-life and laboratory-based screening tests. Their studies reveal a very consistent tendency, in those identified as being at risk, to play down or minimise the severity of the health threat or condition being tested for. Individuals tested positive will typically rate the health threat as less serious than comparison groups who have been tested negative. Shortly after being screened positive, they are also more likely to rate the risk factor as being more common, to perceive the test as unreliable and the health threat as relatively short-term. This "threat minimisation" or "defensiveness" also extends to recall, with test results being remembered as relatively less threatening, particularly at higher levels of risk or threat. Distortions of recall have also been found in recent follow-up studies of people undergoing genetic screening (Axworthy *et al.*, 1996). As Croyle and colleagues point out, the clinical significance of these cognitive biases requires further investigation, particularly since patients' perceptions of risk and recall of past medical information are relied on in many clinical situations.

The chapter by Croyle and colleagues raises the question of the relation between cognition and emotion, and the way responses to screening can be understood within a self-regulatory framework in which independent cognitive and emotional processes may be triggered by a new and threatening health message. While increased vulnerability in the form of a positive screening test result causes emotional activation, threat minimisation, and memory distortion, it can also increase the search for threat-relevant information. In general, illness perceptions research has concentrated more on the cognitive representation than on the representation of emotion, and this limitation is addressed in Linda Cameron's chapter which focuses on screening and preventive behaviour in relation to breast cancer. She acknowledges the role of rational cognitive processes in appraising health threats and in influencing levels of perceived vulnerability, but she extends this to show that vulnerability beliefs serve to activate further cognitive and emotional responses within a dynamic, self-regulatory system. In the latter, vulnerability beliefs trigger the cognitive processes involved in constructing an internal representation of the health threat or actual illness while concurrently giving rise to emotional responses such as fear and worry, which may either motivate adaptive behaviours (e.g. breast self-examination) or result in avoidance as a means of coping. She presents data from two studies, one involving breast cancer screening in "at risk" women and the other investigates the role of symptoms in influencing breast self examination in women in remission from breast cancer. Her results fit well within a self-regulatory framework, in which cognitive and emotional responses are generated by symptoms and other health threats, including increased vulnerability beliefs.

ILLNESS PERCEPTIONS IN ILLNESS AND TREATMENT

The final section of the book contains work that has applied the illness perception approach to clinical problems and populations. For those working in health settings this may be the section that holds the most interest. These papers represent examples of how illness perception models may be used in a wide variety of clinical situations to improve the day-to-day management of physical illness, to minimise the effect of noxious treatment protocols, and to better understand the psychological processes involved in the development and maintenance of chronic illnesses. This section contains contributions from the leading researchers currently doing work in this area.

While the numbers of researchers using an illness perception approach with clinical populations have to date been small, this number is growing rapidly. One of the difficulties in working with clinical populations has been the lack of an efficient means of assessing illness perceptions. The publication of the *Illness Perceptions Questionnaire* (Weinman *et al.*, 1996) has been helpful in facilitating research work with clinical populations. Three of the chapters in the final section report on work that has used this scale. The development of other assessment methodologies designed for specific illnesses or treatments is likely to increase in the future. Examples of this trend in the book are the *Personal Models of Diabetes Interview* developed by Sarah Hampson and her colleagues, and the *Beliefs about Medicines Questionnaire* produced by Rob Horne. We are aware of a growing number of other researchers in many countries who currently have projects underway investigating illness perceptions in patients suffering from physical illness. The time may not be far away when books like this one will be focused entirely on clinical applications of the illness perceptions approach. The final section contains chapters that demonstrate the application of the illness perceptions approach to a wide number of chronic illness groups. Chapters include work on breast cancer, diabetes, arthritis, chronic fatigue syndrome (CFS), and myocardial infarction patients. Also included in this section is a chapter that presents an innovative examination of illness representations by studying the exchanges of support groups for chronic illness on the Internet. This chapter, written by Kathy Davidson and James Pennebaker, examines on-line support groups for arthritis, CFS, heart disease, prostrate cancer, breast cancer and diabetes.

Diabetes is a particularly interesting chronic disease to examine in the context of illness perceptions as a patient's day-to-day perceptions of symptoms are critical in the awareness and self-management of hyper- and hypoglycoemic states. Also, the treatment protocol for managing insulin-dependent diabetes mellitus is in its purest form an example of a self-regulatory process in action. Sarah Hampson, in her chapter describes how the illness representation approach has been used to assess the five components of identity, cause, time-line, control/cure, and consequences. She has used the *Personal Models of Diabetes Interview* to assess differences in personal beliefs in diabetes patients about their illness and to relate these to aspects of self-management. Her review of other studies of health cognitions in diabetes shows that patients' beliefs can influence various aspects of self-management. Her own work demonstrates that personal models of diabetes are related to adherence to recommended dietary restrictions and to levels of physical activity. Perceived treatment effectiveness was found to be the most consistently predictive attribute of illness representations for these two behavioural outcomes.

In recent years a number of psychological interventions have been developed to help people with arthritis manage their illness. Some of these have focused on improving control over specific symptoms, such as pain, but others have taken a broader approach and sought to facilitate coping and self-management with a wider range of symptoms and related problems. John Pimm is currently evaluating a self-management intervention for people with rheumatic disease and is assessing the extent to which therapeutic gains depend on patients' illness perceptions. In his chapter he demonstrates the importance of illness perceptions in determining coping, mood, and well-being in patients with rheumatic diseases. He also reviews a range of psycho-educational interventions and relates their efficacy to different self-regulatory processes, as a basis for outlining his ongoing studies.

Early research on the response of lymphoma patients to chemotherapy by Nerenz, Leventhal, Love and Ringler (1984) was instrumental in the development of the self-regulatory model. Nerenz *et al.* found patients who experienced a rapid reduction in their lymph nodes during chemotherapy to be more distressed than patients who had a more gradual decrease in symptoms. These results, which suggested patients' emotional reactions were the result of a personal illness model in which symptoms defined disease, have been extended by Deanna Buick in her work with breast cancer patients. Buick has been examining the association between illness beliefs and the psychological response to radiotherapy and chemotherapy treatments. She has found interesting differences in causal beliefs between the two treatment groups.

Her study also found that negative illness beliefs were associated with a poor psychological response to cancer treatment. Another important aspect of her work is the striking discrepancy between the stereotypes of women with breast cancer held by both medical staff and lay people and the actual experience of patients. This has significant implications for the information and support services offered to women with breast cancer.

Rona Moss-Morris, in her chapter, examines how illnesses perceptions may play an important role in the development and maintenance of chronic fatigue syndrome (CFS). CFS is a controversial illness that has a devastating effects on the lives of sufferers. This illness has defied satisfactory explanation in terms of either current viral or psychiatric models. In her work, Moss-Morris has investigated the differences in illness perceptions between CFS and clinically depressed patients. She has found quite distinct patterns of illness representations in CFS patients that remain stable and, more importantly, have strong associations with disability. She has also found distinct differences in cognitive errors and distortions between CFS and depressed subjects that may help explain how CFS is maintained over time.

The individual's experience of a heart attack and the later rehabilitation phase offer considerable potential for the application of an illness perceptions approach. In our own chapter we show how illness perceptions can be applied to understand treatment delay after symptoms are first experienced. We also discuss how the relationship of causal beliefs about the illness by both the patient and spouse relate to later changes in health behaviours. Return to work and function have been important concerns for clinicians working with MI patients as many patients remain functionally disabled despite being medically fit. Cardiac rehabilitation programmes have been shown to make a positive impact on many patients following MI. However, a considerable number of patients either do not attend or drop out from courses early. We describe a recently completed study showing that the patient's view of their illness is an important factor in both rehabilitation attendance and in how quickly patients return to work following their MI.

The Internet is changing the way many people access information and has also provided a new gateway of support for patients suffering from chronic illness. Sufferers and their families can ask for advice, share their concerns, and disseminate information to a growing audience of fellow netizens. In their chapter Kathryn Davison and James Pennebaker have looked at what the language used in Internet illness support groups tells us about the generation and maintenance of illness perceptions. Through the use of a text analysis program and a more qualitative examination, they show quite strong differences between different patient illness groups in the way they use language on the Net and the priorities given to various issues. Perhaps more importantly, this chapter presents a new research area to health psychologists interested in how individuals organise and communicate their ideas about illness and its effect on their lives.

Current Issues in Clinical Applications of Illness Perceptions

There are a number of important issues raised by the clinical chapters in the book. The first is a methodological one. That is, what is the most effective way to categorise patterns of illness perceptions in a more global way so as to capture a more coherent picture of the person's view of their illness? Previous research and much of the current work represented in this book indicate that certain patterns of illness perceptions may be associated with better psychological and physical outcomes. However, a difficulty facing researchers is how to efficiently describe recurring patterns of illness beliefs. For example, individuals may view their illness as having serious effects, being long lasting, and being accompanied by a large number of debilitating symptoms. It is likely that the combination of illness beliefs is the most important factor in determining behaviour and adjustment as noted by Sarah Hampson in her studies of diabetic patients. The categorisation of different patterns of illness perceptions has been attempted through the use of cluster analysis by Deanna Buick and also by Rona Moss-Morris. Cluster analysis is used here to separate patients into coherent groups based on the similarity of aspects of their individual illness perceptions. This approach does seem to have considerable potential for capturing differences between individuals. Bishop (1991) used a somewhat related approach, that of multidimensional scaling, to examine the cognitive organisation of diseases.

Perhaps the most intriguing question that comes out of the clinical applications presented in this section is how can we effectively change illness beliefs? It is clear from this research that illness perceptions are important determinants of outcome and adjustment in chronic illness. The next challenge for researchers in this area is to demonstrate that interventions designed to change illness perceptions impact positively on outcome. While there is little work available that has examined this question directly, it is likely many existing effective interventions in the chronic illness area act by influencing illness perceptions. In fact, a number of interventions have been specifically developed to get patients to think differently about their illness. Intervention programmes using cognitive behavioural techniques have now been developed for patients suffering from chronic pain (Williams *et al.*, 1993), chronic fatigue syndrome (Sharpe *et al.*, 1996), arthritis (O'Leary, Shoor, Lorig & Holman, 1988; Pimm, this volume), and other illnesses. Indeed the illness perceptions approach may be able to provide a more adequate explanation for the positive changes occurring after participation in such interventions (Lorig *et al.*, 1989). Rather than re-invent the wheel, researchers developing future interventions directed at changing illness perceptions may be advised to examine previous interventions with illness populations and develop programmes based on established cognitive-behavioural techniques such as cognitive restructuring and behavioural assignments.

Earlier in this introductory chapter we noted the considerable progress which has been made in this area of research and the chapters which follow provide impressive evidence of this. Nevertheless many important questions remain about the cognitive and emotional processes involved in people's perceptions of health and illness. Similarly there are still many unresolved issues concerning the best methods for investigating these perceptions, as well as applying them in clinical settings. If we encourage health care practitioners to be more patient-centred and to pay attention to patients' ideas and beliefs, then the approaches outlined in this book can provide an excellent basis for this. Moreover if we want to make sense of the factors which help and hinder responses to screening and treatment, then many of the insights from the current work will be invaluable. If this can be achieved we will not only be able to gain a greater understanding of health-related behaviour but also be able to use this to provide a more effective delivery of health care.

REFERENCES

Axworthy, D., Brock, D.J.H., Bobrow, M. & Marteau, T.M. (1996) Psychological impact of population based carrier testing for cystic fibrosis: three year follow-up. *The Lancet,* **347**, 1443–1446.

Azjen, I. (1988) *Attitudes, personality and behaviour.* Milton Keynes: Open Univ. Press.

Bandura, A. (1986) *Social foundations of thought and action.* Englewood Cliffs, NJ: Prentice Hall.

Bishop, G. (1991) Understanding the understanding of illness: lay disease representations. In J.A. Skelton & R.T. Croyle (Eds.), *Mental representation in health and illness.* New York: Springer Verlag.

Connor, M. & Norman, P. (Eds.), (1996) *Predicting health behaviour.* Buckingham: Open Univ. Press.

Jensen, M.P., Karoly, P. & Braver, S. (1986) The measurement of pain intensity: a comparison of six methods. *Pain,* **27**, 117–126.

Landrine, H. & Klonoff, A. (1992) Culture and health related schemas: a review and proposal for interdisciplinary integration. *Health Psychology,* **11**, 267–276.

Lorig, L., Seleznick, M., Lubeck, D., Ung, E., Chastain, R.L. & Holman, H.R. (1989) The beneficial outcomes of the arthritis self-management course are not adequately explained by behaviour change. *Arthritis & Rheumatism,* **32**, 91–95.

Meichenbaum, D. & Turk, D. (1987) *Facilitating treatment adherence.* New York: Plenum.

Moss-Morris, R., Petrie, K.J. & Weinman, J. (1996) Functioning in chronic fatigue syndrome: do illness perceptions play a regulatory role? *British Journal of Health Psychology,* **11**, 15–25.

Nerenz, D.R., Leventhal, H., Love, R.R. & Ringler, K.E. (1984). Psychological aspects of cancer chemotherapy. *International Review of Applied Psychology,* **33**, 521–529.

O'Leary, A., Shoor, S., Lorig, K. & Holman, H.R. (1988) A cognitive behavioural treatment for arthritis *Health Psychology,* **7**, 527–544.

Schwarzer, R. (1992) Self-efficacy in the adoption and maintenance of health behaviours: theoretical approaches and a new model. In R. Schwarzer (Ed.), *Self-efficacy: thought control of action.* Washinton DC: Hemisphere.

Sharpe, M., Hawton, K., Simkin, S., Surawy, C., Hackmann, A., Klimes, I., Peto, T., Warrell, D. & Seagroatt, V. (1996) Cognitive behavioural therapy for the chronic fatigue syndrome: a randomised controlled trial. *British Medical Journal,* **312**, 22–26.

Skelton, J.A. & Croyle, R.T. (Eds.), (1991) *Mental representations in health and illness.* New York: Springer Verlag.

Telch, C.F. & Telch, M.J. (1986) Group coping skills instruction and supportive group therapy for cancer patients: A comparison of strategies. *Journal of Consulting and Clinical Psychology,* **54**, 802–808.

Turnquist, D.C., Harvey, J.H. & Anderson, B.L. (1988) Attributions and adjustment to life-threatening illness. *British Journal of Clinical Psychology,* **27**, 55–65.

Weinman, J., Petrie, K.J., Moss-Morris, R. & Horne, R. (1996) The illness perception questionnaire: a new method for assessing the cognitive representation of illness. *Psychology & Health,* **11**, 431–445.

Williams, A.C., Nicholas, M.K., Richardson, P.H., Pither, C.E., Jostin, D.M., Chamberlain, J.H., Harding, V.R., Ralphs, J.A., Jones, S.C. & Dieudonne, I. (1993) Evaluation of a cognitive behavioural programme for rehabilitating patients with chronic pain. *British Journal of General Practice,* **43**, 513–8.

Section 1
Illness Perceptions:
Theory and Measurement

1

Illness Representations: Theoretical Foundations

Howard Leventhal, Yael Benyamini,
Susan Brownlee, Michael Diefenbach,
Elaine A. Leventhal, Linda Patrick-Miller
and Chantal Robitaille*

HISTORICAL BACKGROUND

Can phenomenological data such as reports of feelings, attitudes, goals and procedures be used as process variables in a psychological model? During the years when behaviourism was in its ascendency, the answer to this question was a clear, "No". The experimental studies of fear communications that we began in the early 1960s were in partial accord with this bias. Their objective was to identify the conditions under which threatening communication about diseases elicited fear that led to both more favourable attitudes and to the performance of the action that was recommended for preventing the threat. The central hypothesis was that attitudes and actions would be reinforced when the rehearsal and performance of a

*Preparation of this chapter were supported by grants AG-03501 and AG-12072 from the National Institutes on Aging. Special thanks go to John Weinman, Robert Horne and John Pimm for the stimulus they have provided for continued development of the Illness Representation Model.

recommended response reduced fear by eliminating the person's sense of vulnerability to the threat. This hypothesis, derived from the revised drive reduction theory advanced by Dollard and Miller (1950), postulated that if the actions failed to remove fear and danger, avoidant denial and unrealistic reassurances would remove fear while leaving danger intact (see Janis, 1958; Janis & Feshbach, 1953). In keeping with the behaviourist tradition, we tested for the differential effects of high and low fear messages and of fear reduction on both attitudes and overt action, as we were sensitive to the fact that a subject's post-exposure reports of fear and attitudes were verbal responses that might or might not be related to actual performance.

Our data showed distinct effects of fear that were not, however, in accord with the drive reduction model. First, greater fear led to increased acceptance (i.e., attitude change) of the recommended action; that is, high fear messages provoked more fear and more attitude change whether or not fear was reduced by rehearsal of the recommended action. Both the fear and the attitude effects were transient: they faded away within 24 to 48 hours (Leventhal & Niles, 1965). Second, we rarely found more behavioural change after high than after low fear messages and when it did occur (e.g., more efforts were made to quit smoking after a high than after a low fear message), the effect was short-lived (Leventhal, Watts & Pagano, 1967). Also, higher levels of fear consistently failed to promote more action when the recommended action brought one closer to the threat, e.g., following through on a recommendation to take a chest x-ray (Leventhal & Watts, 1966).

In sum, it was clear that while fear had a variety of short term effects, none of its attitudinal or behavioural effects were durable. Thus, the data were not consistent with the hypothesis that fear reduction reinforces and creates stable attitudes that lead to durable action (see Dabbs & Leventhal, 1966; Leventhal & Singer, 1966). Indeed, all of the effects of fear disappeared as the memory of the threat message and the state of fear faded away (see Leventhal & Niles, 1965). While the failure of the drive reduction hypothesis did not surprise us, the two major features of the model emerging from these data were not fully anticipated. We will briefly describe them and explain how they created the thrust for further theoretical developments.

Parallel Processing of Health Threats

We could account for the data pattern in all of our studies within a framework that we called the parallel response model (Leventhal, 1970). The two major features of this model were: 1) the parallel, that is, relatively independent processing of the cognitive representation of the danger (e.g., the disease threat) and of the processing of fear; and 2) the separation of the representation of the disease threat from the plan and/or procedures for performing the protective response (see Figure 1).

Hot affect and cold(er) "perceived" dangers. The short term, dose dependent effects of fear made clear that fear was indeed at work: it produced effects when "hot" in the mind. The two main negative effects of this "hot" state of mind were: 1) avoidance of actions that moved toward detecting threat (e.g., taking a chest x-ray, Leventhal & Watts, 1966), an effect that has been studied in greater detail by Millar and Millar (1995); and 2) a temporary (24 hour) undermining of willingness to approach a protective act if the act involved minor pain and/or discomfort (e.g., taking a tetanus shot, Kornzweig, 1967). The major positive effect was the activation of statements of

A Descriptive Model for Classifying & Identifying Variables

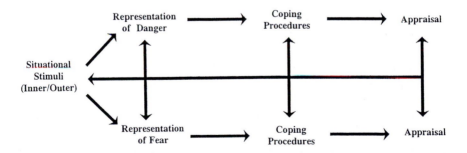

FIGURE 1   A Descriptive Model for Classifying and Identifying Variables. The parallel response model. Situational stimuli, both internal and external, generate both cognitive and emotional representations in response to possible danger. Each representation elicits coping procedures which lead to outcome appraisals that can result in revised outcome criteria, the selection of new procedures, change in the representation and/or change in the eliciting stimuli.

intentions to take protective action. These intentions did not, however, translate into action in the absence of an action plan, that is, an articulated set of procedures for protective action (Leventhal, Singer & Jones, 1965; Leventhal & Trembly, 1968). Adding an action plan to the threat message led to actions such as taking a tetanus shot (Leventhal *et al.*, 1965) and continued efforts to reduce smoking (Leventhal *et al.*, 1967). One critical feature of this behavioural finding was that action was sustained well beyond the point at which fear had dissipated: subjects exposed to a high or low fear message took tetanus shots and/or reported efforts to reduce smoking for weeks post communication if the fear messages were accompanied by a message delineating a clear plan for action (Leventhal, 1970). But a plan alone was ineffective, as action also required a fear message. The probability of action was the same, however, regardless of the level of fear elicited by the message. In short, the motivation for executing plans was something other than the heated state of mind called fear.

Two Types of Representation: Action Plans Translate Representations into Behaviour

Though action plans elicited and sustained behaviour over relatively long time frames when added to a fear message, they were not sufficient to generate action by themselves, either for the short or the long term. This was not surprising as the plan was intended to channel action, not to motivate it. In our studies urging inoculation to prevent tetanus, the plan was a campus map with the student health services clearly marked and instructions asking each student to review his daily class schedule and pick a time when class changes would require that he pass near the health service. That pictorial representations (identifying cues) can effectively channel overt responses had been validated by others (e.g., Hammond & Summers, 1972). The plan generated a procedure that converted a belief about a threat into action, but it did not motivate performance. What was unclear, however, was the nature of the motivating belief. It was clearly not the fear, as all of the post communication effects of fear had faded within a day or two (Leventhal & Niles, 1965). Something else, therefore, had changed. We called this "something" the *cognitive representation* of the disease threat. A label, however, is but the first step toward explanation. The next step was to identify the content and processes subsumed by this construct.

A PERCEPTUAL-MOTOR MODEL FOR SELF AND ENVIRONMENTAL REGULATION

Our search for the nature or attributes of illness representations followed two paths. The first involved a series of experimental studies examining how preparation for noxious experiences affected subjects' emotional reactions and coping procedures. These studies focused on two issues: the link between representations and procedural plans for action and the effects of the meanings assigned to noxious experiences upon emotional behaviour. The second approach relied upon patients' verbal responses to assess the meaning they were assigning to somatic stimuli; that is, we used verbal reports to access the "software" of the mind. Both of these approaches assume a subject's phenomenology and beliefs must be represented as constructs in our psychological theories. Thus, the attributes of illness representations are constructions generated in the minds of our subjects; they are not like traits of personality which are constructions of the investigator.

Dynamics and Content of Illness Representations

Bi-level codes (perceptual and conceptual) to represent disease threats

Observation of individuals' behaviour under stress, studies of the pain system (Egbert *et al.*, 1964; Melzack & Bromage, 1973) and theoretical work on the relationship of language to perceptual categories (Macnamara, 1972), led us to believe that representations of illness threats would be represented both as concrete, perceptual codes and as abstract, linguistic codes. A series of experimental studies designed to identify the factors responsible for emotional distress during medical treatments convinced us that this bi-level hypothesis was indeed valid. Our observations suggested that somatic sensations, such as gagging during endoscopy (Johnson & Leventhal, 1974), and pain sensations during colposcopy and post-surgery (see Johnson, 1975), were key determinants of fear. Our studies were designed to reduce fear by informing patients and encouraging them to monitor the sensations they would experience during stressful episodes. Preparation reduced fear given three conditions: 1) the somatic sensations were described to the patient in clear, concrete language; 2) the sensations were identified as benign and non-threatening: preparation was not beneficial if the sensations were defined as danger cues (Ahles, Blanchard & Leventhal, 1983; Leventhal *et al.*, 1979); and 3) a plan for action was provided in combination with the concrete description of the sensations (Johnson & Leventhal, 1974; E. Leventhal *et al.*, 1989). The monitoring of the objective sensations of a stressful experience could reduce the salience of fear behaviours and increase the probability of problem-focused behaviours (e.g., painful crying versus systematic effort to push and expel the neonate during the final stage of childbirth, E. Leventhal *et al.*, 1989). Thus, by focusing attention upon and developing a clear, perceptual representation of the situation, the individual's behaviour is directed toward realistic problem-solving rather than emotional expression. This suggested that the representation of somatic threats has a perceptual component which ties the patient to situational realities. The role of preparatory information was to redefine the meaning of these perceptual experiences from threatening to benign, which they were, and allow the individual to apply effective coping procedures. The separate effects of the information on sensations and the procedures for coping paralleled the separation of fear and action plans in the fear communication studies.

The second set of studies placed greater reliance on subjects' reports. Influenced by the findings from the studies of preparation for noxious medical procedures, our approach to self-reports assumed that patients perceived somatic sensations as indicators of their underlying disease. For example, in interviews of hypertensive patients, when Meyer (Meyer, Leventhal & Gutmann, 1985) asked, "Can people tell when their blood pressure is up?", 80% of the 50 participants in continuing treatment said, "No". At a later point in time they were also asked, "Can you tell when your blood pressure is up" and "How can you tell?". Surprisingly, 92% of these same patients said that they could tell and they indicated that they did so by monitoring their heart beating, face warming, tenseness, etc. We do not doubt that patients experienced these symptoms. However, neither correlations across subjects ($r = .04$ to $r = .11$) (Meyer *et al.*, 1985) or correlations within subjects over time ($r = .14$) (Baumann & Leventhal, 1985; Pennebaker & Watson, 1988, see page 319), showed significant associations of symptoms to blood pressure.

Levels are linked: The symmetry rule

The results from the hypertension studies indicating that the attributes of illness representations were both perceptual (i.e., symptoms guiding medication taking) and conceptual (i.e., agreement that hypertension {label} is asymptomatic) and the preparation studies showing that the perceptual level played a key role in emotional responding, suggested that representations are bi-level for both their cognitive and affective attributes. These data led to the hypothesis that the linkage of the perceptual and conceptual levels is a product of a pressure toward *symmetry*; i.e., perceptual events create a pressure for labelling and labels generate pressure for a perceptual referent. The often cited study by Schachter and Singer (1962) provides evidence for the symptom(s)-to-label aspect of the symmetry rule, demonstrating that people find specific interpretations or emotion labels for their somatic symptoms. Bishop's studies (Bishop, 1991; Bishop & Converse, 1986) showing agreement among subjects in the categorisation or labelling of defined symptom sets, point to a similar process joining somatic symptoms to illness labels. The potential emotional impact of joining symptoms with an illness label was vividly demonstrated in a study by Easterling and Leventhal (1989). They found that women who regarded themselves as vulnerable to breast cancer reported increasingly higher levels of worry about breast cancer the more they reported somatic symptoms, although none of the symptoms were cancer specific. Thus, neither feelings of vulnerability alone nor symptoms alone generated cancer worry; both were necessary.

The second part of the proposition, that is, that people will seek perceptual evidence (i.e., symptoms) when they are given a disease label, appears to have been at work in the Meyer *et al.* (1985) study of hypertension: hypertensives who were new to treatment in their study were increasingly likely to report that their blood pressure was symptomatic the longer they were in treatment. A similar effect was validated in laboratory studies using undergraduate subjects. Reports of symptoms, similar to those reported by hypertensives (Meyer *et al.*, 1985), increased for those subjects given false feedback that their blood pressure was elevated (Baumann *et al., 1989*). An emotion-to-symptom path has also been identified: the induction of negative mood increases reporting of symptoms for subjects who are ill (Salovey & Birnbaum, 1989) and increases reporting of symptom severity (Croyle & Sande, 1988). Though the symmetry rule assumes that everyone will seek and assign meaning to somatic events, there appear to be both individual (Robbins & Kirmayer, 1991) and cultural (Kirmayer, Young & Robbins, 1994; Kleinman, 1980) differences in readiness to attribute symptoms to illness, to psychological states or to transient environmental conditions.

Content (attributes) of representations

There is more to illness representations than symptoms and labels. Using multi-dimensional scaling of disease labels and symptoms, Penrod and his associates (Penrod, 1980) identified the attributes severity, time-line or duration (acute vs chronic) and cause (Linz *et al.*, 1981). Open-ended interviews have confirmed and added to the list. Five attributes have been identified to date: 1) disease identity (symptoms and label: see also Lau & Hartmann, 1983); 2) time-line (e.g., time to develop and duration); 3) consequences; 4) causes; and 5) controllability (Lau & Hartmann, 1983). Whether these attributes are implicit and identified by inference only (e.g., patients dropping out of hypertension treatment because their symptoms are gone and/or they feel cured (Meyer *et al.*, 1985)), or explicit and identified by direct report, they are part of both the subject's model of disease and of our psychological model of the subject's behaviour in the face of disease threats. The software of the mind and its constructs are part of the conceptual structure of the psychological model designed to represent it.

   Making lists of representation attributes has, however, both benefits and risks, regardless of whether they are compiled by factorial methods or open-ended interviews. We believe that investigators need to be aware of the following. First, models lacking such substantive constructs as cognitive and emotional representation of disease threat, such as the Theory of Planned Behaviour (Ajzen, 1985), are not theories of health behaviour. Models with less differentiated views of disease threats, such as the Health Belief Model (Rosenstock, 1966) and models focused upon the response component, such as the self-efficacy model in Social Learning Theory (Bandura, 1977), are incomplete. The absence of substantive constructs in utility models which propose that behaviour is a function of probabilities multiplied by unspecified values poses a barrier to scientific advance because their quantitative nature creates the illusion of scientific precision. The major shortcoming of such models is that they attempt to explain the process underlying choices in the absence of knowledge of the constituents of the choice process.

Second, any attribute list is likely to be incomplete in at least two respects. New attribute clusters may be found and formerly identified clusters may vanish in future studies. Whether other attributes will appear in other populations depends upon historical factors linked to the social context in which a particular cohort matures and the type of disease-based somatic experience to which it is exposed. Anthropological research has focused upon cultural differences and culture-specific beliefs (e.g., Kleinman, 1980), but we believe that a critical analysis of common-sense beliefs in Western nations will reveal more cross-cultural similarity of disease attributes than might be anticipated. Rather than finding different attributes in different cultures and/or persons, we suspect that cultural differences will affect the amount of variance accounted for by these dimensions. The magnitude of these effects and the importance of their determinants is an empirical question (Kirmayer *et al.*, 1994; Robbins & Kirmayer, 1991).

Another aspect of list making that must not be ignored is that each attribute is subject to further differentiation. For example, Swartzman and Lees (1996) have identified three components of the causal factor, one emphasizing physical or constitutional cause and two emphasizing personal or medical control of the disease. Populations with other salient life experiences (e.g., parents with young children, people living in regions plagued by water-borne infectious diseases, individuals with a familial history of cancer or neurological diseases) might expand the causal attribute to include a wide range of external (e.g., viral or bacterial pathogens, injuries, poisons) and internal factors (e.g., genes, weight, etc.). Furthermore, depending upon their stage in life and the demands they are facing, consequences may be represented by a variety of physical, social and economic effects. As we will suggest momentarily, these differentiations are non-trivial: they have important implications for the selection and maintenance of procedures for prevention and treatment.

The factorial methods that have been used to identify attributes (Bishop, 1991) can create the impression that representations are clusters of independent features. Attributes are organized, however and function as sets. Examination of these clusters suggests that

people have at least three types of disease model: 1) for acute illnesses (e.g., colds, flu, gastrointestinal upset); 2) for cyclic flareups
(allergies, skin problems such as psoriasis); and 3) for chronic illnesses (cancer, cardiovascular disease, arthritis). The models assume
a pattern of identity, causes, time-lines, control and consequences
that vary by disease (e.g., flu = coughs, stuffed nose, fever, fatigue;
viral cause; 2 to 10 days duration; will go away by itself; disrupts
daily life). Protracted experience with a disease, however, may shift
one's model of it from one category to another. For example, in our
study of women with metastatic breast cancer, we found that 29% of
the women regarded their illness as acute and curable (like measles)
during the early cycles in chemotherapy, while only 11% held this
view 6 months later (Leventhal *et al.*, 1986). Although the shift from
an acute to a chronic model of cancer may be most clearly manifest
for an attribute such as time-line, it appears likely that the process
underlying change involves more than one attribute of the representation. Chemotherapy's failure to produce complete remission of a
tumour invalidates the efficacy of the treatment and at least two
attributes of the model of breast cancer: controllability and time
frame. Indeed, we suspect that treatments are always evaluated in
relation to multiple criteria, such as, time and symptom removal, or
time, control of disease and removal of undesired consequences. It
is difficult, if not impossible, to think of the validation process in
terms of a single attribute of the disease representation, as the identity or controllability of a disease is always implicitly, if not explicitly,
linked to a time-line and all three attributes are likely to be linked to
a causal explanation. Few studies have examined these issues.

Are "Ways of Coping" or Procedures Called Upon to Manage Disease Representations?

Although a multitude of studies have been published on coping
with illness, we know precious little about how people select a
coping procedure and how they decide if it merits long term commitment. The reasons for our ignorance are simple: the literature
has been dominated by factor analytic approaches that attempt to
generate factors describing how people cope with their emotions
and ignore how people go about selecting procedures for problem
management, how they define the efficacy of particular procedures
and the dimensions along which they generalize in applying old
procedures to new problems.

There are more procedures than there are ways of coping

There are at least three good reasons for preferring the term "procedure" to "coping". First, it motivates us to look at possible connections between our model of disease management and other formal models of cognitive processing (Anderson, 1990) and at the distinction that has been made between declarative and procedural memory (Anderson, 1983). It is likely that many procedural memories are implicit (i.e.; automated) and their performance relatively independent of conscious processing. Second, laypeople think of coping as positively-valenced, goal directed activity. The term "procedure" is more neutral and does not imply that the response to prevent or control a disease has any special virtue.

Third, the term "procedure" produces a sufficient disconnection from the vast empirical literature on coping and, by doing so, avoids the conceptual pitfalls that are integral to that literature. As we have pointed out elsewhere (E. Leventhal, Suls & Leventhal, 1993) the most egregious of these is the single factor for problem-based coping appearing in the many factorial "validations" of various "ways of coping" check-lists (Endler & Parker, 1990; Lazarus & Folkman, 1984). Analyses such as these tell us that problem-based coping procedures, such as by-pass surgery, dietary change, exercise regimens, diagnostic tests and taking a flu shot, are responses of the same class and will be related to the same underlying process variables. Costa, Somerfield and McCrae (1996) speak to this point when they assert that, "No one would imagine that the same research paradigm would be equally applicable to the processes of deconditioning phobias, forming romantic attachments and learning French verbs" (see pg. 47). Coping with a health threat can be added to the list. We can only believe that investigators satisfied with this level of analysis have never themselves had to choose among alternative procedures for avoiding a threat to life.

The disconnection of procedures from coping avoids a second trap: the distinction between emotion and problem-focused coping, a distinction for which we are partially responsible (Leventhal, 1970). This distinction ignores two critical factors: 1) emotional responses are "coping" procedures, that is, they are ways of expressing distress, of calling for assistance and of manipulating the social environment; and 2) any response, emotional or otherwise, early in a sequence of problem solving may generate new problems and thus require further efforts at problem management.

Representations shape procedures

Because the art of self-care has been part of our socialization, it is difficult for us to recognize the way in which our common-sense representations of disease threats shape our selection and performance of procedures. Every procedure has an associated outcome expectation and a *time frame* (e.g., aspirin is expected to remove a headache within 20 to 30 minutes; antacid is expected to relieve heart burn within seconds; wheat germ is expected to regulate the gastro-intestinal system within days; vitamins to generate an increased sense of vigour and well-being within days and weeks). The route of administration of many, if not all, procedures is also "sensible" or "common-sensical". It assumes *direct contact* of the therapy with the pathogenic irritant. Thus, acid stomach is treated by imbibing antacid; gastro-intestinal problems by ingesting wheat germ; a rash by applying a salve; a cut is treated by applying a topical antiseptic; illness-induced fatigue is treated by resting; injuries by immobilizing the injured limb; etc. Anthropologists have identified procedures for the treatment of commonly observed conditions that have persevered over the centuries. "Molera caida", or fallen fontonelle, a symptom of potentially fatal dehydration caused by gastroenteritis, has been treated by suction on the fontanelle and upward pressure on the soft palate, both futile attempts to save the infant's life by returning the fontanelle to its appropriate position (Kaye, 1993).

While many contemporary medical procedures depart in significant ways from the common-sense notion of *direct contact*, they may compensate for this by taking advantage of a third common-sense rule, the *dose dependent* rule, that is, the notion that the more severe or intractable the symptom the greater the dose or strength of the treatment required. The unavailability of these medications without an expert's prescription, sustains the view of their special power. Still, one might expect that questions about efficacy are more likely to be raised the less common-sensical the route of administration, especially when the time frame exceeds expectations. Rules such as time-line, direct contact and dose dependency, which defines the "fit" between representations and procedures, are similar to the rules identified by Gestalt psychologists for defining good form, or by Garner's (1978) effort to define integral linkages. Identifying these rules may prove a fruitful area for research.

Another reason for changing terminology from "coping" to "procedure" is that it allows us to broaden the way we look at procedures for managing disease threats. Coping responses are conceptualized as actions taken to regulate feelings or actions taken to solve problems, ignoring that these responses typically have multiple functions. For example, if I take an aspirin to relieve a stress-induced headache, I am expecting to eliminate a symptom in a given time frame. By removing the symptom and the emotional distress caused by it, I can avoid the need to call on others for assistance in distress reduction and can turn to more pressing tasks. If the aspirin has its intended effect, it also confirms my representation of the problem as a stress-induced headache. On the other hand, if the response is ineffective, works too slowly, for too brief a period of time, or doesn't work at all, it may both disconfirm the efficacy of aspirin and suggest alternative representations of the problem (e.g., migraine, stroke). The alternatives will stimulate additional monitoring of the features of the self-system (e.g., search for motor deficits, visual changes) thought to be indicators of one or another of these underlying possibilities and may suggest the need for more extensive and potent interventions (e.g., a stronger drug, a visit to the doctor). In sum, procedures have multiple functions, as feedback from them has implications for every facet of the representation as well as for the competence of the individual's support system.

There are representations for procedures

Terms such as "outcome expectations" ignore the complexity of meaning attached to health-related procedures. Procedures exist within a complex representational space whose features are likely similar to those of the diseases they are designed to control. For example, pain killers have each of the five attributes identified with illness representations: time for effectiveness, consequences, cure/control (or efficacy), identity (symptom and illness targets), and cause. Some of these meanings may apply to all members of the class of procedures (pain reduction is expected for all pain killers) and others to only some of its members (e.g., aspirin reduces inflammation and has cardiac protective function which acetaminophen lacks, but aspirin may also cause gastric distress). When these procedures operate within their expected time-lines, they confirm the illness identity.

A class of procedures and its specific members may have other perceived consequences associated with common-sense views of their causal routes and consequences. These perspectives may reflect specific prior experience or they may reflect broader views of causal pathways. Avoiding aspirin in favour of a buffered pain killer may reflect prior experience with the gastro-intestinal effects of the former. Shunning prescribed medication may reflect a broader class-wide fear of drugs based on beliefs that medicines in general are harmful addictive substances. In chronic illness low adherence may be a procedural response to representations of the specific medicine (Horne this volume; Horne & Weinman, 1995). Because pain killers are believed to operate on the brain and affect mood states, they may be perceived as posing the risk of addiction. These views reflect causal (affects brain), time-ordered (after several uses) consequences (addiction) that are experienced symptomatically (stomach burning) and may or may not be controllable, all five of the attributes found in illness representations.

Given the link of procedures to illness representations, it is likely that representations for procedures also are both concrete (perceptual) and abstract (conceptual), such that we can see and perform tasks and feel their consequences and we can describe both how a procedure is performed and what we expect to experience from it. As with disease models, experience and abstract knowledge may be congruent or in conflict. Becker, Drachman and Kirscht (1972) described an instance of this when they found that many mothers stopped the antibiotic regimen that had been prescribed to treat otitis media in their children before it was completed. The children were asymptomatic, so at an experiential level the regimen no longer seemed necessary. Stopping prior to completing the full course of antibiotic therapy could however result in residual pathogens that may result in further flare ups (though to a lay person, these might seem to be due to new infection). Tricyclic treatment for depression is another area in which we have suggested that it could prove fruitful to examine conceptual-perceptual discrepancies (Leventhal, Lambert & Diefenbach, in press). Patients treated with these medications are told that it will take 2 to 3 weeks before they will experience positive changes in cognitions and moods. The time-line for symptomatic experiences such as dry mouth, are much briefer (e.g., one or two days), creating the clear perception that the drug is working and provoking the question, "If it is working, why isn't it affecting my sleep, thoughts and moods?"

In summary, there is more to procedures than the two factors emphasized by social learning approaches, i.e., outcome expectations and the belief that one can perform the required response, or self-efficacy beliefs (Bandura, 1977). Procedures are linked to the definition (representation) of the problem and to a set of beliefs specific to both their class (e.g., medication beliefs) and specific type (e.g., beliefs about aspirin versus beliefs about acetaminophen). In addition, these beliefs and expectations do not exist in isolation and interactions among them can lead to interesting and unexpected outcomes. For example, in many studies of health and behaviour, it is assumed that self-efficacy will lead to positive outcomes such as smoking cessation, weight loss and treatment adherence. This assumption is indeed correct if the representation of the health threat and the procedure are consistent with adherence. Thus, self-efficacy may be an excellent predictor of adherence to anti-hypertensive medications if the medications lead to the expected outcomes (i.e., reduction of symptoms and reduction of blood pressure). On the other hand, if symptom reduction is the patient's criteria for control of an asymptomatic disease, self-efficacy could just as easily lead to non-adherence and seeking of alternative treatment. These issues have been little explored.

The Relationship of Disease Representations and Procedures to the Self-System

Although threats of disease, natural calamity and injury lurk in multiple corners of our world, most such threats remain out of mind. If this was not the case, we would be unable to concentrate on our daily activities. "Out of sight and out of mind" also accounts for the difficulties in motivating health promotive and disease preventive behaviours. Both practice and theory require that we identify the conditions that transform abstract disease threats to personally relevant threats that motivate action.

Overlap of representations of disease and self

Our assumption that a combination of an illness representation (the source of motivation) with an action plan (a concrete image of a series of acts and goals) would lead to motivated behaviour made good sense when we were accounting for the behaviour of patients and/or people who were symptomatic and ill and/or people who thought they were ill (Leventhal, 1970). We face a different situation when trying to enhance health promoting and disease preventing behaviours among well (i.e., asymptomatic) persons. Disease threats in this context are external to the self: they are someone else's problem! What is needed, therefore, is a more complete conceptualization and empirical definition of the conditions that connect disease threats to the self.

Attributes of the self can define risk

Perceptions of vulnerability to disease have been a central variable in the Health Belief Model (Rosenstock, 1966) and the Protection Motivation Model (Rogers, 1983; Sturges & Rogers, 1996) which address health motivation from a utility framework. These models assume that motivation is the product of the scale value of responses to questions of the perceived vulnerability to a disease (e.g., "How likely is it that you will get breast cancer in the next 10 years?") and of perceived severity of the disease ("How serious would it be if you were to get breast cancer?"). Answers to these questions do not reveal, however, the evidence that respondents used in making these judgments, nor do they tell us how the evidence was evaluated. The absence of this information limits our understanding of the judgment process and is a serious barrier to efforts to alter vulnerability appraisals and the health-related actions that may depend upon them (e.g., screening for breast cancer, adopting safe sex behaviour to avoid AIDS, etc).

One way of approaching this problem is to increase the self-relevance of a health practice or a disease threat. For example, Misovich, Fisher and Fisher (in press) found that the adoption of communicators' recommendations to engage in safe sex practices to avoid AIDS is dependent upon the perceived similarity of the communicator's life style to that of the message recipient: personal similarity implies shared exposure to risk. The same approach was used in an early study by Mazen and Leventhal (1972) in which expectant mothers were encouraged to use a "rooming-in" plan for their newborn: the mothers were more likely to have the baby room with them while in the hospital if the communicator delivering the suggestion was also pregnant. Likewise, adoption of the recommendation to breast-feed was dependent upon similarity of racial background. An extensive series of laboratory studies by John Jemmott and Robert Croyle (Croyle & Jemmott, 1991) have also shown that the perceived severity of the consequences of an illness threat are substantially reduced when the risk for the disease is shared by similar others. Their results contribute to our understanding as to how adolescents' perception of smoking among their peers will reduce barriers to experimentation and regular smoking (Leventhal, Glynn & Fleming, 1987).

Rather than focusing on global self-concepts, we have attempted to define attributes of the self that might generate a sense of vulnerability because they are perceived to overlap with the attributes of specific chronic diseases. For example, if older women believe that breast cancer is more likely to strike women in their 40s and 50s, they may feel less vulnerable to that disease as they move into their 70s and 80s (E. Leventhal and Crouch, this volume). The belief is, of course, false, as the rates of breast cancer are highest among women 75 to 80 years of age. By contrast, men feel increasingly vulnerable to prostate cancer as they move into their 60s and 70s, because this cancer is perceived as a disease of the later years.

Many other factors can generate overlap of the representation of disease and the representation of the self. A family history of coronary disease or cancer can increase a sense of personal vulnerability the closer the individual's biological and perceived relationship is to the afflicted, given that heredity is perceived as a central factor in the *causal* component of the disease representation. Other, perhaps less obvious, factors include physical make-up (e.g., if women hold the implicit belief that breast cancer is more likely for large than for small-breasted women, they will be less likely to believe they are vulnerable and less likely to feel the need for screening if they are small-breasted), life stresses and temperament (e.g., people who react strongly to stress and experience high levels of subjective stress will be more likely to see themselves as vulnerable to cardiovascular diseases) and a variety of health related behaviours (e.g., diet: a "heart healthy" diet may reduce feelings of vulnerability to cardiovascular disease; participation in screening: a good result from a colonoscopy may create a sense of safety and invulnerability encouraging future dietary indiscretions). Identifying and understanding how factors such as these become salient and how they are processed and integrated in evaluating personal health will be a major step forward for the elaboration of self-regulation models and the practice of health promotion.

Attributes of the self can moderate procedures for self-regulation

A wide range of personal dispositions, such as beliefs in vulnerability to disease which may change with age and orientations to life such as optimism-pessimism (Carver, Scheier & Weintraub, 1989), can affect both motivation and the strategic procedures used to manage health threats. Our studies of age-related changes in health-enhancing and disease avoidant behaviours show that age moderates the self-regulation process, as older persons appear less willing to tolerate risks and waste scarce physical and psychological resources by delaying seeking health care (E. Leventhal *et al.*, 1993; E. Leventhal & Crouch, this volume). Swiftness in seeking health care makes sense given that advanced age is associated with reductions in physiological (e.g., pulmonary and cardiovascular capacity) and physical strength for all but the most elite elderly, increasing the individual's biological vulnerability to pathognomic processes.

Recent analyses of an extensive longitudinal study examined the affects of an optimistic versus a pessimistic life style on self-assessments of health (Benyamini & Leventhal, 1996; for an overview of the study sample and procedure see E. Leventhal *et al.*, 1996). When participants' outlook on life (optimistic vs pessimistic) was related to their self ratings of health, optimists rated their health more positively than did pessimists. More interesting, was our finding that optimism biased the accuracy of respondents' judgments of their health. Self-assessments of health were excellent predictors of mortality for pessimists (after controlling for age and medical history): there was nearly an 8 times greater mortality five years later among pessimists who rated their health as poor or fair than those who rated their health as excellent or very good. Optimists were far less effective in judging their health status: there was only $1^{1}/_{2}$ times greater mortality five years later among optimists who rated their health as poor or fair than those who rated their health as excellent or very good. In short, optimism moderated people's appraisals of their health status, such that study participants with optimistic dispositions were less accurate in appraising their vulnerability to disease threats and their own mortality, while pessimists were right on target.

THE CONTEXT AND FUTURE DIRECTION FOR THE ELABORATION OF THE SELF-REGULATION PROCESS

We have treated the representation of health threats and the selection and performance of procedures for avoiding and controlling them from an intra-psychic perspective, i.e., the mental operations of the individual as a problem solver. This process does not take place in a social vacuum; rather, it is inter-personal as well as intra-personal. Cultural, institutional, social and personal factors influence each and every one of the variables involved in the representation of health threats and the planning and performance of procedures for their control. Contextual factors are both the initiating sources and the moderators of the mediating factors that participate directly in the problem solving process involved in the prevention and management of disease threats. Treating contextual variables as determinants and moderators of mediating factors does not, however, preclude that they may have direct effects on key outcomes. What distinguishes the illness representation approach to contextual variables from other models, is the conscious effort to identify mediating pathways through representations, procedures and outcome appraisals. A complete model must recognize, however, that contextual factors can have both indirect (mediated) and direct effects on behavioural outcomes.

Current approaches to cultural differences in the anthropological literature focus on the direct effects of cultural factors upon the representations of disease. The belief that bewitchment is a cause of disease would be an example of a culture-bound factor (Koss-Chioino & Canive, 1993). In comparison to psychologists, anthropologists are also more likely to emphasize issues such as the phrasing of questions in terms that are understandable and inoffensive to ethnic minorities. Investigators and practitioners often appear to assume that cultural factors are unique to the group studied and in sharp contrast to the thinking in Caucasian cultures. It is our belief, however, that most of the so-called culture-specific diseases and factors can be found, sometimes in somewhat different form and with somewhat different labels, in all cultures. For example, Logan (1993) argues that the belief that loss of soul, or susto, as a determinant of disease is "... Multicultural in its occurrence ... likely ... very ancient ... as suggested by its wide geographical distribution" (p. 190). While it would be unusual indeed for a native New Yorker or Wisconsinite to attribute chronic disease to soul loss, it would not be surprising to hear talk of "depression", loss of self-esteem or loss of hope, as a common-sense explanation for the death of a grieving loved one. Folk beliefs that belong to the personal world of the investigator are likely to be accepted as "normal" and scientifically reasonable hypotheses of disease causation and progression, rather than the culturally-conditioned or biased views that they are.

The cultural framework is set in bricks and mortar, in language and social relationships as well as in culture-wide myths of cause and control. Hospitals, diagnostic equipment and surgical suites represent models of disease and associated procedures for its management. For example, we recommend quarantine and condom use because we believe that germs cause disease and that disease spreads by contact. Antibiotics are more than medicines: they represent bacteria as a causal factor in disease and the control, cure and removal of symptoms over relatively brief time frames. These medications, along with many other features of the health care system, support an acute model of disease. The model is highly acceptable as it encourages the belief that we can control our fate and avoid painful and untimely injury and deaths.

Many aspects of our common-sense representations of illnesses emerge from our interpretations of the information to which we are exposed during medical encounters. We have previously elaborated upon Blumhagen's (1980) analysis of patients' representations of hypertension. Blumhagen's (1980) main point is that the term "hyper-tension" provides a powerful suggestion that hyper-activity and tension are key symptoms and causes of this disorder. The term, therefore, suggests indicators for monitoring the disorder and suggests that stress is a cause and stress control a potential way of curing and/or controlling the disorder. And the linguistic suggestion is often reinforced during medical encounters as physicians and nurses ask about symptomatology in various organ systems when conducting the standard review of systems. If hypertension is asymptomatic, why is the hypertensive queried about his or her symptoms? In the absence of an explanation for the review (e.g., "This is a standard procedure to detect other problems and is not related to your hypertension."), it is quite reasonable for the "concerned" hypertensive to be attentive to the review and to wonder, "Which of these symptoms is due to my hypertension?".

In our culture, stress is so widely accepted as a cause of disease that the presence of a stressor can affect the interpretation of symptoms and the decision to seek health care. Cameron, E. Leventhal and Leventhal (1995) found that frequency of care seeking was high when an ambiguous symptom occurred in the presence of life stress, but this high level of care seeking appeared only when the stressor was chronic, i.e., present for a minimum of three weeks. When both stressor and ambiguous symptom were new, the symptom was seen as a sign of stress and the frequency of care seeking was low and at the same level as in the absence of stress. By contrast, individuals sought care at relatively high frequency when they experienced symptoms that were clear indications of medical problems and the rates of care seeking were virtually identical whether a stressor was or was not present.

These indirect effects of the cultural and social context on health behaviours (i.e., indirect as they are mediated by changes in representation beliefs and procedures) occur in addition to and in interaction with direct effects. Use of professional services for diagnosis and treatment is often a direct product of social influence: people ask and/or are told by family members and friends to "Go to the doctor and find out what it is", to not be concerned about looking foolish. The representation of disease and treatment by individuals in a person's cohort can generate social pressures and supports encouraging particular representations of a health problem and the adoption of specific procedures for its management. The contextual factors can have direct effects, bypassing or reinforcing the specific, mediating representations and procedures being considered by the target person. As the instigators of social pressure are typically the product of an interaction of the behaviour of the symptomatic, target person with the representations and procedural beliefs of observing members of his or her cohort, we see that we have come full circle. Specifically, the representations and procedural beliefs that we have identified while modelling the factors that have direct effects on an individual's health and illness behaviours, can be used to model the beliefs that have direct effects on the social moderators of these behaviours.

The self-regulation framework needs to be extended into the social context. Doing so will allow us to return to Thomas and Znaniecki's (1918) original conceptualization of attitudes as shared beliefs. More importantly, perhaps, we will be able to examine a host of issues involved in sharing, such as how individuals arrive at common representations of diseases and how the absence of commonality affects care-seeking and the behaviour of the surrounding social network. It will also allow us to begin the interesting task of examining inter-group conflict regarding the cause and treatment of disease as for example, in the case of AIDS. By coming full circle and extending our common-sense framework of self-regulation to the cultural and social domain, we have indirectly addressed

Ogden's (1995) criticism that self-regulation models stay within the head of the individual and ignore the surrounding context. Self-regulation models that emphasize both the perceptual and conceptual structure of the self-regulation system focus upon the individual's way of construing his or her contacts with the environment. The attributes of representations are dimensions extracted from "reality" by these lay bio-medical scientists; they are their common-sense perceptions and conceptions of what is there, what it feels like, what makes it happen, how long it will last, what it has done and will yet do, whether it can be controlled and of the various procedures that can be used to clarify and control various features of the health problem and its somatic expression. By specifying the representations, procedures and procedural beliefs offered by social institutions for defining and resolving health threats, we have taken a step toward defining the environmental inputs to illness representations. While the model uncovers only a corner of the picture, it clearly opens the door for further investigation.

REFERENCES

Ahles, T.A., Blanchard, E.B. & Leventhal, H. (1983) Cognitive control of pain: Attention to sensory aspects of the cold pressor stimulus. *Cognitive Therapy and Research*, **7**, 159–177.

Ajzen, I. (1985) From intentions to actions: A theory of planned behavior. In J. Kuhl & J. Beckman (Eds.), *Action-control: From cognition to behavior* (pp. 11–39). Heidelberg: Springer.

Anderson, J.R. (1983) *The architecture of cognition.* Cambridge, MA: Harvard University Press.

Anderson, J.R. (1990) *The adaptive character of thought.* Hillsdale, NJ: Lawrence Earlbaum.

Bandura, A. (1977) Self-efficacy: Toward a unifying theory of behavioral change. *Psychological Review*, **84**, 191–215.

Baumann, L.J. & Leventhal, H. (1985) "I can tell when my blood pressure is up, can't I?". *Health Psychology*, **4**, 203–218.

Baumann, L.J., Cameron, L.D., Zimmerman, R.S. & Leventhal, H. (1989) Illness representations and matching labels with symptoms. *Health Psychology*, **8**, 449–469.

Becker, M.H., Drachman, R.H. & Kirscht, J.P. (1972) Predicting mothers' compliance with pediatric medical regimens. *Journal of Pediatrics*, **81**, 834–845.

Benyamini, Y. & Leventhal, H. (1996) Optimists and pessimists: How do they evaluate their health status? Manuscript in preparation.

Bishop, G.D. (1991) Understanding the understanding of illness: Lay disease representations. In J.A. Skelton & R.T. Croyle (Eds.), *Mental representation in health and illness* (pp. 32–59). New York: Springer-Verlag.

Bishop, G.D. & Converse, S.A. (1986) Illness representations: A prototype approach. *Health Psychology*, **5**, 95–114.

Blumhagen, D. (1980) Hyper-tension: A folk illness with a medical name. *Culture, Medicine and Psychiatry*, **4**, 197–227.

Cameron, L.D., Leventhal, E.A. & Leventhal, H. (1995) Seeking medical care in response to symptoms and life stress. *Psychosomatic Medicine*, **57**, 37–47.

Carver, C.S., Scheier, M.F. & Weintraub, J.K. (1989) Assessing coping strategies: A theoretically based approach. *Journal of Personality and Social Psychology*, **56**, 267–283.

Costa, P.T. Jr., Somerfield, M.R. & McCrae, R.R. (1996) Personality and coping: A reconceptualization. In M. Zeidner & N.S. Endler (Eds.), *Handbook of coping: Theory, research, applications* (pp. 44–61). New York: John Wiley & Sons.

Croyle, R.T. & Jemmott, J.B. (1991) Psychological reactions to risk factor testing. In J.A. Skelton & R.T. Croyle (Eds.), *Mental representations in health and illness* (pp. 85–107). New York: Springer-Verlag.

Croyle, R.T. & Sande, G.N. (1988) Denial and confirmatory search: Paradoxal consequences of medical diagnosis. *Journal of Applied Social Psychology*, **18**, 473–490.

Dabbs, J.M. Jr. & Leventhal, H. (1966) Effects of varying the recommendations in a fear-arousing communication. *Journal of Personality and Social Psychology*, **4**, 525–531.

Dollard, J. & Miller, N.E. (1950) *Personality and psychotherapy*. New York: McGraw Hill.

Easterling, D. & Leventhal, H. (1989) The contribution of concrete cognition to emotion: Neutral symptoms as elicitors of worry about cancer. *Journal of Applied Psychology*, **74**, 787–796.

Egbert, L., Battit, G., Welch, C. & Bartlett, M. (1964) Reduction of post-operative pain by encouragement and instruction. *New England Journal of Medicine*, **270**, 825–827.

Endler, N. & Parker, J.D.A. (1990) Multidimensional assessment of coping: A critical evaluation. *Journal of Personality and Social Psychology*, **58**, 844–854.

Garner, W.R. (1978) Aspects of a stimulus: Feature dimension and configuration. In E. Rosch & B.B. Lloyd (Eds.), *Cognition and categorization* (pp. 99–133). Hillsdale, NJ: Lawrence Erlbaum.

Hammond, K.R. & Summers, D.A. (1972) Cognitive control. *Psychological Review*, **79**, 58–67.

Horne, R. (this volume) Representations of medication and treatment: Advances in theory and measurement. In J. Weinman & K. Petrie (Eds.), *The patient's perception of illness and treatment: Current research and applications.* London: Harwood Academic.

Horne, R. & Weinman, J. (1995) The Beliefs About Medicines Questionnaire (BMQ): A new method for assessing lay beliefs about medicines. Proceedings of the Special Group in Health Psychology: British Psychological Society.

Janis, I.L. (1958) *Psychological stress.* New York: Wiley.

Janis, I.L. & Feshbach, S. (1953) Effects of fear-arousing communications. *Journal of Abnormal and Social Psychology*, **48**, 78–92.

Johnson, J.E. (1975) Stress reduction through sensation information. In I.G. Sarason & C.D. Speilberger (Eds.), *Stress and anxiety* (Vol. 2, pp. 361–373). Washington, DC: Hemisphere Publishing Corp.

Johnson, J.E. & Leventhal, H. (1974) The effects of accurate expectations and behavioral instructions on reactions during a noxious medical examination. *Journal of Personality and Social Psychology*, **29**, 710–718.

Kaye, M.A. (1993) Fallen fontanelle: Cultural-bound or cross-cultural? *Medical Anthropology: Cross-Cultural Studies in Health and Illness*, **15**, 137–156.

Kirmayer, L.J., Young, A. & Robbins, J.M. (1994) Symptom attribution in cultural perspective. *Canadian Journal of Psychiatry*, **39**, 584–595.

Kleinman, A. (1980) *Patients and healers in the context of culture: An exploration of the borderland between anthropology, medicine and psychiatry*. Los Angeles: University of California Press.

Kornzweig, N.D. (1967) *Behavior change as a function of fear arousal and personality*. Unpublished doctoral dissertation, Yale University.

Koss-Chioino, J.D. & Canive, J.M. (1993) The interaction of popular and clinical diagnostic labeling: The case of embrujado. *Medical Anthropology*, **15**, 171–188.

Lau, R.R. & Hartman, K.A. (1983) Common sense representations of common illnesses. *Health Psychology*, **2**, 167–185.

Lazarus, R.S. & Folkman, S. (1984) *Stress, appraisal and coping*. New York: Springer.

Leventhal, E.A. & Crouch, M. (1997) Are there differences in perceptions of illness. In J. Weinman & K. Petrie (Eds.), *The patient's perception of illness and treatment: Current research and applications*. London: Harwood Academic.

Leventhal, E.A., Hansell, S., Diefenbach, M., Leventhal, H. & Glass, D.C. (1996) Negative affect and self-reports of physical symptoms: Two longitudinal studies of older adults. *Health Psychology*, **15**, 193–199.

Leventhal, E.A., Leventhal, H., Shacham, S. & Easterling, D.V. (1989) Active coping reduces reports of pain from childbirth. *Journal of Consulting and Clinical Psychology*, **57**, 365–371.

Leventhal, E.A., Leventhal, H., Schaefer, P. & Easterling, D.V. (1993) Conservation of energy, uncertainty reduction and swift utilization of medical care among the elderly. *Journal of Gerontology*, **48**, 78–86.

Leventhal, E.A., Suls, J. & Leventhal, H. (1993) Hierarchial analysis of coping: Evidence from life-span studies. In H.W. Krohne (Ed.), *Attention and avoidance: Strategies in coping with aversiveness* (pp. 71–99). Seattle: Hogrefe & Huber.

Leventhal, H. (1970) Findings and theory in the study of fear communications. *Advances in Experimental Social Psychology*, **5**, 119–186.

Leventhal, H., Brown, D., Shacham, S. & Engquist, G. (1979) Effects of preparatory information about sensations, threat of pain and attention on cold pressor distress. *Journal of Personality and Social Psychology*, **37**, 688–714.

Leventhal, H., Easterling, D.V., Coons, H., Luchterhand, C. & Love, R.R. (1986) Adaptation to chemotherapy treatments. In

B. Andersen (Ed.), *Women with cancer* (pp. 172–203). New York: Springer-Verlag.

Leventhal, H., Glynn, K. & Fleming, R. (1987) Is the smoking decision an "informed choice?": Effect of smoking risk factors on smoking beliefs. *Journal of the American Medical Association*, **257**, 3373–3376.

Leventhal, H., Lambert, J. & Diefenbach, M. (in press) From compliance to social self-regulation: Models of the compliance process. In B. Blackwell (Ed.), *Compliance and the treatment alliance in serious mental illness.* Newark, NJ: Gordon and Breach.

Leventhal, H. & Niles, P. (1965) Persistence of influence for varying durations of exposure to threat stimuli. *Psychological Review*, **16**, 223–233.

Leventhal, H. & Singer, R. (1966) Affect arousal and positioning of recommendation in persuasive communications. *Journal of Personality and Social Psychology*, **4**, 137–146.

Leventhal, H., Singer, R. & Jones, S. (1965) Effects of fear and specificity of recommendations upon attitudes and behavior. *Journal of Personality and Social Psychology*, **2**, 20–29.

Leventhal, H. & Trembly, G. (1968) Negative emotions and persuasion. *Journal of Personality*, **36**, 154–168.

Leventhal, H. & Watts, J.C. (1966) Sources of resistance to fear-arousing communications on smoking and lung cancer. *Journal of Personality*, **34**, 155–175.

Leventhal, H., Watts, J.C. & Pagano, F. (1967) Effects of fear and instructions on how to cope with danger. *Journal of Personality and Social Psychology*, **6**, 313–321.

Linz, D., Penrod, S., Leventhal, H. & Siverhus, S. (1981) *The cognitive organization of disease and illness among lay persons.* Unpublished manuscript, University of Wisconsin.

Logan, M.H. (1993) New lines of inquiry on the illness of susto. *Medical Anthropology*, **15**, 189–200.

Macnamara, J. (1972) Cognitive basis of language learning in infants. *Psychological Review*, **79**, 1–13.

Mazen, R. & Leventhal, H. (1972) The influence of communicator-recipient similarity upon the beliefs and behavior of pregnant women. *Journal of Experimental Social Psychology*, **8**, 289–302.

Melzack, R. & Bromage, P.R. (1973) Experimental phantom limbs. *Experimental Neurology*, **39**, 261–269.

Meyer, D., Leventhal, H. & Gutmann, M. (1985) Common-sense models of illness: The example of hypertension. *Health Psychology*, **4**, 115–135.

Millar, M.G. & Millar, K. (1995) Negative affective consequences of thinking about disease detection behaviors. *Health Psychology*, **14**, 1141–1146.

Misovich, S.J., Fisher, W.D. & Fisher, J.D. (in press) Social comparison as a factor in AIDS risk and AIDS preventive behavior. In B. Buunk & R. Gibbons (Eds.), *Health, coping and social comparison*. Hillsdale, NJ: Erlbaum.

Ogden, J. (1995) Changing the subject of health psychology. *Psychology and Health*, **10**, 257–265.

Pennebaker, J.W. & Watson, D. (1988) Blood pressure estimation and beliefs among normotensives and hypertensives. *Health Psychology*, **7**, 309–328.

Penrod, S. (1980) *Cognitive models of symptoms and diseases*. Paper presented at the Annual Meeting of the American Psychological Association.

Robbins, J.M. & Kirmayer, L.J. (1991) Attributions of common somatic symptoms. *Psychological Medicine*, **21**, 1029–1045.

Rogers, R.W. (1983) Cognitive and physiological processes in fear appeals and attitude change: A revised theory of protection motivation. In J.T. Cacioppo & R.E. Petty (Eds.), *Social psychology: A source book* (pp. 153–176). New York: Guilford Press.

Rosenstock, I.M. (1966) Why people use health services. *Millbank Memorial Fund Quarterly*, **44**, 94ff.

Salovey, P. & Birnbaum, D. (1989) Influence on mood on health-relevant cognitions. *Journal of Personality and Social Psychology*, **57**, 539–551.

Schachter, S. & Singer, J.E. (1962) Cognitive, social and physiological determinants of emotional state. *Psychological Review*, **69**, 379–399.

Sturges, J.W. & Rogers, R.W. (1996) Preventive health psychology from a developmental perspective: An extension of protection motivation theory. *Health Psychology*, **15**, 158–166.

Swartzman, L.C. & Lees, M.C. (1996) Causal dimensions of college students' perceptions of physical symptoms. *Journal of Behavioral Medicine*, **19**, 95–110.

Thomas, W.I. & Znaniecki, F. (1918) *The polish peasant in Europe and America*. Boston: Badger.

2

Children's Perceptions of Health and Illness

Christine Eiser and Sheryl J. Kopel*

Children today are very fortunate. Improvements in housing, sanitation and diet mean that they experience fewer episodes of illness than was common in previous generations. Widespread vaccination programmes mean that children are subject to much less in the way of common childhood ailments compared with their parents. Antibiotics control more everyday bouts of illness rapidly. Small wonder that many children have little personal experience of illness.

Yet the progress that has brought about these improvements for some has resulted in greater difficulties for others. A sizeable proportion of children (estimates vary from 10–15%) suffer from chronic diseases (Cadman, Boyle & Offord, 1988). These conditions might once have proved fatal, but now medicine can control many of the symptoms. Cure, however, is not possible. For these children, everyday life can be quite compromised by hospital visits, daily treatments and general difficulties. Interest in children's understanding of health and illness has very much stemmed from the recognition that medical treatment is demanding on family time and relationships. As it has become possible to treat children with more

*The authors are funded by the Cancer Research Campaign, London, United Kingdom (CP 1019/0101).

severe and life-threatening illnesses, the question of how to balance the treatment demands with total quality of life has received much more attention. Increasingly questions are being raised about the wisdom of a policy that emphasizes survival without taking into account the impact of treatment on more general social and psychological development. In writing this chapter, our main purpose has been to consider to what extent academic research about perceptions of health and illness has had any impact on the experience of illness by children and their families.

THEORETICAL BACKGROUND

The early literature was relatively consistent in finding evidence of self-blame in children's understanding of their own illness (Langford, 1948). Anecdotal and clinical evidence in the 1950s and '60s tended to support the idea that small children blame themselves for their illness. However, more recent work is far less conclusive. This may partly be attributed to shifts in theoretical approach. With the decline in importance of psychoanalytic perspectives there is less interest in issues of self blame or recrimination. Perhaps more importantly, the whole atmosphere in children's hospitals has changed. In the 1950s, parents were only allowed to visit their child briefly on a Saturday or Sunday afternoon (Meadow, 1988); open access is now the norm and parents are strongly encouraged to stay and care for their child. As dark corridors have given way to more child friendly environments, it may seem even to a small child that being ill has some compensations and cannot be totally attributable to misbehaviour! In addition, considerable thought has been given to questions of how to explain illness to a child in words they understand. Even so and notwithstanding the efforts which are made by medical staff to persuade them otherwise, some children may still blame themselves and they are not alone. Even today, parents often go through a stage when they blame themselves for their child's illness.

Cognitive

In parallel with other areas of psychology, child development saw a shift to more cognitive theoretical orientations during the 1970s and '80s. Children were seen as active theory builders, not passive recipients of information. They were seen to be individuals who actively sought to understand and make sense of the world in which they found themselves. However, this does not necessarily imply that they share adult perceptions of the world.

Much of the work originally centred on describing how the child developed an understanding of key physical concepts such as space, time or causality (Piaget, 1929). This emphasis on physical concepts was originally seen to lend respectability to the methodological approaches adopted. In the longer-term, it has been the focus of much criticism. Health and illness are socially and culturally defined and as such it may be inappropriate to adopt methods used to study physical concepts by simply substituting "illness" for a concept such as time. In general, Piaget favoured an approach involving quasi-experimental methods and semi-structured interviews. Such methods definitely have advantages in some circumstances, but may also be open to bias. One of the main assumptions made by Piaget was that it was possible to learn as much from studying what children did not know as what they did. This emphasis, on what children do not know, combined with an interviewing style which could be seen as repetitive or misleading (Siegel, Patty & Eiser, 1990), means that much of the early work in this area needs to be interpreted with some caution.

Nevertheless, this theoretical approach has been used extensively in efforts to account for how the child gains an understanding of concepts of health and illness. Following Piaget, it was argued that children's beliefs about these concepts went through a series of stages, paralleling the stages of pre-conceptual, concrete and formal operational thought (Bibace & Walsh, 1981; Perrin & Gerrity, 1981). Others used the same framework to describe children's concepts of sexuality and reproduction (Bernstein & Cowen, 1981), their body (Crider, 1981), health (Kalnins & Love, 1982) and the role of doctors and medicine (Steward & Regalbulto, 1981). More recently and topi-cally, these ideas have been applied to work about children's understanding of smoking (Bibace & Walsh, 1981) and AIDS (Osborne, Kistner & Helgemo, 1993).

These studies point to systematic changes in how children perceive health and illness throughout childhood. In the pre-operational stage (before 7 years of age), there is a confusion between cause and affect and lack of differentiation between ill-nesses. During the concrete-operational stage (7–11 years), children understand the role of contagion and germs in the etiology of illness, though, at least during the early part of this stage, are confused about issues of proximity. More sophisticated understanding of infection and health prevention emerge during the stage of formal operational thought, around 11 years (though Piaget suggested that this stage was not attained by everyone). A number of studies appear on the surface to support this theoretical analysis (Beales *et al.*, 1983; Perrin, Sayer & Willett, 1991). Younger children offer less complex explanations and rely less on internal bodily cues to indicate the presence of illness. Older children offer more restricted definitions of specific illnesses and a more organised description of process and cause.

The purely cognitive approach is not without its critics (e.g. Gellman & Baillargeon, 1983). Along with other work in the Piagetian tradition, these data tend to be based on semi-structured interview procedures. These methods may sometimes be criticised as misleading. In particular the language used can be unnatural and repetitive. There are also indications that children's understanding of their illnesses are predicted better from their developmental level than chronological age. The most serious problems relate to analysis of the interview protocols. Children's responses do not always readily conform to the general pattern described above. There is necessarily some discrepancy between different raters in categorisation of responses. Most importantly, it is not clear that the same response is coded in the same way by different researchers. For example, imminent justice explanations for illness are coded as pre-operational by Brewster (1982) and Perrin and Gerrity (1981), and as concrete-operational by Bibace and Walsh (1980) and Simeonsson, Buckley and Monson (1979).

In addition, contemporary authors increasingly challenge the view that we can understand what children know by studying what they do not know. Alternative cognitive theories have been based on script theory (Nelson, 1985) or conceptual change (Carey, 1985). Nelson (1985) particularly argued that we should focus more on what the child *does* know. According to this view, children develop script-like, sequential representations of everyday common events which include "going to the doctor". Empirical work suggests that both healthy (Eiser, Eiser & Lang, 1990) and chronically sick children (Bearison & Pacifici, 1989) do in fact develop accurate and quite detailed accounts of illness events. In theory, this approach could form the basis of intervention work with sick children, by focusing on any misconceptions or misunderstandings about routine hospital procedures.

Carey (1985) argues that children's ideas about health and illness are unconstrained by structure. The view of health adopted by preschoolers is defined by adult admonitions. Throughout middle childhood, there is a shift to a greater understanding of the role of human body function in the maintenance of life. Overall, Carey argues that children's understanding of the body and health shift from a human (you eat because mum says it's time for dinner) to a more biological basis (you eat to keep your body strong or well).

With changes in method and concern to document knowledge and understanding rather than misconceptions, the message has been consistent that children are more aware and have greater insight in virtually all domains compared with those originally described by Piaget. This applies no less to concepts of health and illness than physical concepts such as space or time. While it may be that children's understanding of illness does evolve in some systematic manner, it is not clear that this is best accounted for in purely cognitive terms. In addition, there is evidence for individual differences in the rate of acquisition of understanding.

Individual Differences

Individual differences in understanding of illness have been considered primarily in relation to two areas: *health motivation* and *perceived vulnerability.*

Health motivation

Social Learning theory has had a major influence, not only on research work but also as a central approach in intervention studies. Issues of self-care and treatment compliance appear relevant to two concepts derived from Social Learning theory. *Locus of control* is a generalised outcome expectancy. Those with an internal locus of control orientation believe that their own behaviour determines outcome, while those with an external orientation believe that outcomes are dependent on chance. There is some evidence that internal locus of control beliefs are associated with better self-care, greater disease related knowledge and better compliance (Moffatt & Pless, 1983; Neuhauser *et al.*, 1978). Other work suggests that additional variables may also be involved and the relationship may be much less simple than originally supposed.

At the least, distinctions must be made between outcome expectancies as measured by locus of control and behavioural expectancies or *self-efficacy* (Bandura, 1977). Individuals may feel responsible for their own health (internal locus of control), but at the same time perceive themselves to be incapable of performing the required activities (low self-efficacy).

While most illnesses may be associated with a lower internal locus of control (in that individuals may feel powerless), diabetes is exceptional in that individuals are encouraged to be responsible for their own disease management. From an early age, children are encouraged to believe that they are responsible for their own health and well-being and the emphasis on self-care reinforces this point of view. Awareness of such potential autonomy might be expected to lead to considerable self-efficacy among children with diabetes.

Havermans and Eiser (1991), therefore, compared locus of control and self-efficacy beliefs in healthy children and those with diabetes. Children with diabetes showed more internal locus of control beliefs compared with the healthy children. However there were fewer differences between the groups in terms of self-efficacy. In fact, healthy children were more confident in their ability to carry out self-care tasks than those with diabetes. Thus, although children with diabetes recognised their own role in self-care (high internal locus of control) they were less confident in their ability to look after their own health (low self-efficacy). As far as interventions are concerned, it may be as important to bolster children's self-confidence and beliefs in their own skills and competencies, as to provide factual information about what should be done.

Perceived vulnerability

In research with adults, there is a relatively large body of work which suggests that, under many conditions, people view their own chances of misfortune as less likely than others. This has been most generally described as *optimistic bias*; optimistic since it is logically impossible for individual risks to be lower than those of everyone else. Despite the amount of work with adults, much less is known about how children and young people perceive their own risks. Early work (Elkind, 1967) suggests that young people do perceive themselves to be less vulnerable compared with others their age. His concept of "adolescent egocentrism" captures the common assumption that young people are more inclined to take risks compared with their parents and see themselves as essentially invulnerable. Until recently, this stereotype was virtually unchallenged.

Whalen *et al.* (1994) adopted a method used extensively in adult work and obtained risk judgments on a range of health, life-style and environmental problems from a relatively large sample of 12 year olds. The strongest levels of optimism emerged for controllable and stigmatising events such as use of illicit drugs, smoking and AIDS. Thus, these young people saw themselves as less likely to succumb to the pressures of smoking or illegal drug use compared with many of their peers. There were few differences in judgment based on gender, challenging the view that boys are more risk oriented compared with girls. While the study suggests similarities between children's and adults' perceptions of risk, methodological differences between this and the methods typically employed in adult work restricts simple extrapolation.

A more direct comparison was reported by Cohn *et al.* (1995). This study very much challenges the view that young people underestimate their vulnerability compared with adults. In this direct comparison, young people were less optimistic about avoiding illness and injury compared with their parents. Most notably, those young people who were at greatest risk (because of their own behaviour) were also less optimistic than others. The implication would be that young people who run risks are well aware of what they do.

Both studies point to a greater need to integrate young people's perceptions of risks into health educational programmes. There is some suggestion that risk perceptions may in fact be an important contributor to risk behaviour. Gladis, Michela and Walter (1992), for example, reported that students' perceptions of their own risk were associated with intentions to change related behaviours. Thus, the success of any health education package may be facilitated through a process of modification of individual risk perception.

IMPLICATIONS

The study of the development of concepts of health and illness has always been justified on the basis of implications for practical and clinical situations. According to Burbach and Peterson (1986), four major applications of the work can be identified:

1. providing age-appropriate health education,

2. reducing fears and anxieties during treatment,

3. involving children in health care decisions,

4. increasing compliance with medical regimens.

Though we fully endorse the first three of these proposed implications, we feel that the fourth should be considered under the more general heading of self-care, that is, of increasing children's ability to be responsible for as much of their own treatment as is possible. In addition, partly as a consequence of the recent interest in quality of life there has been an awareness that the child has different perspectives from the adult. These need to be taken into account when attempting to measure the extent to which a chronic disease compromises normal quality of life. The first of the practical applications presented above, providing appropriate health education, effects the lives of healthy and ill children alike, while the remainder address issues particularly relevant to children with chronic illnesses.

Providing Age-Appropriate Health Education

With some exceptions, attempts to provide systematic health education for children of preschool or primary school age have been minimal. The task is indeed a difficult and demanding one. It is important to provide children with information about complex information, often with the message that any negative consequences are for the future. Implications for the present are invariably not wholly negative and can sometimes be seen as rewarding. For the young person, smoking may be less a long-term threat to health and more a contemporary means of obtaining pleasure or peer acceptance. Information must be provided prior to the time when young people are most at risk and this in itself adds to the challenge facing educators. It is necessary that young people understand the risks involved in sharing needles or engaging in unprotected sex prior to their experience of any situation in which they may be tempted to compromise their health and risk of contracting AIDS. Lack of integration of theoretical research and development of educational packages may be partly a function of the widespread acceptance of cognitive theories of understanding of health and illness, with the implication that children below 11 years of age are unable to assimilate complex, especially relevant biological information. While academic researchers routinely justify their work in terms of the implications for education, they do not generally put the results into practice. In contrast, educationalists are enthusiastic in their efforts to devise educational material and yet may not be aware of research findings. Indeed, research is not always set up in such a way that its findings are readily translated into policy. These criticisms are general and can be made with respect to the majority of smoking, alcohol and safety educational packages.

With the increasing awareness that the adoption of healthy behaviours during childhood is one of the best ways to reduce adult morbidity, interest in health education for the young has flourished. Underlying the development of educational materials is the assumption that information needs to be tailored to the developmental level of the child. Of course, it is clear that care needs to be taken in the selection of appropriate language. More controversial is the question of the content of the information. Most people would probably agree that it would be inappropriate to include information about the risks of lung cancer in a smoking prevention programme for young children. However, the question of when it is appropriate to include information about long term risks is not clear.

Developmental issues have been most clearly taken into account in recent programmes aimed to increase knowledge and understanding about AIDS. Osborne, Kistner and Helgemo (1993) found that children's understanding of AIDS paralleled their understanding of other diseases. Specifically, children of 5 years of age believed that simple proximity to an AIDS victim was sufficient for transmission. This view was disputed by 10–11 year olds, many of whom did believe that casual contact was sufficient; being sneezed on was enough. By 13 years, most children understood that AIDS was contracted through sexual contact, sharing needles, or mixing blood, though again there was misunderstanding about whether the disease could be contracted through kissing and to a lesser extent, sneezing and coughing. The authors suggest that young children would benefit from curricula that reduce their fears, without giving overly complex information. Thus, information not to touch cuts

on others might be important for the younger group, while information to avoid contaminated blood and bodily fluids would only
be appropriate for older children.

In addition to the age differences in children's knowledge of
AIDS, there were also age-related differences in attitudes toward a
peer with AIDS. Since the youngest children believed they could
contract AIDS by being near someone with AIDS, it is not surprising that they were most reluctant to interact with a hypothetical
peer. Older children were also more knowledgeable and were
more likely to be willing to interact. By identifying some of the key
misconceptions held by children of different ages, Osborne and her
colleagues suggest a theoretically based approach to health education, aimed both at increasing knowledge and facilitating social
interactions.

Epidemiological studies suggest that the pattern of accidents that
effect children are partly age-related. For example, most accidents
involving pre-school children take place in the home, suggesting that
effective education should be directed toward alerting parents to the
potential hazards in the child's daily environment. Among school
aged children, accidents are most likely to occur in the immediate
neighbourhood, between home and school and involve traffic accidents. Older school children run greater risks from bicycle injuries.
Recognition of the situations and activities in which children are
particularly vulnerable should be useful in reducing accidents,
especially if this is integrated with an appropriate and sensitive educational programme. Coppens (1986), for example, suggested that
there are age-related differences in children's understanding of safety
and prevention of accidents which parallel cognitive development. In
both preschool and school aged children, an understanding of safety
occurs before children are able to identify appropriate preventative
behaviours. Coppens suggests that helping young children understand cause-effect relationships may be an important precursor of
safe behaviour. While there is much less emphasis on these kind of
interventions compared with smoking or alcohol education, the
number of published reports is increasing. A special issue of the
Journal of Pediatric Psychology (1993) was devoted to this topic and
the articles published represent some of the best available to date.

Diet in childhood plays an important role in development and
has implications for later life. Poor nutrition during childhood seems
to be associated with later risk factors including heart disease and

hypertension (Armstrong, 1989; Gortmaker *et al.*, 1993). Studies have demonstrated that children of various ages are aware that certain foods promote health (Eiser, Patterson & Eiser, 1983) and that others have potentially harmful effects (Oakley *et al.*, 1995), and yet this awareness does not necessarily translate to healthy eating habits. Factors that may influence children to eat a diet of poor nutritional quality are advertising (Liebert & Sprafkin, 1988) and availability in the home (Dennison & Shepherd, 1995). Newman and Taylor (1992) demonstrated that children's food preferences can be shaped through what they called a "means-end contingency". The children in this study (aged 4–7 years old) were presented with two snacks that were ranked to be of approximately equal appeal. They found that the children in the means-end group, who were told to eat one snack as a means of gaining the other, came to devalue the means snack relative to the reward snack. Hence children may come to desire foods of poor nutritional value if they are used as rewards. An additional influential factor for adolescents may be their association of 'junk food' with pleasure, friends and independence from their parents (Chapman & Maclean, 1993).

Tinsley (1992) suggests that the discontinuity of health messages children receive from family, peers and the media burdens children and young people with having to integrate this information as best they can. Nader *et al.* (1982) conducted a study in which 10th-graders (approximately 16 years old) watched a heart disease prevention programme at school and again at home with their parents. Families then discussed ways in which they could reduce behaviours that put them at risk for heart disease. Though the intervention did not yield any evidence of behavioural change, it demonstrated how schools, parents and the media can work together to make consistent the health messages that contribute to children's and young people's health-socialization. Other studies (Harlan, 1989; Stone, Perry & Luepker, 1989) also provide evidence that by making health information consistent across social contexts (e.g. the family and school), young people's health attitudes and behaviour may be more easily modified.

Reducing Fears and Anxieties During Treatment

Bibace and Walsh (1981) quote an example of a healthy child who was highly distressed in a hospital ward. However, inference from the theory, which suggests that children in the concrete-operational stage believe that the most common way in which illness can be contracted is through contamination or contagion, led them to suggest that the child's behaviour was rooted in the fear that more illness would be contracted through such close proximity with sick others. By addressing this fear, the child was able to overcome the distress and remain on a general ward.

In parallel with the work above involving healthy children, there has been an interest in identifying how sick children understand their illness. In part, the interest is theoretical. Any comprehensive account of how children understand illness must be able to accommodate the beliefs of children who have a range of illness experiences. Based on a strict interpretation of Piagetian theory, children with extended illness experience should be more knowledgeable about illness concepts than others (Bibace & Walsh, 1981). However, studies have demonstrated that while chronically ill children may know more than others about their specific illness, they do not necessarily know more about illness in general (e.g. Shagena, Sandler & Perrin, 1988). An explanation for this may be that children with extensive experience of illness practise a form of denial. Perhaps sick children find it easier to cope in their daily lives when they do not allow the often daunting problems associated with illness to preoccupy them and this coping mechanism may impede their understanding of illness concepts (Shagena, Sandler & Perrin, 1988).

The methods used to reveal how children understand their illness are similar to those described above and involve semi-structured interviews. However, general questions about the cause and treatment of minor or everyday childhood illnesses are replaced by questions about the child's own condition. As above, attempts are then made to categorise responses into one of the stages described by Piaget. Using these techniques, it has been argued that the developmental sequence described for healthy children also accounts for development in children with asthma or epilepsy (Perrin, Sayer & Willet, 1991) and arthritis (Beales *et al.*, 1983). In a direct attempt to study how far children with cancer considered themselves to blame for their illness, Springer (1994) compared preschoolers with cancer and healthy controls in terms of their preparedness to accept imminent justice explanations about disease. There were no differences in such beliefs between the groups.

However, the children with cancer differentiated between themselves and others more than the healthy children, i.e., they seemed to believe that there were some causes of illness to which they were more susceptible than other children. Springer (1994) suggests that this has some implications for education, in that it should be explained to children with cancer that they are not more vulnerable to other illnesses compared with healthy children. (This may in fact be too simplistic an interpretation. Children with cancer learn that they are more vulnerable to colds and flu than other children and need to take special precautions in order to avoid contracting chicken pox or measles. To this extent, they are quite right to be concerned that they are differentially vulnerable compared with others.)

For the most part, however, it seems that children are poorly informed about disease and its consequences. In part, this can reflect the questions asked. (It does not matter about the cause of the illness as far as daily management is concerned.) Wider issues about education are also raised. In that children are often diagnosed when they are very young, when information is necessarily directed at the parents, it is not clear how, or when, children routinely obtain formal and systematic information. Children with cystic fibrosis, for example, are normally diagnosed at birth or soon afterwards. As they grow up, it is necessary to explain to them why they need to eat a different diet from the rest of the family, take enzyme replacements with meals and have daily physiotherapy. Later still, they need to learn to do physiotherapy themselves. Boys with this illness are almost always sterile and while education about diet or physiotherapy can often take place on an opportunistic basis, it is not clear how or when the question of infertility should be raised. Staff tend to assume that this is the responsibility of parents, but parents themselves may feel inadequate, poorly informed or too distressed to take on this responsibility themselves. In addition, even where information on diagnosis is adequate, the need to follow up information and provide age appropriate advice as the child grows up is difficult to reconcile with practical arrangements in most clinics. Unfortunately, many children learn about their disease through less than satisfactory sources such as ill-informed friends or relations, other children or the television (Kendrick *et al.*, 1986).

How do sick children find out about their illness?

In an ideal world, children find out about their illness directly, either through information given by their doctor, through their parents, or some joint discussion between the child, parents and doctor (Eiser *et al.*, 1994). However, it is not an ideal world and a distressing number of children find out in less satisfactory circumstances. A friend may let something slip almost casually. It can even happen that a child sees a television programme in which they appear! (We have met children with cancer who have first heard about their illness in this way.)

In the past, open communication with children was not routinely recommended. It was felt that, faced with the knowledge that they had a potentially life threatening disease, children would "give up" or despair. Information was believed to compromise the child's chances of survival. The move toward more open communication has come about through the recognised legal obligations on staff to inform patients about their condition and any possible side-effects of treatment. In addition, many diseases which were once fatal can now be treated, resulting in an increasing number of individuals living with serious illness. Most of these diseases also involve the patients in a degree of self-care; they must learn to be responsible for many aspects of routine health care. The need for patients to manage their own condition also necessitates a good understanding of the nature of the condition and rationale for treatment.

The idea that children should be well informed about their illness is in complete contrast to earlier ideas that knowledge was potentially damaging as far as mental health was concerned. The danger is that we have now swung too far in the other direction and run the risk of failing to recognise that such a policy may be inappropriate for a minority of children.

Some more systematic accounts of how children find out about their illness and integrate this knowledge into their daily lives is very much needed. To date, empirical work in this area is scarce. Perhaps it should not be surprising to find that published work tends to support the idea that there are benefits to children knowing about their disease. However, this work needs to be considered in the light of some criticisms. Broad based measures of general adjustment are used. These measures may lack sensitivity as far as determining how far such knowledge interferes with the child's adjustment. Nevertheless, a number of studies point to the relationship between open and honest communication in the family and the child's adjustment to the disease. Children who adjust well are those who are told about the illness on diagnosis, or, for those diagnosed during infancy or early childhood, by the time they are 6 years old (Claflin & Barbarin, 1991). Despite the current opinion that clinic staff and parents should engage in honest and open communication with the child, there remain areas which seem taboo or not discussed. These most often include discussion of the life-threatening nature of the disease, or possibility of future treatment. Certainly, children do not always report that adults are as honest with them as they think are and this can lead children to feel insecure and unsure about where they can turn for reassurance and answers to their questions.

How do families talk about the illness and its consequences?

Canam (1986) examined how 14 parents communicated with their chronically ill child and any siblings. Parents generally experienced many difficulties talking to their child about the illness and often avoided it. Parents believed they told their children enough about the illness, though most said they answered questions only, did not repeat explanations and gave all their children the same explanation regardless of age. The findings suggest some incongruities between what the children themselves would like and what parents feel comfortable about their child knowing. This includes having more information about the illness and having it repeated.

Poor communication within a family during the treatment of an ill child can cause difficulties not only for the sick child but also for any healthy siblings. Parents may be so preoccupied and dismayed by what is happening that they do not have the resources to keep the rest of the family informed. Often parents may hold back information about the illness and its implications from their healthy children in an attempt to keep their lives as unaffected as possible. However there are often noticeable changes in the ill sibling's appearance and behaviour and in the pattern of the family's activities as treatment progresses. Insufficient explanations for these events may make the healthy child feel excluded from family life. They may see one or both of their parents forming a special relationship with the ill child and in turn perceive that there is a rift between themselves and their parents (Eiser, 1995). Negative attention-seeking behaviour, withdrawal, somatic complaints and a change in academic performance are other difficulties that may arise in children with a chronically ill sibling (Carpenter & Sahler, 1991). Coupled with trying to cope with the illness, these problems can mean quite an escalation in anxiety for the entire family.

There are considerable benefits to informing children about a sibling's illness. First, communication between siblings allows both the ill and the healthy children to express worries about the illness that they may not feel comfortable sharing with parents or doctors (Eiser, 1995). Second, most healthy youngsters who are informed about the illness understand why their sick sister or brother is receiving extra parental care and attention and resign themselves to it (Harder & Bowditch, 1982; Menke, 1987). Third, some illness experience can enhance children's empathy and consideration toward others (Horwitz & Kazak, 1990; Parmelee, 1986).

It is unlikely that parents knowingly alienate their healthy children from themselves or from the family. More likely they underestimate the impact that chronic illness has on their healthy children and may not recognise their considerable anxieties. Encouraging parents to relate more closely with the ill child and any healthy siblings may lead to a reduction of distress during the treatment process for the whole family.

Reducing anxiety during treatment can happen through effective communication within the family and between the family and medical staff. Moreover, ill children may be less distressed if they feel they have a degree of control in the treatment process. This may come through being involved in health care decisions and self-care, though when and how responsibility should be delegated to children in these domains is not a straightforward issue.

Involving Children in Health Care Decisions

Treatment of many chronic conditions involves long and very painful treatment, often with no guarantee of outcome. In the case of young children, parents make the decision about whether or not to continue treatment. As children become older, they rightly become more aware of what is involved and may be less willing than their parents to continue therapy indefinitely. Ellis and Leventhal (1986) reported that children with cancer accepted that their parents and medical staff should make decisions about treatment initially, but felt that they should make any decision to renew chemotherapy if they relapsed. This was part of a wider complaint made by children that they were rarely consulted about treatment-related decisions. These children can present major problems in the clinic. To the extent that they realise what treatment involves, they may be particularly reluctant to undergo therapy in the event of relapse. However, refusal of treatment may result in premature or unnecessary death.

The question arises as to how far young people should be able to make potentially life and death decisions about their own treatment. It is often assumed that the presence of formal operational thought is necessary for an individual to be able to appreciate the nature and consequences of treatments and alternatives, make reasoned choices between alternatives and to reach a decision. Despite the importance of the issue, relatively little work has been concerned with how minors come to understand treatment alternatives and make reasoned decisions. An exception is work by Weithorn and Campbell (1982). These authors developed a series of scenarios involving treatment choice in four situations: diabetes, epilepsy, depressions and enuresis. The scenarios were read to 24 young people at each of four age levels (9, 14, 18 and 21 years). Although 9 year olds were less competent than adults to reason and understand the treatment choices offered, the older groups did not differ. Even so, the 9 year olds did not differ from adults in their expression of reasonable treatment choices, suggesting that the competence of 9 year olds in this respect is quite impressive.

It is of course one thing to consider hypothetical decisions, but quite another to infer from this artificial situation that individuals would make similar treatment choices in real life. Moral and ethical dilemmas mean that this kind of real-life decision making is particularly difficult to study. In practice, some efforts have been made to understand how young people understand the concept of a clinical trial and particularly how they make decisions regarding whether or not to participate.

Progress in treating children with chronic or potentially fatal conditions has advanced through large-scale evaluations of different treatments by means of a clinical trial. In essence, this means that patients are randomly assigned to alternative treatments. Families are often confused and distressed about being asked to participate in a clinical trial. There can seem to be a randomness about the process and anxieties are raised. Therefore, explanations to families need to be thorough and can be expensive in terms of professional time. Efforts need to be made to ensure that families understand the purpose of a trial, as well as the benefits and any disadvantages of participation.

Explanations are especially difficult when the patient is a child. Recent changes in legislation have emphasized the need to consider children's own views about what happens to them. However, evidence as to how well children are able to understand the concept of a clinical trial, or make rational decisions about their treatment is scarce. We do know that adults are often confused when asked to make decisions about their own treatment. In many ways, the decisions for a child are even more complex.

Postlethwaite *et al.* (1995) interviewed 30 children with short stature as a consequence of chronic renal failure and who were to be entered into a trial to determine the effects of growth hormone therapy. While short stature is a consequence of the illness, it is not life-threatening. Treatment involves daily injections of growth hormone and is intrusive and expensive. Nevertheless, for some families, a degree of discomfort may seem to be acceptable in order to achieve a more acceptable height. Children were aged between 9 and 18 years. All but one felt that they had been actively involved with the decision-making process with their parents. Nevertheless, only 36% were able to recall any details of the information about the trial that they had been given.

This study highlights the considerable dilemmas which face families in making complex medical decisions of this kind. Postlethwaite *et al.* (1995) point out that the more obvious factors such as child's height deficit, age, concern about growth or awareness of risks of treatment did not seem more important than the views of paediatricians, or emotional factors in determining how families reach a decision to participate in such a trial. Neither is it clear how far parents, faced with difficult decisions, delegate responsibility for decision-making to the children. How do families then apportion blame if the treatment fails? Given trends in legislation which emphasize the need to take into account children's views on treatment, more research in this area is urgently needed.

Encouraging Self-Care and Compliance with Medical Regimens

Perhaps the most important reason why children need to have a clear and accurate understanding of their disease is that they are frequently required to be responsible for many aspects of their own treatment. Diabetes is the classic example. Children need to be aware that their illness involves some metabolic dysfunction, to the extent that they must balance their food intake, exercise and meet insulin requirements. For the youngest children, little more is expected than an understanding that certain foods are taboo. With increasing age, they must slowly take responsibility for the whole range of self-care activities required.

Good self-care is dependent on a number of variables, including appropriate knowledge of procedures and understanding of medical instructions and agreement about who is responsible for any aspect of the treatment. A failure of research is that there has often been a focus on rather theoretical aspects of illness at the expense of more practical skills. For example, knowledge question-naires typically include questions about the cause or incidence of a disease. This information may have relevance for a child's attitude to treatment, including whether the illness is seen to be very rare or something that is experienced by many people. This information has little relevance for whether or not children are able to look after themselves. Where authors have attempted to measure these different components of knowledge (e.g. Johnson *et al.*, 1982) it seems that children typically lack the basic knowledge necessary to manage their own self-care.

It is often assumed that adolescents are less compliant with medical treatment compared with younger children (Lemanek, 1991). However, this seems to be dependent on adolescents' per-ceptions of the severity of their condition. Where adolescents are aware of the severity of their condition (e.g. following a bone-marrow transplant) they were reported to be more compliant than younger children (Phipps & DeCuir-Whalley, 1990). Poor compli-ance in adolescents may also be the result of a methodological arti-fact. Clinic staff, who make the judgments about the extent of poor compliance, may have unrealistically high expectations for adoles-cents, assuming that their behaviour should be more like adults than is reasonable. Perhaps we have also underestimated the extent to which adolescents have control over their own health. Certainly in diabetes there is increasing evidence that poor blood-sugar control may be dependent partly on hormonal changes which influence the body's insulin metabolism (Amiel *et al.*, 1986).

To some extent, the poor control that characterises adolescence has been attributed to a lack of communication within families, particularly the failure to clarify aspects of care that remain the responsibility of parents and those that have become wholly the responsibility of the adolescent (Anderson *et al.*, 1990).

Transfer of responsibility can happen slowly, with the child initially being enthusiastic about self-care, only to lose interest as soon as competence is achieved. Parents, however, may be slow to realise that the child has become bored. The novelty of independence soon wears thin!

Parents can be a significant influence also on how well children adhere to medical treatment. With regard to chronic illness, adherence can be assessed in relation to 1) satisfactory appointment keeping, 2) prompt reporting of adverse symptoms and 3) competent implementation of home based treatments (mouth care, central access line care[1]).

Among children with cancer, the younger ones had more difficulties in adhering to procedural demands, including mouth care, or cleaning the central line. For all ages, though, better adherence (appointment keeping and prompt report of treatment reactions) was related to parenting styles which were sensitive, less restrictive and more nurturant (Manne *et al.*, 1993).

THE ROLE OF PARENTS

So far, a very child-centred approach has been adopted. However, children do not develop their ideas about health or illness out of a hat. There may be a number of influences, among which parents, teachers, other children, brothers and sisters are obvious contenders. Not surprisingly, the most systematically researched of these is the influence of parents.

Parents undoubtedly do influence their child's attitudes and behaviour. Where a parent has a chronic or on-going health problem, children are more likely to present with unexplained paediatric pain

(Walker, Garber & Greene, 1991). The most parsimonious explanation for this centres on a social learning model; children model their own illness behaviour on that of key adults in their lives.

Parents play an important role in determining the child's behaviour during medical procedures. Chronic conditions frequently require painful and invasive treatments. While some children adopt a very stoic approach, others are more open in their fear and disapproval. Children who are repeatedly noisy are difficult, upset other children and parents and considerably add to the burden of staff. Children's behaviour does seem to depend at least in part on the way in which parents handle the situation. Parents who use distraction (e.g. read to their child while waiting for appointments) have children who are less disruptive than if parents appear agitated and uneasy (Melamed, 1992).

Parents can also influence their children's ability to cope during painful medical procedures. Based on observations of children undergoing bone-marrow aspirations and lumbar punctures and their parents, Blount *et al.* (1991) classified children into high- and low-coping groups. They found that high-coping children tended to have parents who engaged in more coping-promoting behaviours, such as non-procedural talk, humour directed at the child and commands to engage in coping behaviours (such as directions to breathe deeply). Children's distress behaviours in both groups (e.g. crying, screaming, verbal resistance) were associated with distress-promoting behaviours by the parents, such as apologies and criticism.

Other studies (Powers *et al.*, 1993; Manne *et al.*, 1994) have demonstrated the utility of training parents to coach their children to use appropriate coping strategies before and during painful medical procedures. Manne *et al.* (1994) found that children coped better when their parents gave them direct and specific coping commands as opposed to more general encouragement.

INTERVENTIONS

We have stressed throughout that one of the aims of work concerned with children's understanding of illness is to direct interventions, to guide the practice of caring for a sick child. This may involve directing the content of intervention programmes, i.e. ensuring that the information provided is appropriate and of concern to children of different ages. Second, the work can direct the kind of intervention, or the methods used.

With regard to content, there have been some attempts to teach children the social consequences of their disease, rather than focus on the facts. Varni *et al.* (1993) for example developed a social skills programme for work with children with cancer. A common problem for these children is that they are teased on return to school. Before returning to school, children were therefore encouraged to think about the ways in which others might respond to them. Part of the educational package therefore involved teaching the children different ways in which they might respond when teased as well as making them feel that their experience was not unique! They were encouraged to draw on the experiences of children in similar situations. This study demonstrates that for children, knowledge of the disease process is not an integral part of daily coping with disease. Much more important are the social skills necessary to facilitate reintegration with peers.

Despite this, most education focuses on increasing knowledge. Rarely, however, do methods stand up to close scrutiny or fulfil basic criteria for facilitating learning. Mostly, work focuses on school-aged children. Yet in many cases, preschool children are in some need of help. Several conditions require changes in diet which require that children know of the need to avoid certain foods. This can include asthma, diabetes or cystic fibrosis. Children with eczema can make their condition worse by playing in the playschool sand-pit. In all such cases, some basic advice to preschool children about their own self-care needs is essential. Yet education of this age-group is particularly daunting and few have made any attempt to develop methods particularly appropriate.

An exception is a study by Holzheimer, Mohay and Masters (1995) who have shown that preschoolers can learn appropriate use of an inhaler in the control of asthma. These authors compared a teaching video, instruction booklet and opportunities to rehearse the skill. Greater success was achieved when the video was used in combination with opportunities to rehearse the skill compared with a video or asthma information booklet alone. What is most important, however, was the fact that they demonstrated that preschool children could be taught a skill which had previously been considered too complex and developmentally inappropriate. The use of

video in patient education may have considerable potential, especially when part of a package which includes opportunities to
rehearse the chosen skill (Eiser & Eiser, 1995).

CONCLUSIONS

Despite the increasing interest in these issues, there remains a void
in work which really attempts to link research and practice. As a
consequence, theoretical work has had limited influence on practice and vice versa.

Of particular significance is the failure to develop reliable
methods of assessment for younger children, especially those with
limited language and reading skills. Very little work has been conducted in which alternative methods to the semi-structured interview have been adopted. Key questions which have not been
addressed include; can illness understanding in young children be
reliably assessed? Can we develop child-centred instruments, less
dependent on language which are reliable and lend themselves
readily to work with sick or handicapped children? Very few studies
have adopted techniques based on children's more everyday experiences, including stories, pictures or videos. The search for creative measures, which also satisfy conventional statistical criteria
has far to go.

The most significant concession in work with young children has
been the development of ratings based on "faces" rather than the
conventional Likert scales. Some greater innovation has occurred
where workers attempt to quantify children's pain experiences. In
these cases, the use of vertical ladders rather than horizontal scales
or "squeezy" pumps may have some potential.

A major criticism is that almost all work in this area is based on
the views of children from predominantly white backgrounds. Yet
illness and health are socially, as much as cognitively, defined and
therefore it is important to recognise ethnic and racial differences in
the development of these concepts. Lack of attention to this factor
seriously limits our potential to develop appropriate health education for these groups. Nowhere is this need as apparent than in
efforts to inform young children about AIDS and its prevention.
Children from some ethnic and racial groups are at much greater
risk from AIDS than others (Miller, Turner & Moses, 1990). Yet

work typically does not include children from multi-ethnic backgrounds and when it does, fails to account satisfactorily for socioeconomic status. Thus, we are not in a position to develop health education materials which truly target the concerns of groups most at risk. Similar criticisms can be made of work concerned with chronically sick children. Groups are invariably drawn from prestigious medical centres, with poor representation of ethnic groups. Yet some conditions are more prevalent in some cultures than others. Sickle cell disease, for example, predominantly effects children from Afro-Carribean backgrounds. Failure to acknowledge the specific meaning of the disease within the culture again limits efforts to help these children or their families.

In this chapter we have written more at length about the perceptions and experiences of ill children than about those of healthy children. This imbalance reflects the literature. As healthy children represent the ideal state of affairs, their perceptions and experiences are not frequently investigated outside the areas of health promotion and education and their experiences with ill relatives or friends. More common are studies that concentrate on ill children, though this in no way reflects a grim outlook for this population. On the contrary, the types of questions we ask, such as how to increase compliance with treatment and when self-care is appropriate, have to do with the most effective ways of improving the health and quality of life for these children. This health-oriented bias reflects a very optimistic outlook for children with chronic illnesses.

NOTES

1. Central access lines are used in order to facilitate withdrawal of blood and delivery of medication and avoids use of repeated injections.

REFERENCES

Amiel, S.A., Sherwin, R.S., Simonson, D.C., Lauritano, A.A. & Tamborlane, W.V. (1986) Impaired insulin action in puberty: A contributing factor to poor glycemic control in adolescents with diabetes. *The New England Journal of Medicine,* **315**, 215–219.

Anderson, B.J., Auslander, W.F., Jung, K., Miller, J.P. & Santiago, J.V. (1990) Assessing family sharing of diabetes responsibilities. *Journal of Pediatric Psychology*, **15**, 477–492.

Armstrong, N. (1989) Children's physical activity patterns and coronary heart disease. In *Coronary Prevention Group, Should the prevention of heart disease begin in childhood?* (pp. 37–44). London: Coronary Prevention Group.

Bandura, A. (1977) *Social learning theory*. Englewood Cliffs, NJ: Prentice-Hall.

Beales, J.G., Lennox, Holt, P., Keen, J. & Mellor, V. (1983) Children with juvenile chronic arthritis: Their beliefs about their illness and therapy. *Annals of Rheumatic Diseases*, **42**, 481–486.

Bearison, D.J. & Pacifici, C. (1989) Psychological studies of children who have cancer. *Journal of Applied Developmental Psychology*, **5**, 263–280.

Bernstein, A.C. & Cowen, P.A. (1981) Children's conceptions of birth and sexuality. In R. Bibace & M.E. Walsh (Eds.), *Children's conceptions of health, illness and bodily functions*. San Francisco: Jossey-Bass.

Bibace, R. & Walsh, M.E. (1980) Development of children's concepts of illness. *Pediatrics*, **66**, 912–917.

Bibace, R. & Walsh, M.E. (1981) Children's conceptions of illness. In R. Bibace & M.E. Walsh (Eds.), *Children's conceptions of health, illness and bodily functions*. San Francisco: Jossey-Bass.

Blount, R.L., Landolf-Fritsche, B., Powers, S.W. & Sturges, J.W. (1991) Differences between high and low coping children and between parents and staff behaviors during painful medical procedures. *Journal of Pediatric Psychology*, **16**, 795–809.

Brewster, A.B. (1982) Chronically ill hospitalized children's concepts of their illness. *Pediatrics*, **69**, 355–362.

Burbach, D.J. & Peterson, L. (1986) Children's concepts of physical illness: A review and critique of the cognitive developmental literature. *Health Psychology*, **5**, 305–327.

Cadman, D., Boyle, M. & Offord, D.R. (1988) The Ontario Child Health Study: Social adjustment and mental health of siblings of children with chronic health problems. *Journal of Developmental and Behavioural Pediatrics*, **9**, 117–121.

Canam C. (1986) Talking about cystic fibrosis within the family: What parents need to know. *Issues in Comprehensive Pediatric Nursing*, **9**, 167–178.

Carey, S. (1985) *Conceptual change in childhood.* Cambridge, Ma: MIT Press.

Carpenter, P.J. & Sahler, O.J.Z. (1991) Sibling perception and adaptation to childhood cancer: Conceptual and methodological considerations. In J.H. Johnson & S.B. Johnson (Eds.), *Advances in child health psychology.* Gainesville: University of Florida Press.

Chapman, G. & Maclean, H. (1993) 'Junk food' and 'health food': meanings of food in adolescent women's culture. *Journal of Nutrition Education,* **25**, 108–113.

Claflin, C.J. & Barbarin, O.A. (1991) Does telling less protect more? Relationships among age, information disclosure and what children with cancer see and feel. *Journal of Pediatric Psychology,* **16**, 169–174.

Cohn, L.D., Macfarlane, S., Yanez, C. & Imai, W.K. (1995) Risk-Perception: Differences between adolescents and adults. *Health Psychology,* **14**, 217–222.

Coppens, N.M. (1986) Cognitive characteristics as predictors of children's understanding of safety and prevention. *Journal of Pediatric Psychology,* **1**, 189–202.

Crider, C. (1981) Children's concepts of the body interior. In R. Bibace & M.E. Walsh (Eds.), *Children's conceptions of health, illness and bodily functions.* San Francisco: Jossey-Bass.

Dennison, C.M. & Shepherd, R. (1995) Adolescent food choice: an application of the Theory of Planned Behaviour. *Journal of Human Nutrition and Dietetics,* **8**, 9–23.

Eiser, C. (1995) *Growing up with a chronic disease: The impact on children and their families (2nd ed.).* London: Jessica Kingley Publishers.

Eiser, C., Eiser, J.R. & Lang, J. (1990) How adolescents compare AIDS with other diseases: Implications for prevention. *Journal of Pediatric Psychology,* **15**, 97–103.

Eiser, C., Parkyn, T., Havermans, T. & McNinch, A. (1994) Parents' recall of the diagnosis of cancer in their child. *Psycho-Oncology,* **3**, 197–203.

Eiser, C., Patterson, D. & Eiser, J.R. (1983) Children's knowledge of health and illness: implications for health education. *Child: Care, Health and Development,* **9**, 285–292.

Eiser, J.R. & Eiser, C. (1995) Effectiveness of video on psychology health education: A review. Unpublished report for the Health Education Authority, London.

Elkind, D. (1967) Egocentrism in adolescence. *Child Development*, **38**, 1025–1034.

Ellis, R. & Leventhal, B. (1986) Information needs and decision-making preferences of children with cancer. *Psycho-Oncology*, **2**, 227–284.

Gellman, R. & Baillargeon, R. (1983) Review of some Piagetian concepts. In J.H. Flavess & E.M. Markman (Eds.), *Handbook of child psychology*, New York: Wiley.

Gladis, M.M., Michela, J.L. & Walter, H.J. (1992) High school students' perceptions of AIDS risk: Realistic appraisal or motivated denial? *Health Psychology*, **11**, 307–316.

Gortmaker, S.L., Must, A., Perrin, J., Sobol, A. & Dietz, W.H. (1993) Social and economic consequences of overweight in adolescence and young adulthood. *The New England Journal of Medicine*, **329**, 1008–1012.

Harder, C.F. & Bowditch, A. (1982) The impact of cystic fibrosis on siblings. *Children's Health Care*, **14**, 141–145.

Harlan, W.R. (1989) A perspective on school-based cardiovascular research. *Health Education Quarterly*, **16**, 151–154.

Havermans, G.M.F.A. & Eiser, C. (1991) Locus of control and efficacy in healthy children and those with diabetes. *Psychology and Health*, **5**, 297–306.

Holzheimer, L., Mohay, H. & Masters, B. (1995) A comparison of written versus video taped materials for teaching young children about asthma management. *Proceedings of the seventh national health promotion conference*, Brisbane.

Horwitz, W.A. & Kazak, A.E. (1990) Family adaptation to childhood cancer: Sibling and family system variables. *Journal of Clinical Child Psychology*, **19**, 221–228.

Johnson, S.B., Pollak, T., Silverstein, J.H., *et al.* (1982) Cognitive and behavioral knowledge about insulin-dependent diabetes among children and parents. *Pediatrics*, **69**, 708–713.

Journal of Pediatric Psychology (1993) Special Issue: Interventions in Pediatric Psychology, 18.

Kalnins, I. & Love, R. (1982) Children's concepts of health and illness — and implications for health education: An overview. *Health Education Quarterly*, **9**, 104–115.

Kendrick, C., Culling, J., Oakhill, T. & Mott, M. (1986) Children's understanding of their illness and its treatment within a paediatric oncology unit. *Association for Child Psychology and Psychiatry* (Newsletter), **8**, 16–20.

Langford, W.S. (1948) Physical illness and convalescence: Their meaning to the child. *Journal of Pediatrics,* **32**, 242–250.

Lemanek, K. (1991) Adherence issues in the medical management of asthma. *Journal of Pediatric Psychology,* **15**, 437–458.

Liebert, R.M. & Sprafkin, J. (1988) *The early window: effects of television on children and youth (3rd ed.).* New York: Pergamon.

Manne, S., Bakeman, R., Jacobsen, P.B., Gorfinkle, K. & Redd, W.H. (1994) An analysis of a behavioral intervention for children undergoing venipuncture. *Health Psychology,* **13**, 556–566.

Manne, S., Jacobsen, P.B., Gorfinkle, K., Gerstein, F. & Redd, W.H. (1993) Treatment adherence difficulties among children with cancer: The role of parenting style. *Journal of Pediatric Psychology,* **18**, 47–62.

Meadow, R. (1988) Time past and time present for children and their doctors. In J.O. Forfar (Ed.), *Health in a changing ward* (pp. 198–214). Oxford University Press, Oxford.

Melamed, B. (1992) Family factors predicting children's reactions to anesthesia induction. In A.M. LaGreca, C.J. Siegel, J.L. Wallander & C.E. Walker (Eds.), *Stress and coping in child health* (pp. 140–156). New York: Guilford Press.

Menke, E.M. (1987) The impact of a child's illness on school-aged siblings. *Children's Health Care,* **15**, 132–140.

Miller, H.G., Turner, C.F. & Moses, L.E. (Eds.) (1990) *AIDS: The second decade.* Washington, DC: National Academy Press.

Moffatt, M.E.K. & Pless, I.B. (1983) Locus of control in juvenile diabetic campers: Changes during camp and relationship to camp assessments. *Journal of Pediatrics,* **103**, 146–150.

Nader, P.R., Perry, C., Maccoby, N., Solomon, D., Killen, J., Telch, M. & Alexander, J.K. (1982) Adolescent perceptions of family health behavior: A tenth-grade educational activity to increase family awareness of a community cardiovascular risk reduction program. *Journal of School Health,* **52**, 372–377.

Nelson, K. (Ed.) (1985) *Event knowledge: structure and function in development.* Hillsdale, N.J.: Lawrence Erlbaum.

Neuhauser, C., Amsterdam, B., Hines, P. & Steward, M. (1978) Children's concepts of healing: Cognitive development and locus of control factors. *American Journal of Orthopsychiatry,* **48**, 335–341.

Newman, J. & Taylor, A. (1992) Effect of a means-end contingency on young children's food preferences. *Journal of Experimental Child Psychology,* **53**, 200–216.

Oakley, A., Bendelow, G., Barnes, J., Buchanan, M. & Husain, O.A. (1995) Health and cancer prevention: knowledge and beliefs of children and young people. *British Medical Journal*, **310**, 1029–1033.

Osborne, M.L., Kistner, J.A. & Helgemo, B. (1993) Developmental progression in children's knowledge of AIDS: Implications for education and attitudinal change. *Journal of Pediatric Psychology*, **18**, 177–192.

Parmelee, A.H. (1986) Children's illnesses: Their beneficial effects on behavioural development. *Child Development*, **57**, 1–10.

Perrin, E.C. & Gerrity, P.S. (1981) There's a demon in your belly: Children's understanding of illness. *Pediatrics*, 841–849.

Perrin, E.C., Sayer, A.G. & Willett, J.B. (1991) Sticks and stones may break my bones ... Reasoning about illness causality and body functioning in children who have a chronic illness. *Pediatrics*, **88**, 608–619.

Phipps, S. & DeCuir-Whalley, S. (1990) Adherence issues in pediatric bone-marrow transplantation. *Journal of Pediatric Psychology*, **15**, 459–475.

Piaget, J. (1929) *The child's conception of the world*. New York: Harcourt Brace.

Postlethwaite, R.J., Reynolds, J.M., Wood, A.J., Evans, J.H.C., Lewis, M.A. & Eminson, D.M. (1995) Recruiting patients to clinical trials: lessons from studies of growth hormone treatment in renal failure. *Archives of Disease in Childhood*, **73**, 30–35.

Powers, S.W., Blount, R.L., Bachanas, P.J., Cotter, M.W. & Swan, S.C. (1993) Helping preschool leukemia patients and their parents cope during injections. Special Issue: Interventions in pediatric psychology. *Journal of Pediatric Psychology*, **18**, 681–695.

Shagena, M.M., Sandler, H.K. & Perrin, E.C. (1988) Concepts of illness and perception of control in healthy children and in children with chronic illnesses. *Developmental and Behavioral Pediatrics*, **9**, **5**, 252–256.

Siegal, M., Patty, J. & Eiser, C. (1990) A re-examination of children's conceptions of contagion. *Psychology and Health*, **4**, 159–165.

Simeonsson, R.J., Buckley, L. & Monson, L. (1979) Conceptions of illness causality in hospitalized children. *Journal of Pediatric Psychology*, **4**, 77–84.

Springer, K. (1994) Beliefs about illness causality among preschoolers with cancer: Evidence against imminent justice. *Journal of Pediatric Psychology*, **19**, 91–102.

Steward, M. & Regalbulto, B.A. (1981) Do doctors know what children know? *American Journal of Orthopsychiatry*, **45**, 146–149.

Stone, E.J., Perry, C.L. & Luepker, R.V. (1989) Synthesis of cardiovascular behavioral research for youth health promotion. *Health Education Quarterly*, **16**, 155–169.

Tinsley, B.J. (1992) Multiple influences on the acquisition and socialization of children's health attitudes and behavior: An integrative review. *Child Development*, **63**, 1043–1069.

Varni, J.W., Katz, E.R., Colegrove, R. & Dolgin, M. (1993) The impact of social skills training on the adjustment of children with newly diagnosed cancer. *Journal of Pediatric Psychology*, **18**, 751–768.

Walker, L.S., Garber, J. & Greene, J.W. (1991) Somatization symptoms in pediatric abdominal pain patients: Relation to chronicity of abdominal pain and parent somatization. *Journal of Abnormal Child Psychology*, **19**, 379–394.

Weithorn, L.A. & Campbell, S.B. (1982) The competency of children and adults to make informed treatment decisions. *Child Development*, **53**, 1589–1598.

Whalen, C.K., Henker, B., O'Neil, R., Hollingshead, J., Holman, A. & Moore, B. (1994) Optimism in children's judgments of health and environmental risks, *Health Psychology*, **13**, 319–325.

3
Are There Differences in Perceptions of Illness Across the Lifespan?

Elaine A. Leventhal & Melissa Crouch*

INTRODUCTION

The behaviours that we adopt to maintain health and avoid and control disease reflect our medical and psychosocial histories. These histories are stored as memories of events (e.g., memories of illness in ourselves, family members and friends and socially derived information about health and disease from teachers and mass media), and knowledge and skills for avoiding and treating illness (e.g., dietary practices, exercise, use of over the counter preventives and medications and seeking medical care and using prescribed treatments). The schemata in this knowledge base in combination with new somatic sensations and information about illness in other persons, generate *illness representations* whose attributes define the *cause, identity* (symptoms & label), potential *consequences*, possibility for *control* and *time-lines* associated with each of these attributes (time for development: for cure, disability and/or death). These representations point to specific coping procedures for avoiding and managing the defined threat and generate

*Preparation of this chapter and the results were supported by grants AG-03501 and AG-12072 from the National Institutes on Aging. We would like to thank Howard Leventhal for critical readings of early drafts.

goals for evaluating coping outcomes. Thus, illness representations vary over settings and over time, and shape how we cope with illness and treatment.

The question addressed in this chapter is whether specific components of illness representations and coping strategies evolve across the lifetime. This question defines a particular approach to investigations of the relationship of age to health and to health and illness behaviours. Rather than treating chronological age as a direct determinant of health and health behaviour, chronological age is entered as a moderating factor in our *self regulation* framework (Figure 1). This approach leads us to ask whether the relationship of age to health behaviours is mediated by differences in the way older persons in these cohorts represent illnesses and select strategies and specific procedures to cope with potential and current health threats. Thus, if we find differences in health or health behaviours among samples of old-old, young old, middle-aged and young adult study participants, we are not satisfied to restrict ourselves to the question of whether these differences are a direct effect of chronological age (or cohort). We are now concerned as to whether age (or cohort differences) has led to changes in how the threat is represented and whether age has affected the overall strategies or specific coping tactics for detecting, preventing and treating the threat. If age acts through these mediating factors and if we can identify the factors through which it operates, we will have both a more complete understanding as to how age affects health and illness behaviour and most important, we will be better able to intervene to optimize behaviour to enhance health and improve the individual's quality of life.

Figure 1 suggests at least two additional sets of factors that affect health and illness behaviours: both involve age-related changes in the self. First, differences in age produce differences in the information people are exposed to and in experience in responding to and managing such factors. An obvious factor is the age related increase in morbidity and mortality among members of one's immediate cohort. This factor is likely to be common across cohorts and cultures: the older one gets the more one finds family and peers talking about and managing chronic illness and the greater the mortality among these persons. These age-related changes in morbidity and mortality are reflected in two types of statistics: the objective data collected by epidemiologists and the subjective data compris-

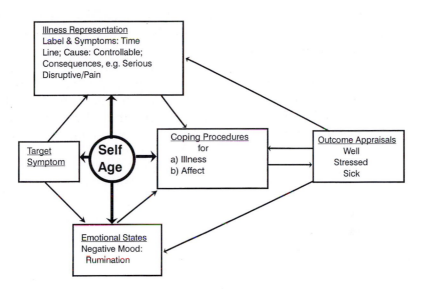

FIGURE 1 Age as a moderating factor in the illness representation model. Age can affect the target symptoms, the way the symptoms are represented, emotional responses, coping procedures and appraisals. Data indicate a shift in age-related coping strategies to optimize adaptation and compensate for risk inducing changes in symptoms and representations.

ing what we have called "common-sense epidemiology" of older persons (H. Leventhal, Nerenz & Strauss, 1982).

A second set of factors affects self identity. It consists of age related changes in the biological self and age related changes in work and social roles affecting economic and social status. Aging related physiological changes alter the way specific diseases behave both in symptom manifestation and in response to treatment. For example, it is often said that age leads to a blunting of disease symptoms (slower rate of emergence and less severity) encouraging the identification of disease related symptoms as symptoms of normal aging. Inappropriate self diagnoses of this type can occur because the opportunity to experience, seek treatment and learn how to correctly label blunted symptoms will lag behind the occurrence of these physiological changes. Inappropriate responses to illness symptoms because of this lag may increase risk to health and result in unnecessary morbidity. Thus, our premise is that it is the variables that accompany chronological age, not chronological age itself, that are responsible for age related changes in health and illness behaviours. The expression "*self age*" in Figure 1 stands for the change in self identity that arises from the individual's observation of mortality and morbidity in others and the experience of the physical signs of aging in him or herself. The facet of an individual's self identity that may change as a function of these life span related experiences is an increasing sense of vulnerability to illness and susceptibility to harm, which may affect older persons' decisions to act to prevent, diagnose and treat physical illness.

Because changes in the strategies and tactics adopted for managing illness threats may reflect variables in either of the two broad sets of factors discussed above (i.e., changes in procedures generated by modifications of the representations of disease threats and changes in procedures generated by modifications of the representation of the self and its resources), it may be difficult to isolate the determinants of age related differences in health and illness behaviours. It may also prove difficult to separate the contribution of ethnic, social, economic status and history (cohort) from age related changes in the representation of disease and self. In the remainder of this chapter, we will examine these issues drawing upon existent data whenever possible. Because the investigation of the effects of age upon illness representations and self identity is in its infancy, we will be forced at times to engage in speculation about the ways in which these age related changes may alter health and illness behaviours.

SYMPTOMS AND THEIR REPRESENTATION

Many illnesses reveal themselves symptomatically in their early stages. Thus, the first notice of a somatic change can initiate a period of time during which the individual is faced with the need to identify or appraise the meaning of a somatic change. Understanding the process that unfolds during this initial period of "self diagnosis" is critical as its conclusion, the establishment of a tentative identity of the somatic change, is critical for subsequent behaviour. The decision that symptoms such as soreness and emission of fluid from the breast are a sign of breast cancer rather than a sign of injury-caused infection, will likely generate a sharply contrasting set of expectations respecting consequences (life threatening vs not life threatening), control (uncertain versus treatable), time-line (last for life vs a few days), causes (genetics, injury) and procedures for control (surgery and chemotherapy versus antibiotics). Age related changes in this appraisal process and changes in beliefs about the strategies and tactics relevant for threat management, can have important consequences for the selection of coping procedures and for health outcomes. Our investigations and those of others have attempted to identify rules guiding the symptom appraisal process that may change over the life span. One of three such rules that have been identified involves retrospective self-comparisons (i.e., the *age-illness rule*); the two others involve scans of the external environment that may change over the life span (i.e., the *stress-illness rule* and the *shared-benign/singular-serious rule*). As all three of these rules allow the individual to discount the medical meaning and potential seriousness of somatic changes, they could create health risks if used to excess by older, more frail persons.

Discounting Via Historical Self-Comparison

Comparisons of current with prior body schema form the core of the evaluation of all somatic changes. These comparisons can be made against the prior perception or "feel" of the body schema (e.g., noticing an asymmetry, lump, pain or ache in a previously unattended to and benign region of the soma) or against prior conceptual knowledge of the body (e.g., I can't recall ever feeling/having anything like that before). While establishing the identity of a somatic change, whether it is an illness or something else, is the core issue for a person of any age, it is an issue that is compounded for the elderly. "Wait and see", a widely used strategy or rule for evaluating the direction and meaning of initially ambiguous symptoms, may be less effective for older than younger persons for two reasons. First, older persons often report experiencing more bodily symptoms than do younger persons (Hale *et al.*, 1986; NCHS, 1970). Hence older persons have to notice and evaluate new symptoms against a larger and more complex background of somatic activity. Second, both the biological changes associated with normal aging and the chronic conditions that are common in later life, develop only gradually. In addition, symptoms that depend upon a vigorous immune response such as fever and symptoms of pain in response to various factors such as cardiovascular disease appear to present in blunted form with increasing age. Thus, the older individual has the difficult task of evaluating the significance of symptoms that are slow to change and that appear against an increasingly complex background of age related somatic changes.

Aging or illness: An attribution rule

Because the symptoms in the elderly are often slow to develop, less severe and longer lasting, and because they appear against a more complex background of somatic sensations, older persons may have difficulty distinguishing illness specific symptoms from those attributed to normal aging, creating unnecessary risk for morbidy and mortality. Indeed, Kart (1981) has suggested that physicians, as well as the elderly themselves, overestimate the changes that are caused by biological aging, physicians often assuming that physical and intellectual debilitation necessarily come with age and that pain should be expected as a consequence of aging. One consequence of older persons, acceptance of symptoms as signs of aging is that they fail to report these symptoms to friends and medical practitioners (Brody & Kleban, 1981). For example, 60% of the participants in Brody and Kleban's study failed to tell their physicians of difficulties passing urine and 71% failed to report swelling of feet or ankles. These substantial failures of reporting do not seem to reflect inhibition due to embarrassment at reporting somatic changes as only 39% failed to report on constipation. This type of misattribution could be important if it leads to the discounting and ignoring of treatable symptoms that impact negatively upon quality of life and delay of diagnosis and treatment of potentially life-threatening disorders (Leventhal & Diefenbach, 1991). Haug, Wykle and Namazi's (1989) data showing that aging attribution increased self-care rather than seeking medical care supports this concern even though the effect is slightly more reliable for symptoms that older persons perceive as less serious, as the lay-persons' perception of seriousness will not necessarily agree with medical evaluation.

Experimental evidence of the existence of an *age-illness rule* was reported by Prohaska *et al.* (1987). They presented participants with scenarios depicting symptoms of varying severity and duration and found that the likelihood of attributing symptoms to aging was greater for mild than severe symptoms. Attributions of symptoms to age rather than illness also occurred more frequently for older than younger participants regardless of the severity and duration of the symptoms. Participants who attributed symptoms to age also reported less emotional distress and more delay in care-seeking than participants who attributed symptoms to illness — this held for participants of all ages. The results with the scenarios were replicated in a field study where middle-aged (40 to 55 years of age) and older participants (65 years and over) were interviewed prior to seeing their physician at a medical clinic and asked to report on their attributions and delay in seeking care with respect to the symptoms for which they were seeking care. Participants' responses showed both stimulus and age effects. Symptoms with gradual onset were more likely attributed to age (41%) than symptoms with sudden onset (23%), and older patients were somewhat more likely to attribute their symptoms to aging than were middle-aged patients, although this latter difference was not statistically significant. The data were also clear in showing that all patients were more likely to delay care-seeking when they initially attributed symptoms to aging. Extrapolation from these data suggests that older individuals may be at greater risk because they are somewhat more likely to make aging attributions and because older persons are less robust and resistant to pathogens and may suffer more if they do delay in seeking care for a serious illness. Thus, while stimuli, such as gradual onset of symptoms, that lead to aging attributions and their behavioral consequences are similar for younger and older persons (Keller *et al.*, 1989), negative health consequences of errors induced by such attributions are more likely for the elderly.

Attributions Based Upon Environmental Scanning

Safety in sharing

While comparing self now to self yesterday is a familiar route for gathering information and establishing the identity of a somatic change or a medical test, the meaning of a symptom can also be clarified by identifying possible environmental causes. Other persons are a particularly valuable source of information depending on their similarity or relevance to the comparing person. For example, Kulik and Mahler (1987) found that coronary by-pass patients were less fearful and rehabilitated more rapidly postoperatively if their preoperative roommates were patients who had completed surgery. The concrete or perceptual evidence that others are alive and looking well, countered the images of mutilation, death and pain that may fill the mind during this anticipatory period. Contrary, however, to social comparison theory (Festinger, 1954) and Schachter's (1959) work on emotional comparison in which undergraduates anticipating exposure to the threat of electric shock preferred to wait with others in a similar situation, Kulik and Mahler's data suggest that the greatest benefit occurred with comparison to non-similar others. Thus, preoperative patients benefited more from comparison with roommates who had completed and survived surgery than from comparison with roommates who were in a similar, preoperative and expectant frame of mind. The healthy and non-distressed appearance of a postoperative roommate was more relevant to countering the fear provoking cognitions of the preoperative patient. There is no way of knowing whether the difference in response is partially attributable to differences in the participants' ages (Kulik and Mahler's participants in their 40s to 70s, Schachter's in their late teens) or entirely due to differences in the situation.

A series of elegant studies by Jemmott and his collaborators (summarized by Croyle and Jemmott, 1991), show how information generated by monitoring the social environment can substantially reduce the perceived threat of a positive result from a diagnostic test when the observation demonstrates that risk is shared. The targeted participants in these studies were given (false) feedback (a change of colour of a paper strip exposed to the participants' saliva) suggesting they were deficient for a pancreatic enzyme. Participants rated the enzymatic deficiency as less severe if they were one of several individuals within the group given positive test results (e.g., 4 of 5 having colour change) while participants rated it as more severe if they were the only person in the group with a positive test. Although we have no data to indicate whether similar findings would be obtained with older persons, the participants in these studies were Princeton undergraduates, there is no shortage of evidence indicating that older persons converse about medical topics (e.g., symptoms, treatments and physicians). For example, we compared the responses of 111 symptomatic participants who were interviewed immediately prior to seeing their doctors on a patient driven visit, to the responses of 33 participants who also were symptomatic but did not visit a doctor, and found that 92% of the patient group had discussed their symptoms with another person in comparison to 61% of the controls (Cameron, Leventhal &

Leventhal, 1993). While most of these 45 to 90 year old participant care-seekers said they "simply wanted to talk about the problem" (56%), many wanted to find out what to do and whether the symptom was something to worry about. In addition, a substantial number of the care-seekers were told to go to the doctor (50%) while few controls were so advised (9%). The reports of care-seekers suggest that social information emphasizes the seriousness of symptoms (i.e., over half of the care-seekers who talked about their symptoms were advised to see a doctor). But one could also conclude that social information downplays severity from the fact that only 9% of the controls were advised to seek care, though 61% had talked to someone about their symptoms (1 in 7 ratio). As the number of symptoms reported increases with age, it is reasonable to suppose that in comparison to younger persons, the elderly are more likely to share information with symptomatic others and, therefore, downplay the seriousness of their symptoms.

Stress-illness rule

Studies showing that life stress increases the use of medical care, appear to support the common-sense observation that stress is a major cause of illness (Mechanic, 1974). Not surprisingly, the studies supporting this simple hypothesis are counterbalanced by studies showing only a very weak effect or showing no effect at all (Berkanovic, Hurwicz & Landsverk, 1988; Sarason *et al.*, 1985). Disagreements of this sort are often responded to with methodological criticisms and improved replications, which we believe is insufficient. Our response to inconsistency of main effects is to turn to theory in a search for relevant moderators. Our basic proposition, that people are "common-sense" medical scientists who search for the meaning of somatic events, as well as the suggestion by Pennebaker (1982), led Baumann *et al.* (1989) to reason that the presence of life stress may lead people to attribute symptoms to stress rather than to illness when searching for the cause of a somatic event. They also reasoned that stress attributions would be more likely for sets of symptoms that were unfamiliar rather than familiar. A laboratory simulation was designed in which different groups of participants were asked to imagine how they would react to a set of five symptoms if they were to experience them the following morning. Approximately half the participants were studied the day before a mid-term examination (a stressful morning ahead) and the other half on a Friday before a stress free weekend. The participants responding the day before a mid-term were more likely to regard the symptoms as signs of stress (73.5% made stress and 46.3% made illness attributions), than those completing the task on a pleasant Friday afternoon (34.5% made stress and 71.4% made illness attributions). The effect was strong for two of the three sets of symptoms used in the study: an ambiguous set and the unfamiliar set of symptoms of diabetes. There were no effects for the set that represented mononucleosis, a syndrome that was frequently discussed and well known among the university students.

With this experimental information in hand, Cameron, Leventhal and Leventhal (1995) examined the effects of the presence of this contextual factor, life stress, on both the interpretation of symptoms and the seeking of medical care in a sample of 361 patients whose ages ranged from 45 to 90 years of age. The hypothesis was that the presence of life stress would encourage participants to interpret symptoms as signs of stress rather than signs of illness, but that this effect would occur only for ambiguous symptoms such as fatigue, headaches and others that might reflect either illness or stress. For each participant, a single symptom episode was selected at random from a group of five symptoms reported during five interviews which she or he had completed over the span of a year. The questions about this symptom focused on participants' perceptions of its cause and specifically if the symptom was caused by stress. Participants were also queried about factors such as the perceived seriousness of the symptom, its duration, how they coped with it and whether they sought medical care and the emotional distress caused by the symptom. Ratings by four internists of each of the symptoms on scales pertaining to the likelihood of psychophysiological origin and to the need for follow-up testing were used to classify the symptoms as clearly disease specific or as of uncertain or ambiguous cause.

The results were clear: when a stressor was present, one third to half of the participants attributed ambiguous symptoms to stress, while less than 10% of the participants with symptoms that were clear indicators of illness made this attribution. More importantly, the presence of life stress had virtually no effect on seeking medical care for symptoms that were clear indicators of illness. Participants sought medical care for these symptoms whether they had no life stress (43%), a chronic life stress (51%) or a new life stress (52%). But when symptoms were ambiguous, participants were much less likely to seek care. Approximately 20% of the participants sought care for ambiguous symptoms when there was no life stress or a new stressor in their lives. Not all stressors are the same however. Care-seeking is low (22%) when the stressor is new, defined as appearing in the prior week, but care-seeking is increased (40%) when the stressor is three or more weeks old and was creating distress well before the appearance of the symptom. A moderately complex mental operation, evaluating symptom ambiguity and relating ambiguity to the presence and duration of life stress (if brief stress then attribute symptom to stress, if longer term stress then attribute symptoms to illness), appears to underlie older persons' decisions to seek care.

It is clear, therefore, that life stress can either decrease or increase care-seeking depending upon the causal attribution given the symptoms, which depends in turn upon the nature and duration of both the symptoms and the stressor. We can expect the details and outcome of such processes to vary, however, as a function of the specific disease and, perhaps, as a function of the age of the individual. For example, in their experiments conducted with university students, Baumann *et al.* (1989) demonstrated that students reported the very same symptoms characteristically reported by hypertensives if they were told their blood pressures were high after having it taken. Students not given such false feedback did not report such symptom experiences. Further studies showed that the effect of labelling (high blood pressure) on somatic experience, which was seen as evidence for a "symmetry" rule (i.e., given symptoms seek label, given label seek symptoms) is moderated by the individual's representation of hypertension. Specifically, individuals who believe hypertension is a stress-induced disorder report more symptoms after they are given a high blood pressure reading (i.e., they assume they may have the disease) if they also believe they are under high levels of life stress. In contrast, individuals who believe high blood pressure is due to systemic, constitutional factors, report more symptoms after they receive feedback showing a high reading if they also believe their life situation is not stressful: a high reading in the absence of stress means hypertension.

Similar effects have been observed in a sample of 45 to 70 year old African American men and women (Contrada *et al.*, 1996).

These investigators assessed two critical attributes of the representation of hypertension, causes and control, and grouped participants on the basis of their models of hypertension: those holding a behavioral model (that hypertension is caused by life stress and risky life-style and controlled by stress reduction and life-style changes) and those holding a biological or constitutional model of the disease (that hypertension is caused by genes, family history, etc. and controlled by medication). As participants could be high on both or neither, four groups were formed: behavioral model only, behavioral and biological, biological only and neither. Comparisons revealed that the behavioral group's systolic and diastolic blood pressures were statistically and clinically higher than the values of the other three groups combined (behavioral systolic = 157.3 and diastolic = 92.5, versus 140 and 84.4 mm of mercury for the three remaining groups, there were no significant differences among the three remaining groups). While we assume that intermittent rather than continuous use of medication may be responsible for the elevated pressures of participants holding a behavioral model, it is possible, of course, that the model is a product of variation in pressure. The direction of causation is unclear in these correlational data.

Strategies, tactics and risk to the self

The data for aging and stress attributions as well as those for social comparison, suggest that the elderly appear to be more likely to misattribute symptoms to benign causes or to downgrade the seriousness of their symptoms and to put themselves at risk for health crises. The increased risk caused by aging attributions is relatively easy to understand as is the downgrading of seriousness due to social sharing. The former leads to increased delay in care-seeking and is somewhat more common among the elderly, and the latter reflects the higher prevalence of symptoms among older persons. Although there is no clear evidence to suggest that delay in care-seeking due to stress attributions is more common among the elderly, there is a factor that may increase the potential risk to the elderly from both age and stress attributions and social sharing. Specifically, many symptoms of the life threatening chronic diseases that strike in the later years, are gradual in onset and ambiguous. They are, therefore, more susceptible to both aging and stress attributions. In addition, medical folklore suggests that old age tends to be associated with a blunting of symptoms, which may be a product of reductions, in older age, of the intensity of emotional reactions (Diener, Sandvik & Larsen, 1985) that play a key role in the amplification of pain sensations (H. Leventhal & Everhart, 1979). The greater use of medical care by the elderly seems inconsistent with the presence of these risk enhancing attributions and suggests that some other factor may affect health behaviours in the later years.

VULNERABILITY AND BOLSTERING THE SELF-SYSTEM

The Risk Aversion, Resource Conservation Hypothesis

What might change in the later years to account for the greater use of health care and the vigor and survival of the elderly despite the risk that seems to be entailed by age and stress attributions? Phrased differently, is there a change in strategy with increasing age that compensates for the risk created by these tactics?

The data that we collected during the late 1970s through the mid 1980s supported the hypothesis that in comparison to middle-aged and younger persons, the elderly are less willing to take risks with their health and are increasingly motivated to conserve and protect their physical, social and economic resources (H. Leventhal, Nerenz & Strauss, 1982; Prohaska *et al.*, 1985; Prohaska *et al.*, 1987). Thus, while the rules guiding the generation of illness representations may favor discounting and minimization of threat, a set of broadly based strategies may emerge which exert an over-arching influence on the procedures selected for health maintenance and disease avoidance. Because these strategies are focused on the procedural/action component of our model (Figure 1), they are independent of and can compensate for the possibility of risk that emerges from the minimization procedures involved in the interpretation of symptoms and the construction of illness representations.

What might be responsible for risk aversion and energy conservation by elderly persons and what evidence do we have to support this hypothesis? First, we can repeat the points made at the opening of this chapter respecting age-related changes in the self. People in the seventh decade of their lives will observe increases in morbidity and mortality among members of their cohort and the complete or near disappearance of the parental generation and will experience the transition to the role of family seniors. The increase in morbidity and mortality among peers is paralleled by physical changes in the self: changes in sleep patterns and sensory losses (hearing, sight, somatic sensations associated with bodily functions, etc.) that result in more time spent talking about chronic conditions and their management. In concert with these age-related biological changes are changes in work and social roles affecting economic and social status. The individual's psychological age is likely to include, therefore, an increased sense of human frailty and the transitory nature of life leading to a growing sense of vulnerability to illness and susceptibility to harm. This increased sense of vulnerability, in conjunction with a lifetime of successful self and medical management of a variety of controllable ills, would be the source of a strategic shift toward increased promotion of physical health and swifter and more efficient use of expert care for the diagnosis and treatment of potential disease. Indeed, placing the burden of illness management on the health care professional reduces distress accompanying uncertainty and effort involved in self-care. The pattern is completely concordant with the increased selectivity, optimization and compensation in responding that Baltes and Baltes (1990) proposed as the mechanisms involved for adapting to age related cognitive changes and that Carstensen (1992) has proposed as the adaptive process underlying social relationships.

Evidence for risk aversion in treatment and preventive action

A series of studies from our laboratory provided increasingly strong support for the risk aversion hypothesis. A review of the health behaviour literature by H. Leventhal, Prohaska and Hirschman (1985), showed that performance of many health promoting behaviours increase with age and suggested that increased health behaviours are due to increased sensitivity to potential vulnerability to illness. If people are generally more vulnerable to diseases as they age and their ability to distinguish symptoms of disease from other bodily symptoms is lost by changes in symptom presentation or obfuscated by aging attributions, increases in health promotive behaviours driven by a general sense of vulnerability may partially compensate for the risk generated by inaccuracies in symptom interpretation. Thus, the increase in care-seeking and preventive behaviours could be interpreted as adaptive coping strategies.

In accord with the vulnerability hypothesis, a study by Prohaska *et al.* (1985) found a number of age-related differences in reported vulnerability to diseases such as heart attack, high blood pressure, lung cancer, colon-rectal cancer, senility and colds. Older participants (60 years and older) felt more vulnerable to high blood pressure, heart attack and senility than did younger participants (20 to 39), and middle-aged participants (40 to 59) felt more vulnerable to lung cancer in comparison to younger participants. Younger participants, however, felt more vulnerable to non-life threatening ills such as colds and were more likely than older participants to associate weakness and aches with illness. Participants of all ages agreed upon and were accurate in identifying symptoms associated with the specific illnesses asked about in the survey, and they also agreed upon effective health promoting behaviours. But the older participant's feeling of vulnerability to several of the illnesses was a likely candidate for reporting that they were careful to maintain a nutritional diet, get sufficient sleep, take moderate exercise and medical checkups on a regular basis, stay mentally alert, think positively and avoid the emotional upset of anger and depression. While reported performance of these behaviours increased with age, the three age groups agreed on the potential benefit of these behaviours with one exception. Regular, aerobic and strenuous *exercise* was not seen as more valuable and was less likely to be performed by older participants. Younger adults attributed significantly more health benefits to exercise than did middle-aged or older participants.

In general, therefore, older persons report higher levels of performance of all health behaviours with the exception of vigorous *exercise*. It is difficult to determine whether this is an aging or a cohort effect as there has been a dramatic interest in exercise in current young, middle-aged and young-old Americans. There is no doubt, however, about the physiological and psychological benefits of exercise for the elderly (Hagberg, 1994; Holloszy, 1990; Netz & Tamar, 1994). Unfortunately, participants in such studies are a highly select group and investigators have often failed to report whether their participants have a past history of regular exercise or other athletic activities and we do not know whether the beneficial results of exercise would replicate on a broader, as yet unsampled population of the elderly. Studies which used community samples were often plagued with very low inclusion rates (see sample description in Judge, Whipple & Wolfson, 1994) and many of the studies cited to support the benefits of exercise were conducted with nursing home residents whose sedentary life-style might have led to greater benefits than those that would be seen in an active elderly population. In addition, there has been no evaluation of the effects of exercise on the health beliefs or perceived importance of exercise by the participants.

Changes in illness representations can also result in other procedures that have positive therapeutic effects. Studies of patient populations show that older patients use symptom monitoring less than do young or middle-aged patients (Prohaska *et al.*, 1987). As symptom monitoring can lead to inappropriate, episodic use of medication, older patients who use less symptom monitoring are less likely to stop or drop out of treatment. Thus, in comparison to young and middle-aged adult samples, older patients (65 to 80) were more compliant with antihypertensive medication and were less likely to consider dropping out of cancer chemotherapy. Reanalysis of the data reported by Meyer, Leventhal and Gutmann (1985), which showed that patients receiving treatment for hypertension who mentioned symptoms of hypertension at the first treatment session were more likely to drop out of treatment than those who did not, showed that older patients were also less likely to drop out of treatment. Presumably, their health behaviour is less influenced by their symptom experience so they are more likely to follow the prescribed treatments. Finally, Myers *et al.* (1994) found that regardless of the intensity of efforts to encourage participation, participants over 65 years of age were more likely to return fecal occult blood tests in the second year of a screening study than were younger adults.

Work now in progress suggests there may be some situations in which advanced age leads to decreased feelings of vulnerability and decreased health behaviour. Declines in feelings of vulnerability with advancing age may occur for illnesses which people represent as having a young age of onset. Unfortunately, such lay perceptions of age of onset may be incorrect, leading to the abandonment of beneficial health behaviours and screening practices. A preliminary analysis of data from our current program on minority health points to an instance of inaccurate perceptions of breast cancer on part of elderly African American women. Our data suggest that as women age, the difference between their own age and the age that they think breast cancer occurs increases. In this sample of 62 year old to 93 year old women, virtually all of the women believed that breast cancer occurred at an age lower than their own (the average of the responses to the question, "At what age does breast cancer usually occur", was 46 years). Use of mammography also declines with age. One explanation for these results is that many older women believe there is no need for screening because they have passed the age at which they are most vulnerable to breast cancer. The misperception that breast cancer happens to younger women may be attributed to vivid memories of cases of breast cancer among younger women. For example, stories about a friend's 40 year old daughter, newly diagnosed with cancer, will make a greater impression and may lead to inaccurate expectations about cancer's typical age of onset. Hearing about breast cancer in a 70 or 80 year old woman is less surprising and less dramatic and will not be as influential on a woman's beliefs about age of onset. Thus, while women overestimate the occurrence of highly memorable events, an example of the availability heuristic (Tversky & Kahneman, 1974), the actual incidence of the disease increases with age, with the highest incidence occurring in the 8th decade of life. It is important that individuals accurately judge their personal vulnerability and take appropriate self-protective behaviours.

Risk aversion and seeking medical care

Our data on the use of primary health care provided what is perhaps the clearest evidence for health-related risk aversion among the elderly. Our basic finding was that older participants delayed significantly less than middle-aged participants in seeking care for newly arising symptoms. Our first such study compared delay in two groups of patients seeking medical care: one 45 to 55 years of age (n = 80), the other 65 (n = 83) and over (E.A. Leventhal *et al.*, 1993). Participants were patients who presented with symptoms at a medical clinic at a large university hospital who were interviewed prior to seeing the doctor (interviews took place only for patient-driven appointments and not for follow ups or regularly scheduled exams). The early section of the interview asked for the time-line of the episode: the day the symptom was first noticed, the time they decided they were ill and the time at which they contacted the medical care system for an appointment. Participants were asked to focus on each time point and to recall their assessment of the cause, seriousness and familiarity of the symptoms for each, along with their coping behaviours and emotional reactions to the symptoms. Delays from symptom onset until contacting the medical care system were shortest for symptoms that participants rated as definitely serious when first noticed than for symptoms rated as possibly serious or mild at that same point in time. In addition, the delay was less for older than for the middle-aged patients regardless of the perceived symptom severity at onset.

Insight into the nature of the age differences in delay emerged from a more detailed analysis in which delay was divided into two different time periods: appraisal delay (temporal period from first notice till deciding one was ill) and illness delay (from the decision one was ill till calling for care). Delay for each of the time periods was examined for three levels of judged symptom severity (mild, possibly serious, definitely serious) by both the elderly and middle-aged samples. Appraisal delays (first notice to decide ill) were shorter for the elderly at every level of judged seriousness. In short, the elderly are swifter than the middle-aged in deciding they have an illness and potential medical problem. The data for the illness delay were striking. There were no differences among the elderly and middle-aged for either mild or serious symptoms: time from deciding one was ill until calling for an appointment was longer for mild than for serious symptoms. Illness delay for possibly serious symptoms was substantially longer, however, for the middle-aged than for the elderly. In fact, the middle-aged patients had longer illness delays for symptoms they judged as possibly serious when first noticed than for symptoms they judged as mild. When questioned regarding as to what led to this delay, the middle-aged participants did not talk about lack of time and/or conflict with work. Their most common-reports focused on issues such as "... not wanting to know the bad news, thinking of something else, waiting to see what it might be ...", etc. We argued, therefore, that middle-aged patients are more likely to engage in avoidance behaviours than are older participants. They respond to threat with avoidance as they have sufficient strength to both worry and go about their daily business and they are less certain about their ability to control the potential risk. The elderly, on the other hand, are more eager to reduce both stress and risk by putting the threat in their physicians' hands.

With but one exception, the above findings were replicated in a second study by E.A. Leventhal *et al.* (1995) which included three important methodological refinements. The first was the use of an event history analysis which allowed us to examine the rates of utilization over time for the entire delay period as well as for its two component periods, that of initial appraisal followed by illness delay. The method also allowed us to up-date the predictors. We could examine the effects upon delay of perceived severity, emotional distress, etc., as reported upon first noticing the symptom and as reported at the point the individual decided that he or she was ill. The third, most important and most difficult to describe of the methodological refinements, was an experimental design that allowed us to interview both the individuals seeking care and their matched controls who might not be seeking care at that very same time. We were able, therefore, to compare delays for over 65 and under 65 year old participants with knowledge of the rate of symptoms and health care use (or non use) among control cases as well as index cases, or users. This allows us to address questions such as the following, "Is the swifter care-seeking by the older cohort due to the fact that very ill and slow to react elderly fail to seek care, (i.e., remain at home and not appear in the sample)?" Given these important refinements, it was satisfying to note that the overall pattern of results replicated our prior findings. The elderly cohort was swifter to seek care than that under 65 years of age: Its members were especially quick during the initial, appraisal phase. The cohorts did not differ in the illness phase (from deciding one is ill till calling for care) and emotional upset increased illness delay as was found in the first study (E.A. Leventhal *et al.*, 1993) and in our very first study of delay, which was not focused on elderly respondents (Safer *et al.*, 1979). Emotional upset did not, however, increase illness delay to a greater extent for the middle-aged than the older cohort for possibly serious symptoms. While we were disappointed by the absence of this effect, complex, three-way interactions (age by seriousness by time period) of this type are undoubtedly less stable than simple effects.

The overall picture, therefore, is one of swifter, more efficient health behaviours by the older cohorts. Whether the issue is one of prevention, response to treatment, or the diagnosis and treatment of new symptoms, the elderly optimize their situation and compensate for reduced resources and increased vulnerability by making quick and efficient use of a familiar source of assistance: medical care to reduce risk and conserve resources. This important strategic change will over-ride many of the risks that would otherwise emerge from changes in the way symptoms present and illnesses are represented in the later years of life.

Gender and Health Behaviour

In addition to observing differences in illness representations over the life span, we also regularly encounter *gender* differences similar to those reported by The National Health Survey conducted by the National Center for Health Statistics (1982). These parallel the differences between the sexes in longevity and disease presentation as well as other biological, psychological and social gender distinctions in illness and health behaviours. For example, in adolescence and early adulthood, there are gender differences in diet and exercise practices that reflect current standards of attractiveness and assumptions regarding activities that are life extending. Body building, intense physical exercise, steroid use and increased dietary intake are adopted for these purposes by males, and fasting and exercises to attain anorectic slimness are frequently adopted by females. These behaviours may persist throughout the life span for women, while they appear to decline with age for males (E.A. Leventhal, 1994).

We have looked at the relationship of age and gender and found significant sex and age differences in illness burden (index of the number of serious illnesses and morbidity) and number of symptoms reported in our longitudinal study conducted in Wisconsin (see Cameron, Leventhal & Leventhal, 1993; E.A. Leventhal *et al.*, 1993). Gender effects were clear: Women had a greater total number of symptoms than men, with a significant rise for the middle-aged female, an effect not seen in males, probably consistent with menopausal symptoms. Females also reported more somatic symptoms of depression and more cognitive and somatic symptoms of anxiety than did the male participants. Age affected these variables for both sexes with both illness burden and symptom reporting increasing with age. There was, however, a cross-over with increasing age. Whereas younger females had higher illness burdens than younger males, males more than 75 years of age had greater illness burdens and more severe illnesses than did the females of similar age. These differences produced a significant sex-by-age interaction and a significant contrast in the oldest old group: The illness burden was greater for the oldest old males than for the oldest old females. Gender differences in symptom reporting paralleled the differences in illness burden as the total number of symptoms increased with age for both sexes and the escalation of symptoms with age was significantly greater in the males. That the females in our sample report more morbidity, more worry about getting sick, have greater physical impairment (morbidity) and make greater use of health care, replicate findings reported in the medical literature over the centuries. The cross-over effect, the increase in morbidity among elderly males, is what is different in our findings as it suggests that biological factors and not merely socialization, play an important role in gender differences in morbidity and self reporting of symptoms.

It is also interesting to note that there are significant relationships between affect and age. The somatic symptoms of depression are more common in the oldest participants, while the cognitive and somatic symptoms of anxiety are more common in the younger participants. Both the decline in reports of an activating emotion such as anxiety and the increase in reports of depression, an emotion consistent with resource depletion, are consistent with our interpretation that the risk aversion of the elderly reflects an underlying motive to compensate for declines in vigour and optimize existent resources. It also appears that older women are the more effective than older men in this process of optimization and compensation, as they seem more effective in the utilization of both illness and wellness behaviours to maintain their own health and appear to be more vigilant and open to seeking care (Cameron, Leventhal & Leventhal, 1993; E.A. Leventhal *et al.*, 1993).

SUMMARY

Transitions across the lifespan are reflected in changing patterns of health and illness behaviours. These patterns are moderated by biological aging, by pathologies and life experiences and also by the changing personal affective coping strategies, the psychosocial milieu, the family and the social network. These complex interrelationships have implications for illness representations and for selection of coping responses to preventive and therapeutic treatments. In addition, there are different expectations and response patterns anticipated from different disease entities across the adult lifespan. The self-regulation or common-sense model has contributed to our understanding of these changes in three major areas. First, it is clear that a variety of specific tactics or procedures for symptom evaluation, may encourage benign attributions and delay in seeking care. These include attributing slow-to-develop symptoms to aging, ambiguous symptoms to stress and the minimization of perceived severity of shared symptoms, an effect more likely among the elderly who are multi-symptomatic and discuss health with peers. These changes are potentially risk inducing as many of the life threatening diseases which are most prevalent during the later years are slow to develop and ambiguous in presentation.

The elderly optimize their situation and compensate for reduced resources and increased vulnerability by care-seeking. An important change in strategy for self regulation in the health domain, rapid, efficient and sustained use of a familiar source of assistance or medical care, appears to over-ride many of the risks that emerge from changes in the way symptoms present and illnesses are represented in the later years of life. This optimization and compensation in the health domain appears to reflect a broadly based strategy to reduce risk and conserve resources, the need for which is consistent with the age related changes in reports of negative affect: the elderly reporting less intense anxiety, an activating emotion and more depression, a sign of depletion.

While it is possible to express satisfaction with the insights achieved to date, it is also necessary to state our frustration and disappointment at the necessarily slower pace demanded for the empirical verification of the multitude of hypotheses suggested by the self regulation model. The opportunity for research in specific disease domains is vast and limited only by the ability of the researcher to attend to clinical clues and to devise methodologies to gain insights into the psychological processes accompanying the biological and social changes associated with aging. The self regulation model has an added power lacking in many alternative social-psychological models. Its conceptual structure and data base are readily translated into interventions that can be used in the clinical setting to improve the health and quality of life of patients. The illness representation model provides a framework to understand how individuals move from an acute perception of illness to a chronic model of learning appropriate types of monitoring with "just enough" vigilance to adjust to a continuous appraisal of symptoms and necessary self protective procedures. The model can be used to develop paradigms for practitioner-patient interaction that will generate shared perceptions of disease and treatment congruent with respect to symptom causation, time-lines for both symptoms and treatments, consequences of treatment or of lack of treatment and maladaptive behaviour and strategies for effective self appraisal and efficacy in self management. The challenges are many.

REFERENCES

Baltes, P.B. & Baltes, M.M. (1990) Psychological perspectives on successful aging: The model of selective optimization with compensation. In P.B. Baltes & M.M. Baltes (Eds.), *Successful aging: Perspectives from the behavioral sciences* (pp. 1–34). New York: Cambridge University Press.

Baumann, L.J., Cameron, L.D., Zimmerman, R.S. & Leventhal, H. (1989) Illness representations and matching labels with symptoms. *Health Psychology*, **8**, 449–469.

Berkanovic, E., Hurwicz, M. & Landsverk, J. (1988) Psychological distress and the decision to seek medical care. *Social Science & Medicine*, **11**, 1215–1221.

Brody, E.M. & Kleban, M.H. (1981) Physical and mental health symptoms of older people: Who do they tell? *Journal of the American Geriatrics Society*, **29**, 442–449.

Cameron, L.D., Leventhal, E.A. & Leventhal, H. (1993) Symptom representations and affect as determinants of care seeking in a community-dwelling, adult sample population. *Health Psychology*, **12**, 171–179.

Cameron, L.D., Leventhal, E.A. & Leventhal, H. (1995) Seeking medical care in response to symptoms and life stress. *Psychosomatic Medicine*, **57**, 37–47.

Carstensen, L.L. (1992) Social and emotional patterns in adulthood: Support for socioemotional selectivity theory. *Psychology and Aging*, **7**, 331–338.

Contrada, R.J., Lambert, J.F., Jahn, N., Leventhal, E.A. & Leventhal, H. (1996) *Illness representations among African-American hypertensives: Relationship to adherence and blood pressure control.* Manuscript in preparation.

Croyle, R.T. & Jemmott, J.B. (1991) Psychological reactions to risk factor testing. In J.A. Skelton & R.T. Croyle (Eds.), *Mental representation in health and illness* (pp. 85–107). New York: Springer-Verlag.

Diener, E., Sandvik, E. & Larsen, R.J. (1985) Age and sex effects for emotional intensity. *Developmental Psychology*, **21**, 542–546.

Festinger, L. (1954) A theory of social comparison processes. *Human Relations*, **7**, 117–140.

Hagberg, J.M. (1994) Physical activity, fitness, health and aging. In C. Bouchard, R.J. Shephard & T. Stephens (Eds.), *Physical activity, fitness and health: International proceedings and consensus statement* (pp. 993–1005). Champaign, IL: Human Kinetics Publishers.

Hale, W.E., Perkins, L.L., May, F.E., Marks, R.G. & Stewart, R.B. (1986) Symptom prevalence in the elderly: An evaluation of age, sex, disease and medication use. *Journal of the American Geriatrics Society*, **34**, 333–340.

Haug, M.R., Wykle, M.L. & Namazi, K.H. (1989) Self-care among older adults. *Social Science and Medicine*, **29**, 171–183.

Holloszy, J.O. (1990) The roles of exercise in health maintenance and treatment of disease in middle and old age. In M. Kaneko (Ed.), *Fitness for the aged, disabled and industrial worker. International series on sport science: Vol. 20*, (pp. 3–8). Champaign, IL: Human Kinetics Publishers.

Judge, J.O., Whipple, R.H. & Wolfson, L.I. (1994) Effects of resistive and balance exercises on isokinetic strength in older persons. *Journal of the American Geriatrics Society*, **42**, 937–946.

Kart, C. (1981) Experiencing symptoms: Attribution and misattribution of illness among the aged. In M.R. Haug (Ed.), *Elderly patients and their doctors* (pp. 70–78). New York: Springer Publishing Company Incorporated.

Keller, M.L., Leventhal, H., Prohaska, T.R. & Leventhal, E.A. (1989) Beliefs about aging and illness in a community sample. *Research in Nursing and Health*, **12**, 247–255.

Kulik, J.A. & Mahler, H.I. (1987) Effects of preoperative roommate assignment on preoperative anxiety and recovery from coronary by-pass surgery. *Health Psychology*, **6**, 525–543.

Leventhal, E.A. (1994) Gender and aging: Women and their aging. In D.M. Reddy, V.J. Adesso & R. Flemming (Eds.), *Psychological perspectives on women's health* (pp. 11–35). New York: Hemisphere Publishing Co.

Leventhal, E.A., Easterling, D., Leventhal, H. & Cameron, L. (1995) Conservation of energy, uncertainty reduction and swift utilization of medical care among the elderly: Study II. *Medical Care*, **33**, 988–1000.

Leventhal, E.A., Leventhal, H. Schaefer, P. & Easterling, D. (1993) Conservation of energy, uncertainty reduction and swift utilization of medical care among the elderly. *Journal of Gerontology: Psychological Sciences*, **48**, 78–86.

Leventhal, H. & Diefenbach, M. (1991) The active side of illness cognition. In J.A. Skelton & R.T. Croyle (Eds.), *Mental representation in health and illness* (pp. 247–272). New York: Springer-Verlag.

Leventhal, H. & Everhart, D. (1979) Emotion, pain and physical illness. In C.E. Izard (Ed.), *Emotions and psychopathology* (pp. 263–299). New York: Plenum Press.

Leventhal, H., Nerenz, D. & Strauss, A. (1982) Self-regulation and the mechanisms for symptom appraisal. In D. Mechanic (Ed.), *Monograph series in psychosocial epidemiology 3: Symptoms, illness behaviour and help-seeking* (pp. 55–86). New York: Neale Watson.

Leventhal, H., Prohaska, T.R. & Hirschman, R.S. (1985) Preventive health behaviour across the lifespan. In J.C. Rosen & L.J. Solomon (Eds.), *Prevention in health psychology* (pp. 191–235). Hanover, NH: University Press of New England.

Mechanic, D. (1974) Discussion of research programs on relations between stressful life events and episodes of physical illness. In B.S. Dohrenwend & B.P. Dohrenwend (Eds.), *Stressful life events: Their nature and effects* (pp. 87–97). New York: Wiley.

Meyer, D., Leventhal, H. & Gutmann, M. (1985) Common-sense models of illness: The example of hypertension. *Health Psychology*, **4**, 115–135.

Myers, R.E., Ross, E., Jepson, C., Wolf, T., Balshem, A., Millner, L. & Leventhal, H. (1994) Modeling adherence to colorectal cancer screening. *Preventive Medicine*, **23**, 142–151.

National Center for Health Statistics. (1970) *Selected symptoms of psychological distress* (Series 11, No. 37). Washington, DC: U.S. Government Printing Office.

National Center for Health Statistics. (1982) *Current estimates from the National Health Interview Survey. Vital and health statistics* (Series 10, No. 150). Washington, DC: U.S. Government Printing Office.

Netz, Y. & Tamar, J. (1994) Exercise and the psychological state of institutionalized elderly: A review. *Perceptual and Motor Skills,* **79**, 1107–1118.

Pennebaker, J. (1982) *The psychology of physical symptoms.* New York: Springer-Verlag.

Prohaska, T.R., Keller, M.L., Leventhal, E.A. & Leventhal, H. (1987) Impact of symptoms and aging attribution on emotions and coping. *Health Psychology,* **6**, 495–514.

Prohaska, T.R., Leventhal, E.A., Leventhal, H. & Keller, M.L. (1985) Health practices and illness cognition in young, middle-aged and elderly adults. *Journal of Gerontology,* **40**, 569–578.

Safer, M., Tharps, Q., Jackson, T. & Leventhal, H. (1979) Determinants of three stages of delay in seeking care at a medical clinic. *Medical Care,* **17**, 11–29.

Saranson, I.G., Saranson, B.R., Potter, E.H. & Antoni, M.H. (1985) Life events, social support and illness. *Psychosomatic Medicine,* **47**, 156–163.

Schachter, S. (1959) *The psychology of affiliation.* Stanford, CA: Stanford University Press.

Tversky, A. & Kahneman, D. (1974) Judgment under uncertainty: Heuristics and biases. *Science,* **185**, 1124–1131.

4

Measurement of Illness Perceptions in Patients with Chronic Somatic Illness: A Review

Margreet Scharloo & Adrian Kaptein

INTRODUCTION

Research shows that lay theories of illness today are based on essentially the same explanatory framework of health and illness as they were 300 years ago (Schober & Lacroix, 1991). People appear to regulate their health-related behaviour according to these frameworks: lay theories guide interpretations of and coping with health events, entry into and use of medical treatment, as well as evaluations of treatment effects. Illness perceptions are an important factor in how patients manage their illness (Bradley *et al.*, 1987; Hampson, Glasgow & Zeiss, 1994; Jensen & Karoly, 1992; Lacroix *et al.*, 1991; De Valle & Norman, 1992; Williams & Keefe, 1991).

Research into the structure of lay theories has been consistent in finding five dimensions according to which experiences of illness are cognitively organised. These dimensions are: identity, cause, consequences, time-line and controllability. This chapter reviews the literature on assessing these five dimensions and reviews research literature on relations between illness perceptions and psychological and medical characteristics. On the basis of this overview, research and clinical implications are discussed.

From an original concern with "fear", Leventhal and co-workers (Leventhal, Meyer & Nerenz, 1980) began to consider how lay people perceive illness as a threat. They developed a theoretical model, the "self regulating processing system" (Leventhal, Nerenz & Steele, 1984), describing a system for the mental and emotional activity involved in the construction of a representation of illness. This model guided their research into how people interpret and cope with current and potential health events (Leventhal, 1992; Leventhal & Diefenbach, 1991; Leventhal, Nerenz & Steele, 1984). The assumptions underlying this model are that people have an active information processing system which leads them to generate both a representation of illness and an emotional reaction to this illness. This processing system consists of three recursive stages: representation, coping and appraisal. Throughout these stages the system is hierarchically organised, which creates the possibility of conflict between the concrete (e.g. somatic sensations) and the abstract (e.g. memories about past illnesses) operating levels.

Based on the work of Pennebaker (1982), who proposed a theory of symptom perception emphasizing patients' cognitive models or "schemata", Lacroix (1991) defined an illness schema as

> *a distinct, meaningfully integrated cognitive structure that encompasses (a) a belief in the relatedness of a variety of physiological and psychological functions that may or may not be objectively accurate, (b) a cluster of sensations, symptoms, emotions and physical limitations in keeping with that belief, (c) a naive theory about the mechanisms that underlie the relatedness of the elements identified in (b) and (d) implicit or explicit prescriptions for corrective action (Lacroix, 1991, p. 197).*

Although there are differences in emphasis, methodology and terminology (terms also used instead of illness schemata are: illness perceptions, illness representations, illness beliefs and illness cognitions), studies on the structure of illness schemata are consistent in finding five dimensions according to which experiences of illness are cognitively organised (Baumann *et al.*, 1989; Bishop *et al.*, 1987; Lau, Bernard & Hartman, 1989; Lau & Hartman, 1983; Leventhal, Meyer & Nerenz, 1980; Meyer, Leventhal & Gutmann, 1985):

(a)   The first dimension is the individual's perception of the *identity* of the problem: the label placed on the disease by the patient and the symptoms associated with it. Illnesses can be identified by labels (e.g. rheumatoid arthritis), concrete signs (e.g. deformations, affected joints) and by concrete symptoms (e.g. pain, stiffness).

(b)   The second dimension is based on the individual's ideas about the *causes* of the problem: ideas about how one gets the disease, for example as a consequence of genetic factors or of environmental pollution.

(c)   The third dimension reflects the individual's ideas about possible *consequences* of the problem: the perceived short-term and long-term effects of the disease; the perceived physical, social, economic and emotional consequences of the disease.

(d)   The fourth is that of *time-line*: expectations about the duration of the disease and its characteristic course, perceptions about whether the disease will be acute, chronic or episodic/cyclical.

(e)   The fifth is concerned with the individual's ideas about *cure* or *controllability*: patients' ideas about what they themselves, or providers of medical care can do to bring about recovery or to exert influence on the course of illness.

Research shows that lay peoples' ideas with regard to the five dimensions are important since they regulate their health-related behaviour according to these ideas. Lay theories guide coping (Crisson & Keefe, 1988; Jensen, Karoly & Huger, 1987; Lacroix *et al.*, 1991; Nerenz & Leventhal, 1983; Nerenz, Leventhal & Love, 1982; Williams & Keefe, 1991), entry into (Jensen & Karoly, 1992; Meyer, Leventhal & Gutmann, 1985) and use of medical treatment (Hampson, Glasgow & Zeiss, 1994; Leventhal, Meyer & Nerenz, 1980; Leventhal, Nerenz & Steele, 1984), as well as evaluations of treatment effects (Lowery & Jacobsen, 1985; Nerenz & Leventhal, 1983; Timko & Janoff-Bulman, 1985).

We are currently studying the relationships between illness perceptions and medical and behavioural outcomes in patients with chronic illness. The purpose of our chapter is (a) to review how the dimensions of illness perceptions have been assessed in recent empirical studies and (b) to present an overview of the empirical literature on the relations between illness perceptions and course of illness. In line with Kaplan (1990), who proposed that outcome measures in health and medicine should be anchored in their relations with behaviour, course of illness is understood to encompass both behavioural and medical outcomes.

METHOD

Since it was our purpose to review recent studies on the assessment of illness perceptions in chronic somatic patients, we identified a set of articles by a search of the National Library of Medicine's MEDLINE database from 1985 up to September 1995 using the medical subject headings and single concepts "chronic illness" and "chronic disease". To make sure we would be tracking down studies on *perceptions* of patients and not studies on actual diagnoses, duration of illness, etc., we avoided using the main terms for the five dimensions and connected "chronic illness" and "chronic disease" to the key words: cognitions, beliefs, lay, representations, theoretical, concepts, attributions, schemata, perceptions, knowledge, idea, causal, "common sense" and meaning. The same key words were used in a search of the APA PsycINFO's PSYCLIT articles databases, also from 1985 up to September 1995. The Social and Behavioral Sciences Current Contents was used to identify the most recent studies — up to November 1995. Reference lists of the studies which explicitly mentioned the dimensions were used to identify articles which may have been ignored.

Studies had to meet the following criteria to be included in the review:

- The study described the development or use of an instrument intended to measure illness perceptions, measuring one or more dimensions.
- The study listed the assessed dimension as a separate concept in the result section of the article.
- The publication was written in English, French, German or Dutch.
- The study included only adult patients with chronic physical illnesses.

Studies on illness perceptions of children are not included since many of these use methods based on the cognitive developmental stages of Piaget, consequently the measurement methods are very different from those used in adult patients. A recent literature review in German (Schmidt & Lehmkuhl, 1994), classified studies on illness concepts of children on the basis of their underlying theoretical models. Studies on illness perceptions of psychiatric patients are not included since many of these are either comparing illness perceptions within families of psychiatric patients, or are measuring solely the perceptions of spouses, parents or siblings.

Information on the studies which were identified will be presented according to illness, assessment instrument and method, assessed dimension and main results involving illness perceptions and associations between the dimensions of illness perceptions and psychological, medical and/or behavioural outcome. Illnesses will be presented separately only if the number of subjects with a particular illness was mentioned in the study. If a study utilized more than one measurement instrument to assess the same dimension, all instruments are described and the matching dimensions are reported. Measurement instruments were identified as established when previous data were cited. Novel ones were those specifically designed for the study.

RESULTS

The search resulted in 101 studies that fitted the criteria, 98 were published in English, 3 in German. Appendix 1 at the end of this chapter provides details about the samples, methods, illness schema and main findings of the studies which have been included here.

The year of publication for the 101 studies ranged from 1985 to 1995, with most studies on illness perceptions published in 1992 (n = 16). Studies came from a total of 47 different journals. The largest numbers of studies were obtained from *Pain* (18), *Psychology & Health* (7), the *Journal of Behavioral Medicine* (6) and *The Clinical Journal of Pain* (6). In 62% of the studies previously used measures were employed. The remaining ones used interviews and scales created by the investigator or adapted versions of existing questionnaires.

Most frequently investigated (46 times) were groups of patients suffering from various chronic pain complaints: 28 with unspecified pain, 14 with (low) back pain, 2 with headache, 1 with malfunctioning temporomandibular joints of the jaw and 1 with pelvic pain. The second most investigated group of patients were

Table 1   Overview categories of illness, illness groups and number of studies investigating illnesses (101 empirical studies)

Category of illness	Illness	Investigated in ... studies*
Chronic pain	unspecified pain	28
	(low) back pain	14
	headache	2
	malfunctioning temporomandibular joints of jaw	1
	pelvic pain	1
Rheumatic diseases	arthritis	17
	ankylosing spondylitis	2
	fibromyalgia	2
	systemic lupus erythematosus	2
	coxarthrosis	1
	sarcoidosis	1
	scleroderma	1
Cardiovascular diseases	hypertension	5
	myocardial infarction	5
Chronic respiratory conditions	asthma	5
	chronic obstructive pulmonary disease	4
Malfunctioning of the endocrine glands	diabetes	9
Unspecified		8
Nervous diseases	multiple sclerosis	4
	epilepsy	1
	amyotrophic lateral sclerosis	1
	vertigo	1
Other	cancer	6
	chronic fatigue	4
	renal disease	4
	AIDS	1
	lung tuberculosis	1
	sickle cell disease	1

* If a study encompassed more than one illness group, or two sub-studies investigating different subjects with the same disease, all groups were counted separately.

those with rheumatic diseases (Table 1). If a study encompassed more than one illness group (12 studies), or two sub-studies investigating different subjects with the same disease (2 studies), all groups were counted separately. Acute illnesses were not included.

Most frequently researchers used semi-structured or open-ended interview approaches to obtain data on illness perceptions; there were 20 studies using these approaches. Researchers in the majority of these studies initially recorded the responses verbatim, employed judges to develop codes or categories for the open-ended responses and examined the frequencies of the categories (Ailinger & Schweitzer, 1993; Fry, Crisp & Beard, 1991; Hampson, Glasgow & Toobert, 1990; Hampson, Glasgow & Zeiss, 1994; Jones, Jones & Katz, 1991; Lowery & Jacobsen, 1985; Lowery, Jacobsen & McCauley, 1987; McDonald *et al.*, 1993; Meyer, Leventhal & Gutmann, 1985; Weaver & Narsavage, 1992; Williams, 1986). In some of these studies combinations of open-ended interview-questions and rating scales were used (Hampson, Glasgow & Toobert, 1990; Hampson, Glasgow & Zeiss, 1994; Lowery & Jacobsen, 1985; Lowery, Jacobsen & McCauley, 1987; Westbrook, Gething & Bradbury, 1987). All of the studies investigated beliefs about the causes of the different illnesses; common causes mentioned were self (personality), heredity, stress, self (physical), fate and environment.

Some researchers using interview approaches reported all of the patients' responses and their frequencies or counted how many patients did respond (Kleinman *et al.*, 1995; Reinert & Steurich, 1990; Westbrook, Gething & Bradbury, 1987; Raleigh, 1992). Others instructed patients to select responses from a range of predetermined alternatives and to comment on their choices (Ray *et al.*, 1992; Timko & Janoff-Bulman, 1985).

Beliefs about control were most frequently assessed using the "Multidimensional Health Locus of Control Scales" (MHLOCS) (in 17 studies) or the version adapted for patients with chronic pain, the "Multidimensional Health Locus of Pain Control Scales" (in 6 studies). The "Pain Beliefs and Perceptions Inventory" (measuring "causes" and "time-line") was used in 8 and the "Survey of Pain Attitudes" (measuring "consequences" and/or "control") was used in 7 studies.

Beliefs about control were assessed in 59 of the 101 studies, using 22 different instruments. Beliefs about causes, consequences, identity and time-line were assessed in 44, 39, 22 and 17 studies, respectively (Table 2). Most studies only measured 1 or 2 dimensions and did so using separate instruments for separate dimensions. In only a few studies (Edwards *et al.*, 1992; Skevington, 1993; Turk, Rudy & Salovey, 1986) did researchers use just one instrument to assess several dimensions. Turk, Rudy and Salovey (1986) factor-analysed

Table 2 Overview of assessed dimensions, number of studies in which the dimension was assessed, number of instruments, measurement instrument and number of studies in which a particular instrument is used (101 empirical studies)

Assessed dimension	Measured in .. studies[a]	Number of instruments	Measurement instrument	Number of studies[b]
Control	59	22	Multidimensional Health Locus of Control Scales	17
			Semi-structured or open-ended interview	11
			Survey of Pain Attitudes	7
			Multidimensional Health Locus of Pain Control Scales	6
			Self-made questionnaires	6
			West Haven-Yale Multidimensional Pain Inventory	5
			Respiratory Illness Opinion Survey	3
			Beliefs about Pain Control Questionnaire	2
			Implicit Models of Illness Questionnaire	2
Causes	44	11	Semi-structured or open-ended interview	19
			Pain Beliefs and Perceptions Inventory	8
			Self-made questionnaires	8
			Implicit Models of Illness Questionnaire	2
			Pain Beliefs Questionnaire	2
			Schema Assessment instrument	2
Consequences	39	17	Semi-structured or open-ended interview	9
			Survey of Pain Attitudes	6
			West Haven-Yale Multidimensional Pain Inventory	6
			Pain Impairment Relationship Scale	3
Time-line	22	6	Semi-structured or open-ended interview	10
			Pain Beliefs and Perceptions Inventory	8
Identity	17	11	Semi-structured or open-ended interview	5
			Schema Assessment Instrument	2

[a]If a study employed different instruments to assess one dimension, the study is counted only once.
[b]Only instruments that were used in more than one study are listed.

ratings on the 38-item Implicit Models of Illness Questionnaire, revealing a four-dimensional structure of illness, composed of (a) Seriousness, (b) Personal Responsibility, (c) Controllability and (d) Changeability. Skevington (1993) redesigned Abramson, Seligman and Teasdale's (1978) dimensions to gather data on attributions of painful symptoms. She asked patients to rate on 7-point scales:

if they thought their pain would go away completely (stable) (1), come and go (unstable) (4), or be continuous (stable) (7) (…). For internality they reported whether they believed the pain to be the result of their own actions (1) (internal), the result of the actions of others (7) (external), or neither (4). (…) The global-specific dimension assessed whether they thought their symptom affected every area of their lives (1) (global) or only a small part (7) (specific). Controllability was evaluated by asking whether the pain was believed to be controllable (1) or not at all controllable (7) (uncontrollable) (Skevington, 1993, pp. 55–56).

All five dimensions are only measured in studies using interviews (Garro, 1994; Hampson, Glasgow & Toobert, 1990; Hampson, Glasgow & Zeiss, 1994). Possible relations between dimensions were examined in research by De Valle and Norman (1992). In their study health locus of control beliefs were related to the endorsement of certain causes. Causal attributions were related to reported lifestyle changes, but health locus of control beliefs were not. Jensen, Turner and Romano (1994a) found that changes in patients' beliefs in control over pain and beliefs in oneself as disabled were associated with changes in depressive symptoms and physical functioning. Research by Schiaffino and Revenson (1992) shows the moderational effect of the interaction of perceived control and causal attributions on depression and disability. When arthritis was perceived as less controllable, internal and stable causal attributions were associated with greater depression, but lower disability. When arthritis was seen as more controllable, level of depression did not vary as a function of causal attributions, but disability increased as more internal, stable and global attributions were made.

In 14 studies the (main) purpose of the investigators was to test validity and reliability of a new measurement instrument, 64 studied associations between illness perceptions and medical and/or behavioural outcome. "Identity" was related to outcome in 5 out of 5 studies, "causes" in 10 out of 11 studies, "time-line" in 3 out of 6 studies, "consequences" in 17 out of 17 studies and "control" in 26 out of 36 studies.

Studies assessing the control dimension show that perceived internal control is positively related to various indices of medical, psychological and behavioural well-being. In three of the studies that did not find associations between control beliefs and outcome, the authors (Barlow, Macey & Struthers, 1992; Linton *et al.*, 1989; Wassem, 1992) stated this was due to methodological problems (e.g. ceiling effect, insensitive measurement instrument, comparing two groups of patients who did not differ in their scores on internal control). Primavera and Kaiser (1994) found only a trend in the expected direction and Fowers (1994) found significant associations only when level of life stress was also taken into account. Westbrook, Gething and Bradbury (1987) reported that although members of the perceived control group did not differ from the helpless group on indexes of severity and handicap, perceived health changes occurring in the previous year were described as being "somewhat better" by the perceived control group and "much worse" by the helpless group. In a study by Jensen *et al.* (1994b) significant associations between internal control beliefs and physical disability disappeared when the order of entry of the variables in a regression analysis was changed and control was forced into the equation after demographic and pain-related variables, but before consequences.

Research shows that relations between internal health locus of control beliefs and outcome measures are mediated by situational factors, such as age (Buckelew *et al.*, 1990), illness status (Jensen & Karoly, 1991; Tennen *et al.*, 1992), stressful life-events (Fowers, 1994) and previous treatment. In a study by Christensen *et al.* (1991) the belief in internal personal control was associated with less depression for patients who had not previously experienced a failed renal transplant, but with greater depression for those who had returned to dialysis following an unsuccessful transplant. This effect was found only among severely ill patients. Health locus of control was unrelated to depression among patients with less severe disease. Andrykowski and Brady (1994) showed similar results in patients with leukemia: disease severity and treatment history moderated the relationship between locus of control beliefs and psychological adjustment. In this study however, patients with a history of failure of prior therapy and high "powerful others" control belief evidenced the greatest distress and this association was most pronounced at low levels of disease severity.

Affleck *et al.* (1987) emphasize the need to distinguish among aspects of control beliefs to enhance outcome predictions. Their research shows that both greater perceived personal control over *treatment* and greater perceived personal control over *symptoms* (only for patients experiencing moderate and severe symptoms) were related to positive mood and psychosocial adjustment, whereas greater perceived personal control over *course of disease* was associated with negative mood and less positive adjustment (only for patients experiencing severe symptoms).

Research on the time-line dimension shows it may not be the perceived duration of the illness that is related to pain ratings, discomfort during activities and psychological well-being, but rather the perceived constancy of the illness (Herda, Siegeris & Basler, 1994; Williams, Robinson & Geisser, 1994) and its perceived impact on life (Heidrich, Forsthoff & Ward, 1994; Ireys *et al.*, 1994). Williams, Robinson and Geisser (1994) have shown that perception of *pain constancy* (as opposed to intermittency) was the only temporal pain belief that had an association with pain ratings. Believing pain would *persist* did not appear to be associated with intensity ratings.

A number of authors warn of the possibility that significant relationships found between the beliefs in the consequences of illness and self reports of physical dysfunctioning could be due to conceptual overlap and suggest research should include objective measures of functioning. Sacks, Peterson and Kimmel (1990) included such measures and their research shows that the perception of interference of illness with personal and social behaviour is a better predictor of depression than objective severity of illness. Also in research by Riley, Ahern and Follick (1988), a belief that pain implies disability was associated with actual impairment, independent of the contribution of actual pain (measured with a seven-day set of daily pain diaries).

DISCUSSION

Major Results

In conclusion, illness perceptions (especially perceived consequences and perceived control) are important factors influencing medical (e.g. pain severity, glycaemic control), psychological (e.g. depression, self-esteem, anxiety, life satisfaction) and behavioural (e.g. working time, impairment, activity levels) outcome.

Over the past five years the number of studies on illness perceptions are increasing. The use of a reliable and valid measurement instrument, the "Multidimensional Health Locus of (Pain) Control Scales" (MHLOCS) and the consistent results on the control dimension in terms of predictions of behavioural and medical outcome may account for this increase.

The most studied and most successful dimension in predicting positive outcome is the control dimension. In several studies relations between internal health locus of control and positive outcome are mediated by situational factors (Andrykowski & Brady, 1994; Buckelew *et al.*, 1990; Christensen *et al.*, 1991; Fowers, 1994; Jensen & Karoly, 1991; Tennen *et al.*, 1992). These studies provide evidence that research should also take into account the moderating effects of contextual factors. Several research reports emphasize the need to distinguish among aspects of beliefs to enhance predictions about the adaptive significance of beliefs in chronic diseases (Affleck *et al.*, 1987; Williams, Robinson & Geisser, 1994).

The most frequently investigated groups of patients in the studies reviewed were those suffering from chronic pain. This may be due to the widespread prevalence of pain patients as well as the number of available instruments for these patients and the systematic use of the MHLOCS in this clinical population. Interview approaches have been the most widely used method for obtaining data on illness perceptions. The most frequently used single questionnaire was the MHLOCS.

The majority of studies measured only one or two dimensions of illness perception and very rarely examined possible relations between dimensions. In a recent overview on cognitive representations of health and illness Lau (in press) calls "for better measurement of health and illness representations (…) and (…) for better theory and evidence explaining how (or whether) cognitive representations of health and illness interact and mutually affect each other" (p. 35). Leventhal (1992) stresses the existence of five dimensions, describing patterns of these dimensions. One may speculate that certain combinations of illness perceptions are more functional predictors of medical and/or behavioural outcome than single beliefs (Jensen, Turner & Romano, 1994a; Schiaffino & Revenson, 1992; De Valle & Norman, 1992).

In only a few studies have researchers used just one instrument to assess several dimensions. In most of these cases (semi-structured) interviews were employed and results were analysed at an individual level. In a study by Moss-Morris, Petrie and Weinman (1996) illness perceptions were measured using one instrument that has been specifically designed to measure the five dimensions. Illness perceptions, as measured with the "Illness Perception Questionnaire", explained a greater percentage of the variance in levels of disability and psychological well-being than did the coping strategies used by the patients with chronic fatigue syndrome. The instrument appears to be a valid measure (Weinman *et al.*, 1996).

Most studies on associations between illness perceptions and illness outcome use indices of behavioural and emotional well-being. Only a few also considered medical data. A favourable course of illness seems to be associated with high scores on "internal control" (e.g. Dalal & Singh, 1992; Flor & Turk, 1988; Gilutz *et al.*, 1991; Jensen, Turner & Romano, 1994a; Kerns, Turk & Rudy, 1985; Lipchik, Milles & Covington, 1993; Marshall, 1991; Pastor *et al.*, 1993; Schüssler, 1992; Tennen *et al.*, 1992). High accuracy ratings on the "identity" and the "causes" dimension showed a similar relation (e.g. Gillespie & Bradley, 1988; Lacroix *et al.*, 1991; Lacroix *et al.*, 1990; Millard, Wells & Thebarge, 1991; Reesor & Craig, 1988). Also a belief that the illness will be intermittent or discontinuous (e.g. Herda, Siegeris & Basler, 1994; Skevington, 1993; Williams & Thorn, 1989; Williams, Robinson & Geisser, 1994) and a low level of perceived disability or seriousness of the illness (e.g. Hampson, Glasgow & Zeiss, 1994; Jensen & Karoly, 1992; Jensen, Karoly & Huger, 1987; Jensen, Turner & Romano, 1994a; Jensen *et al.*, 1994b; Kerns, Turk & Rudy, 1985; Pollock, 1993; Riley, Ahern & Follick, 1988; Rudy, Kerns & Turk, 1988; Sacks, Peterson & Kimmel, 1990; Strong *et al.*, 1990; Yardley, 1994) appear to be associated with a favourable course of illness.

In a study by Flor and Turk (1988) cognitive variables (e.g. perceptions of control) explained much more variance in pain and disability levels than disease related variables (duration of pain, amount of degenerative change on spinal X rays, amount of disease activity, number of surgeries). Many studies, however, do not employ objective measures of severity, thus making it difficult to predict the causality of relationships between illness perceptions and outcome.

Limitations

The purpose of this chapter was to review how the dimensions of illness perceptions have been assessed. Overviews of this area of research (e.g. Skelton & Croyle, 1991) confirm the existence of five dimensions, but most of the research reviewed in our chapter incorporates different underlying models and therefore examines only one or two dimensions at a time. For example, pre-existing concepts like "Coping" and "Locus of Control" are included. According to Leventhal and Nerenz (1985) the control dimension could also be defined as a summary of expectations with respect to coping (response effectiveness and self-effectance). The many different perspectives make it difficult to make a detailed comparison in the results of the various studies.

The distinction between temporary illness and chronic illness is not always easy to make. We have tried to identify patients with chronic illnesses by searching only under the heading "chronic illness" and by skipping first-time patients, but we are aware of the fact this sometimes may have led to somewhat arbitrary decisions, for example in the case of patients with myocardial infarction.

Also, as shown in recent studies on the adequacy of MEDLINE searches, our MEDLINE literature search may not be covering all studies on assessing illness perceptions (Adams *et al.*, 1994; Gill & Adams, 1995).

Future Research

In order to answer the many questions that still remain, future research should be designed to allow for unambiguous statements about the direction of causality between perceptions and outcome. Measurement methods should allow for studying possible relations between dimensions, not only to examine if combinations of illness concepts are better predictors of outcome but also to clarify questions about conceptual overlap of the dimensional constructs. Our review indicates that on the time-line dimension it may not be the perceived duration of the illness that is related to outcome, but rather the perceived constancy of the illness and its perceived impact on life (see also the chapter by Hampson in section three of this book). Also some research reports on the causal dimension suggest the causal search for reasons/meaning could be called an attempt to gain secondary control (Lowery, Jacobsen & McCauley, 1987; Tennen *et al.*, 1992; Williams & Thorn, 1989). Further research on the possible overlap of the time-line and the consequences dimension and the causal and the control dimension is needed. Future research should also take into account contextual (e.g. treatment history and severity of illness) and personal (e.g. age and sex) variables and should employ medical, psychological and behavioural indices of outcome.

Interventions

With regard to future aims for intervention studies involving illness cognitions, it should be noted that the majority of studies on changes in illness beliefs (mainly control beliefs of patients with chronic pain) show promising results. In a study by Linton *et al.* (1989) positive effects on behavioural outcome after intervention (a physical and behavioural therapy package for nurses with back pain) were not mediated by subjects' beliefs in increased ability to control their pain problem. Informal interviews though, indicated improvements in patients' beliefs concerning self-efficacy. In a study by Flor, Behle and Birbaumer (1993) improvement in therapy (reduced pain severity) was associated with lessening of negative internal control cognitions. Lipchick, Milles and Covington (1993) showed that treatment in a short-term inpatient multidisciplinary pain management unit programme produced significant increases in the sense of personal control over pain and also significant reductions in subjective pain intensity. In research by Rainville, Ahern and Phalen (1993) changes in beliefs about the consequences of pain (after intensive physical reconditioning) showed a high degree of correlation with changes in disability. Post-treatment pain measures and depression were much less important as correlates of disability than were pain beliefs. Also Jensen, Turner and Romano (1994a) found that change in the belief in oneself as disabled by pain was associated with improvement in depressive symptoms and physical functioning after multidisciplinary pain treatment. Increased belief in internal control was also associated with a decrease in number of pain-related physician visits. The data from these intervention studies are encouraging and should result in more effective interventions from health-care professionals and in improved self-management packages for people with chronic illnesses. At the same time it will be necessary to develop the theories and methods, not only to increase our understanding of the nature and role of schemata in chronic illness but also as a basis for psychological interventions.

Appendix 1 Overview of studies on assessment of illness schemata (101 empirical studies)

First author (year)	Subjects	Assessment instrument	Assessed schema dimension	Results
Gaston-Johansson (1985)	–31 Pts. with primary chronic fibromyalgia (PCF) –30 Pts. with rheumatoid arthritis (RA)	Pain preoccupation-circle, shade part of life affected by pain + Beliefs about causes of pain, 16 items, 2 subscales, yes-no + Pain/Ache/Hurt (PAH), 3 parts, identifying meaning and intensity of pain experience, score 1–3	Conse-quences, causes, identity	Pts. with PCF selected higher intensity affective descriptors, reported a greater portion of their life was preoccupied by pain, believed to a higher degree that physical heavy or stressful work, repetitive movements and accidents were responsible for pain than patients with RA
Kerns (1985)	–120 Pts. with chronic pain	West Haven-Yale Multidimensional Pain Inventory, 12 scales, 3 parts, part 1: interference, self-control, 7-point scales.	Conse-quences, control	Self-control inversely related to general affective distress and positively with activity level. Interference correlated with pain
Kutner (1985)	–86 Pts. receiving haemodialysis at center –22 Pts. receiving haemodialysis at home –54 Pts. using continuous ambulatory peritoneal dialysis (CAPD)	Multidimensional Health Locus of Control Scales, assessing the orientation of subjects' health locus of control beliefs (Internal, Powerful Others, Chance), 18 items, 6-point Likert scale	Control	In-center haemodialysis group had significantly more external locus-of-control than the home-haemodialysis groups
Laborde (1985)	–160 Pts. with osteo arthritis	Health Locus of Control Scales, 11 items, 6-point Likert scale, agreement	Control	Present life satisfaction was related to higher internal locus of control and less joint pain

Appendix 1 *(cont.)*

First author (year)	Subjects	Assessment instrument	Assessed schema dimension	Results
Lowery (1985)	–77 Pts. with arthritis –113 Pts. with diabetes –106 Pts. with hypertension	Open and close-ended interview questions about causes, 5-point scales, importance + 10 reasons (internal/external) for outcome, 5-point scale, importance + "How do you expect your illness to do?", 4-point scale, very-not well	Causes, control, timeline	If pts. perceived their current illness-outcome as successful, perceived causes were internal and controllable. The successful pts. rated possible causes as more important than the failure group. Most pts. expected future success, regardless of stability of perceived cause for current outcome
Meyer (1985)	–65 Pts. with hypertension, newly treated –50 Pts. with hypertension in continuous treatment –65 Pts. with hypertension, returned drop-outs –50 normotensive controls	Semi-structured interview, questions about perceptions of causes mechanisms and symptoms of high blood pressure, coded afterwards	Identity, causes, timeline	Illness duration was related to perceived identification of symptoms. Pts. in continuing treatment reported more compliance and made more linkages between physiological hypotheses, perceived causes, symptoms and treatment
Timko (1985)	–42 Pts. with breast cancer	Structured interview, questions about perceived causes (others, environment, chance, self) and control over future recurrence, 11 point scales, not at all-completely	Causes, control	Causal beliefs about others or own personality were associated with a disbelief in success of mastectomy. Own behavior and control over recurrence were positively associated with psychological adjustment

Appendix 1   *(cont.)*

First author (year)	Subjects	Assessment instrument	Assessed schema dimension	Results
Kuckelman-Cobb (1986)	–2 Pts. with amyotrophic lateral sclerosis	Open-ended interviews, questions focused on ideas of causation	Causes, consequences	Qualitative analysis of interviews. Causal beliefs stable and view of worst consequences changing over time
Turk (1986)	–55 Pts. with diabetes –55 diabetes educators –55 college students	Implicit Models of Illness Questionnaire, 9-item seriousness, 8-item personal responsibility, 5-item controllability, 2-item changeability scales, 9-points, agreement	Consequences, control, causes, timeline	Pts. and nurses perceived illness as serious but controllable. Both groups did not believe cause or cure is a result of own behavior
Williams (1986)	–29 Pts. with arthritis	Semi-structured, open-ended interview questions. Thematic checklist of topics, e.g. causal beliefs	Causes	Perceived causes involved combinations of genetic, viral and environmental factors, long-term social stress, serious life-events and personality type
Affleck (1987)	–9 Pts. with rheumatoid arthritis	Structured questions about perceptions of control, 11-point scale, no-extreme control	Control	Personal control over *treatment* was related to positive mood and psychosocial adjustment. More severe pts. who expressed control over *course of illness* reported more negative mood and less positive adjustment Severe pts. expressing more control over *symptoms* reported less negative mood

Appendix 1 *(cont.)*

First author (year)	Subjects	Assessment instrument	Assessed schema dimension	Results
Bradley (1987)	–116 diabetics with continuous subcutaneous insulin infusion (CSII) –169 diabetics with intensified conventional therapy (ICT) –97 diabetics with conventional therapy (CT)	2 composite scales measuring personal (5 subscales) and medical (2 subscales) control, 42 items, 7-point scales	Control	CSII pts. perceived more medical control than CT pts. and less personal control than ICT or CT pts., CSII pts. with poorer glycaemic control after one year were found to have perceptions of greater medical control
Jensen (1987)	–33 Pts. with chronic pain	Survey of Pain Attitudes (SOPA), beliefs about pain control, disability, medical cure, solicitude, medication, 24 items, true-false	Control, consequences	More perceived disability was related to less self-reported working time and more self-reported rest. Pain self-control was positively related with active coping strategies
Lowery (1987)	–296 Pts. with various chronic diseases –83 Pts. with first-time myocardial infarction	2 interview questions: "Have you ever thought about why me?" "How well do you expect to do in the future ?", 4-point scale, very-not at all well	Causes, timeline	Most frequent mentioned causes in chronic pts. were: fate and stress. Pts. who did not ask why me? had lower depression and anxiety scores and higher expectations for recovery
Maes (1987)	–397 Pts. with asthma	Respiratory Illness Opinion Survey (RIOS), 36 items relating to shame, optimism and external control, 5-point scale, agreement	Control	Control did not explain variance in well-being, days absent from work during last year, hospital admissions and amount of medicine taken per day

Appendix 1 *(cont.)*

First author (year)	Subjects	Assessment instrument	Assessed schema dimension	Results
Westbrook (1987)	–156 Pts. with scleroderma	Questions about symptoms, 12 areas (yes-no); difficulties in 9 areas of life, 4-point scale (no problem-need much help), and in social life, 5 statements, 7-point scales (agreement); perceptions of control over relapses, perceived causes, open-ended questions	Identity, consequences, control, causes	Perceived control group made more causal attributions, finding meaning in their illness. They did not differ from helpless pts. in severity of symptoms and handicaps. Perceived health changes in the previous year were related to pts.' perceptions of control
Crisson (1988)	–62 Pts. with chronic pain	Multidimensional Health Locus of Control Scales, modified for pain, 18 items, 6-point scale, agreement	Control	Chance-control pts. felt more helpless, used more diverting attention and praying/hoping strategies and reported more psychological distress
Flor (1988)	–30 Pts. with chronic back pain –40 Pts. with rheumatoid arthritis –50 Pts. with various chronic pain complaints	Pain Related Control Scale (PRCS), cognitive schemata influencing perception of pain, 15 statements, agreement + Multidimensional Health Locus of Control, 18 items, 6-point scales + West Haven-Yale Multidimensional Pain Inventory, 2-item life-control, 9-item interference, 3-item pain severity scales, 7-point scales	Control, control, control, consequences	Pain related perceptions of control were highly related to reports of pain severity and disability in both samples. Cognitive variables explained much more variance in pain and disability levels than disease related variables

Appendix 1 (*cont.*)

First author (year)	Subjects	Assessment instrument	Assessed schema dimension	Results
Gillespie (1988)	–54 Pts. with diabetes	Perceived control, 3 composite 7-point scales: patient, medical external control, importance + Problem Congruence and Causal Congruence Rating Scale, congruence between pt. and doctor scored by judges, 6-point scale, similarity	Control, identity, causes	Lowest problem and causal congruence scores and many discrepancies between perceived control ratings in group having an unstructured consultation. Tendency for glycaemic control to improve with increased causal congruence
Kerns (1988a)	–97 Pts. with chronic pain	West Haven-Yale Multidimensional Pain Inventory, 3 subscales: 3 items pain severity, 9 items interference, 7-point scales, 30 items activity level, 6-point scale, none-extreme	Consequences	Self-monitored pain intensity correlated positively with perceived interference and with decreased satisfaction with important areas of functioning
Kerns (1988b)	–131 Pts. with chronic pain	West Haven-Yale Multidimensional Pain Inventory, 7-point scales: pain severity, interference, self control, negative mood, support (none-extreme)	Consequences, control	Declines or deficits in coping, instrumental activity and self control perceptions are related to the experience of depression
Kraaimaat (1988)	–441 Pts. with chronic headache	The Attribution Inventory, 20 items, 4 factors: psychological distress, stimulants and foods, inborn somatic and physical causes, 4-point scales, not at all-very much so	Causes	Perceived causes explained <2% of the variance in coping. Belief in stimulants and foods associated with duration and external physical causes with frequency of headache

Appendix 1 *(cont.)*

First author (year)	Subjects	Assessment instrument	Assessed schema dimension	Results
Laffrey (1988)	−29 Pts. with cardiovascular disease −29 Pts. healthy controls	Perceived Health Status, 4 dimensions: clinical, functional/role performance, ability to adapt, self-actualization, and an overall score, 10-rung Cantril ladder, worst–best health imaginable	Conse-quences	Cardiovascular pts. perceived themselves less healthy on the overall measure and on the clinical dimension of perceived health. Conceptions of health not significantly different
Maes (1988)	−19 Pts. with asthma	3 Scales of the Respiratory Illness Opinion Survey (RIOS), cognitive attitudes towards asthma; optimism, locus of control, shame/stigma, 36 items, 5-point scales, agreement	Control	No significant effects of the cognitive-educational intervention programme on optimism, locus of control and shame
Pfeiffer (1988)	−53 Pts. with systemic lupus erythematosus (SLE)	Multidimensional Health Locus of Control scales, assessing the orientation of subjects' health locus of control beliefs (internal, powerful others, chance), 18 items, 6-point scales	Control	Those who had SLE longer had less belief in powerful others and less belief in internal control. Pts. who could predict flares in SLE had significantly higher internal control
Reesor (1988)	−80 Pts. with chronic low back pain (CLBP)	Inappropriate Symptom Scale, 7 vague, ill localized symptoms. Non-organic physical signs: pain reports deviating from anatomical principles. Pain drawing: non-anatomical or exaggerated features of pts' drawings depicting quality and location of pain	Identity	Incongruent CLBP pts. displayed more maladaptive and dysfunctional cognitions (more catastrophizing, less perceived control). Their pain experience tended to be perceived and judged as more disturbing, distressing and debilitating

Appendix 1 (*cont.*)

First author (year)	Subjects	Assessment instrument	Assessed schema dimension	Results
Riley (1988)	~56 Pts. with chronic pain	Pain and Impairment Relationship Scale (PAIRS), 15 thoughts, attitudes and opinions about pain, 7-point Likert scale, agreement	Consequences	Belief that pain implies disability is associated with actual impairment, independent of the contribution of actual pain
Rudy (1988)	~100 Pts. with chronic pain	West Haven-Yale Multidimensional Pain Inventory, 3 subscales: 3 items pain severity, 9 items interference, 2 items self control, 7-point scales + Multidimensional Health Locus of Control internal control subscale	Consequences, control, control	Association between pain and depression was significantly mediated by perceived interference and lack of self-control
Turk (1988)	Study 1: ~122 Pts. with chronic pain Study 2: ~100 Pts. with chronic pain	West Haven-Yale Multidimensional Pain Inventory, 5 subscales: 3 items pain severity, 9 items interference, 2 items self control, 3 items support, 3 items affective distress, 7-point scales	Consequences, control	Three subgroups of pts.: interpersonally distressed (no supportive friends or family), dysfunctional and minimizers or adaptive copers (respectively high/low severity of pain, high/low interference scores, high/low degree of psychological distress, low/high activity level, low/high perceived self-control)
Bertolotti (1989)	~19 Pts. with chronic respiratory failure ~60 Pts. with chronic obstructive lung disease	Respiratory Illness Opinion Survey, six attitude categories, e.g. SIA (specific internal awareness), EC (external control), scale 1-100	Identity, control	No significant differences between the two groups of patients for either dimension

Appendix 1 *(cont.)*

First author (year)	Subjects	Assessment instrument	Assessed schema dimension	Results
Bobo (1989)	–48 Pts. with sickle cell disease (SCD) –60 Pts. with asthma –50 Pts. healthy siblings	General Health Perceptions Battery (subscale of the Rand Health Insurance Study), 90 items, Likert scales, score 1–5, true-false	Consequences	Low health perceptions in adults with chronic medical conditions, lowest for persons with SCD
Deshields (1989)	–19 Pts. hypertensives –12 Pts. diabetics –11 Pts. healthy persons	Perceptions of Personal Health Status, 2 Likert type items, scale 1–5, (no-very severe problems, doesn't bother me at all-causes major changes in my life)	Consequences	More disruptions in pts. with diabetes than in healthy persons. Disease impact related to trait anger and total anger expression
Gallon (1989)	–300 Pts. with chronic pain	Perception of Disability Scale, 18 items, perceived change in condition (increase, same, decrease)	Consequences	Only 29% of the pts. perceived themselves as improving, whereas over half of the sample reported themselves working, no longer receiving compensation, having no medical treatment
Linton (1989)	–66 Pts. with low back pain	Modified version of 15-item Arthritis Helplessness Index. Control over pain symptoms, 5-category scale, agreement	Control	Positive effects of intervention not mediated by subjects' beliefs in increased ability to control
Williams (1989)	–87 Pts. with chronic pain	Pain Beliefs and Perceptions Inventory, 16 items, Likert scale, score 1–4, agreement + Multidimensional Health Locus of Control Scale, 18 items	Causes, timeline control	Belief in long endurance of pain associated with: increased subjective report of pain intensity, lower compliance with physical therapy, less improvement on measure of somatization, negative perceptions of self, diminished sense of internal personal control

Appendix 1 *(cont.)*

First author (year)	Subjects	Assessment instrument	Assessed schema dimension	Results
Buckelew (1990)	–160 Pts. with chronic pain	Multidimensional Health Locus of Control Scale, 18 items, 6-point Likert scale, assessing the orientation of subjects' health locus of control beliefs (Internal, Powerful Others, Chance)	Control	Younger men relied more on "internal control", older men on both "chance" and "powerful others". Women with high "internal" control beliefs were more likely to use cognitive self-management techniques than women with both "internal" and "powerful others" beliefs
Hampson (1990)	–46 Pts. with diabetes mellitus	Personal Models of Diabetes Interview (PMDI), 5 components of personal models explored with open-ended questions, 5-point scales	Identity, causes, timeline, consequences, control	Personal models were generally consistent with medical views. Perceived importance of treatment and perceived seriousness of the condition enhanced the prediction of diet level and exercise
Lacroix (1990)	–100 Pts. with low back pain	Schema Assessment Instrument (SAI), pts.' knowledge about medical condition, symptoms, relatedness of symptoms, causes and physiological basis, and prognosis rated by physician on 7-point scales	Identity, causes	The SAI was the only variable to significantly predict return to work
Powell (1990)	–58 Pts. with unexplained fatigue –33 Pts. depressed patient control group	Self-assessment questionnaire, 2 questions about attribution of symptoms, 5-point scales	Causes	Fatigue pts. with major depression having an external attributional style ("a virus") experienced less guilt and preserved their self-esteem

Appendix 1   *(cont.)*

First author (year)	Subjects	Assessment instrument	Assessed schema dimension	Results
Reinert (1990)	–21 Pts. with asthma (new patients) –41 Pts. with asthma (in treatment)	Semi-structured interview, 20 questions about pts.' ideas about diagnosis and treatment of asthma	Identity, causes, timeline	Half of the new pts. had no ideas about mechanism of asthma and believed treatment sufficed, 75% believed asthma was curable
Sacks (1990)	–73 Pts. with renal disease	Illness Effects Questionnaire, perception of interference with personal and social behavior, 20 items, Likert scale, score 1–7	Conse-quences	Perception of illness better predictor of depression than objective severity of illness
Shutty (1990)	–100 Pts. with low-back pain	Multidimensional Health Locus of Control Scale (MHLOC)	Control	Association between internal control and pts.' beliefs about applicability of treatment small and nonsignificant, LoC not predictive of treatment outcome
Skevington (1990)	–29 Pts. with rheumatoid arthritis –60 Pts. with cancer –34 Pts. with various types of illnesses –158 Non-patients	Beliefs about Pain Control Questionnaire (BPCQ), 6-point Likert scale, 15 items, agreement + Multidimensional Health Locus of Control Scale (MHLOC)	Control, control	Pts. with poorest health tended to have stronger external beliefs in both powerful doctors and chance than more healthy groups. Chronic pain pts. scored lowest on internal scale
Strong (1990)	–50 Pts. with chronic low back pain	Pain Beliefs and Perception Inventory (PBPI), 16 items, 4-point Likert scale, agreement + Survey of Pain Attitudes (SOPA), 35 items, 5 subscales, 5-point Likert scale, agreement	Timeline, causes, control, conse-quences	Self-reported dysfunction positively associated with belief that pain is a mystery and pain is disabling. Increase in dysfunction associated with decrease in belief that one can control one's pain

Appendix 1 *(cont.)*

First author (year)	Subjects	Assessment instrument	Assessed schema dimension	Results
Vlayen (1990)	–188 Pts. with chronic back pain	Pain Cognition List (PCL), 50 statements, 5-point Likert scale, agreement + Multidimensional Health Locus of Control Scale	Conse-quences, control, control	PCL intended for identifying pain patients whose pain problem is mainly controlled by cognitive factors. High scores on perceived pain impact associated with depression and pain
Christensen (1991)	–66 Pts. receiving haemodialysis –30 Pts. receiving haemodialysis after failed transplant	Internal Health Locus of Control and Powerful Others Health Locus of Control scales from the Multi-dimensional Locus of Control Scale (MHLOC), 5-point Likert scale, agree-disagree	Control	Belief in internal control associated with less depression among pts. who did not have a transplant and more depression among pts. with a failed one, but only for severely ill pts.
Fry (1991)	–64 Pts. with chronic pelvic pain	8 Open-ended questions (modified version of series proposed by Kleinman), responses grouped in categories afterwards	Causes, timeline, conse-quences	Pts. do not appear to have clear schemata about causes, models are flexible, worries focused on interminability of illness and effects on sex and work
Gilutz (1991)	–194 Pts. with myocardial infarction	2 Central questions: — Why me? — What will help to recover? Q-sort items, 20 possible answers, grade answers into 3 groups in order of importance	Causes, control	Sense of internal personal control correlated positively, and sense of external control negatively with return to work and functioning

Appendix 1   *(cont.)*

First author (year)	Subjects	Assessment instrument	Assessed schema dimension	Results
Härkäpää (1991[a])	–476 Pts. with chronic low-back pain (LBP)	Multidimensional Health Locus of Control scales, 11 items, 3 subscales, range 1–6	Control	Use of more active coping strategies was more frequent in pts. with internal control beliefs. Pts. with more severe LBP reported higher levels of psychological distress, lower levels of internal and stronger beliefs in external control
Härkäpää (1991[b])	–459 Pts. with chronic low back pain (LBP)	Multidimensional Health Locus of Control scales, 11 item + 2 items beliefs in back pain control, 4 subscales: chance, others, internal, internal back pain	Control	Stronger LBP internal control associated with more frequent exercising. Tendency that LBP internal control predicte positive changes in self-assessed LBP disability, irrespective of initial LBP severity
Jensen (1991)	–118 Pts. with chronic pain	Pain control scale from the Survey of Pain Attitudes (SOPA), belief in one's ability to control pain, 6 statements, true-false + 3 Interview questions about beliefs in controllability of pain, administered by telephone, 7 point scale	Control, control	Feeling of control over pain correlated positively with psychological functioning (non-significant after controlling for coping). Positive relation between activity level and perceived control for pts. reporting low levels of pain

Appendix 1 *(cont.)*

First author (year)	Subjects	Assessment instrument	Assessed schema dimension	Results
Jones (1991)	–172 Pts. with chronic illnesses: 74 with asthma 72 with hypertension 26 with diabetes –670 Pts. with various acute illnesses	Interview and/or chart review, questions about knowledge about illness and the degree to which the patient regarded the illness as serious	Causes, consequences	Chronic pts. are generally more compliant, more likely to regard the potential consequences as serious, more accurate in assessment of cause
Lacroix (1991)	–31 Pts. with chronic respiratory conditions	Schema Assessment Instrument (SAI), accuracy of pts. knowledge about symptoms, medical condition, prognoses, relatedness of symptoms, causes and physiological basis, rated by physician on four 7-point scales	Identity, causes	Accuracy rating correlated positively and significantly with ratings of adaptive functioning, no relationship was observed between severity and prognosis of pts.' medical condition and functioning
Loomis (1991)	–19 Pts. with various chronic illnesses	List of NANDA-diagnoses, pts.' choices compared with nurses diagnoses	Identity	Nurses identified 212 diagnoses, 46 more than those selected by pts., rate of agreement: 78%
Marshall (1991)	–181 Pts. with various chronic illnesses	Mailed Questionnaire containing questions about internal control over health, 5 items illness management, 4 items self-mastery, 3 items self-blame, 2 items illness prevention, 6 point scale, agreement	Control	Only perceptions of self-mastery were independently associated with indexes of physical health and well-being

Appendix 1 *(cont.)*

First author (year)	Subjects	Assessment instrument	Assessed schema dimension	Results
Millard (1991)	~179 Pts. with chronic pain	Physiological Responsivity factor of the Biobehavioral Pain Profile, perceptions and reports of physical symptoms, 5 items, 8-point scale	Identity	The frequency of reporting physical symptoms was more useful than pain intensity in predicting reported activity interference
Robbins (1991)	~100 Pts. attending a hospital family practice centre (self-initiated)	Symptom Interpretation Questionnaire, 13 symptoms, pick one attribution most clearly fitting probable explanation (somatic, psychological, normalizing) for symptom	Identity, causes	Psychological attributions, more common in pts. with a history of chronic psychiatric problems, were predictive of the number of psychosocial complaints presented. Somatic attributions, more common in pts. with acute or chronic physical illness, predicted the number of somatic complaints
Slater (1991)	~31 Pts. with chronic low back pain	Pain and Impairment Relationship Scale (PAIRS), 15 personal statements reflecting thoughts, attitudes and opinions about pain, 7-point Likert scale, agreement	Consequences	Scores on PAIRS significantly related to measures of physical impairment but not to physicians' ratings of disease severity
Williams (1991)	~120 Pts. with chronic (mainly low back) pain	Pain Beliefs and Perceptions Inventory, 3 basic dimensions: Time, Mystery, Self-blame, 16 items, 4-point Likert scale, agree-disagree	Timeline, causes	Pts. believing that pain was enduring and mysterious were more likely to use cognitive coping strategies and to catastrophize, and less likely to rate their strategies as effective

Appendix 1   *(cont.)*

First author (year)	Subjects	Assessment instrument	Assessed schema dimension	Results
Barlow (1992)	~161 Pts. with ankylosing spondylitis (111 members of self-help groups, 50 non-members)	Multidimensional Health Locus of Control Scales, perceived control (personal, external, chance) over health	Control	Members of self-help groups placed significantly less reliance on powerful others. No significant differences were found on personal or chance control. The two groups did not differ in health status
Dalal (1992)	~70 Pts. with lung tuberculosis	Questionnaire on: causal beliefs, 6 items, 5-point scale, least-most responsible; recovery beliefs, 8 factors, 5-point scale, very low-very high contribution; perceived control, 2 items, 5-point scale, very little-very much	Causes, control	Causal attribution to external factors (others' carelessness and family conditions) and recovery beliefs of a cosmic nature (God and fate) correlated negatively with psychological adjustment. Perceived control was linked with better adjustment
Edwards (1992)	Study 1: ~194 Controls ~100 Pts. with chronic pain	Pain Beliefs Questionnaire (PBQ), beliefs about the cause and treatment of pain, 20 sentences, choice of qualifying adverbs at appropriate place, 6-point scale, always-never	Causes, consequences, control	Organic Beliefs scale (8 items), and Psychological Beliefs scale (4 items) accounted for 68% of the variance on the BPQ. Chronic pain pts. are more likely than controls to endorse items on the Organic Beliefs scale
	Study 2: ~40 Pts. with chronic pain (subsample of study 1)	PBQ, 12 items + Multidimensional Health Locus of Control scale	Causes, consequences, control	Organic Beliefs scale was significantly associated with the belief that powerful others and chance or fate control health status. Belief in psychological factors was significantly associated with belief in internal control

Appendix 1   *(cont.)*

First author (year)	Subjects	Assessment instrument	Assessed schema dimension	Results
Jensen (1992)	–118 Pts. with chronic pain	Survey of Pain Attitudes (SOPA), administered by telephone, beliefs about: medical cure, solicitude, disability, medication, emotion, 15 statements, true-false	Control, conse- quences	Pts. with low and medium pain levels who believed themselves to be disabled demonstrated significantly lower levels of activity and psychological well-being and higher levels of professional services utilization
Muthny (1992)	–70 Pts. with myocardial infarction (MI) –66 Pts. with cancer –108 Pts. with end stage renal disease (ESRD) –207 Pts. with multiple sclerosis (MS)	Persönliche Ursachen und Gründe für die Erkrankung (PUK), personal causes, 20 items, 5-point scale (not at all-very much appropriate) + Erkrankungsbezogene Kontrollattributionen (EKOA), 9 control dimensions	Causes, control	Predominant causal attributions: heredity in MS, pollution in cancer, stress in MI and mistakes of doctors and somatic models in ESRD. Main perceived influences on course of illness in all groups: progress of medicine, internal cognitive and behavioural factors. Highest scores on internal control: MI and cancer. Less influence of powerful others: MS
Raleigh (1992)	–45 Pts. with cancer –27 Pts. with diabetes –4 Pts. with multiple sclerosis –2 Pts. with arthritis –1 Pt. with emphysema –11 Pts. with various chronic illnesses	2 Questions from the Sources of Support Interview Schedule. "Do you believe there is a purpose/reason for your illness?" and "What do you believe the purpose/reason is?"	Causes	No significant variance existed between the chronic illness and oncology groups

Appendix 1 *(cont.)*

First author (year)	Subjects	Assessment instrument	Assessed schema dimension	Results
Ray (1992)	–208 Pts. with chronic fatigue syndrome	Questionnaire, rate extent of experience with symptoms, 5-point scale, not at all–extremely +	Identity,	Fatigue, somatic symptoms and cognitive difficulty were associated with general illness severity. Emotional distress did not contribute directly to pts.' perceptions of illness severity
		Perceptions of: illness onset, severity, variability, causes, outcomes, select response from ranked alternatives, comment	causes, conse-quences, timeline	
Remien (1992)	–53 Pts. with AIDS (longterm survivors, >3 years)	Health Locus of Control Scales (HLOC), perceived control (personal, external, chance) over health, 18 items, 6-point scales, agree–disagree +	Control,	Longterm survivors believed more in "chance" and less in "powerful others" than control groups of HIV+ and HIV-. Almost 40% stated positive outlook as important factor in longer survival
		open-ended question, belief about causes of surviving	causes	
Schiaffino (1992)	–64 Pts. with rheumatoid arthritis	Implicit Models of Illness Questionnaire, 2 items about control, 5-point scale, agreement +	Control,	When perceived controllability was low, internal, global and stable attributions for the cause of a symptom flare were linked to greater depression but less disability
		Causal attributions, 3 scales: internality, stability, globality, 7-point scales	causes	
Schüssler (1992)	–50 Pts. with rheumatoid arthritis –44 Pts. with sarcoidosis –59 Pts. with coxarthrosis	Illness concepts assigned according to pts.' answers on interview, 10 categories, 3-point scale, not applicable–applicable	Control	Internal/external control beliefs differentiated between a group with a favourable course of disease, and a group with marked deterioration

Appendix 1 *(cont.)*

First author (year)	Subjects	Assessment instrument	Assessed schema dimension	Results
Sharpe (1992)	–144 Pts. with unexplained fatigue	Postal questionnaire, beliefs about the cause of illness, 3-point scale, not a cause–definitely a cause	Causes	Functional impairment was associated with belief in a viral cause of the illness
Strong (1992)	–100 Pts. with chronic low back pain	Survey of Pain Attitudes-Revised (SOPA-R), 35 items, 5-point Likert scale, agree–disagree + Pain Beliefs and Perception Inventory (PBPI), 16 items, 4-point Likert scale, agree–disagree	Control, consequences, timeline, causes	Results of the comparison between the SOPA-R and the PBPI provide strong support for the SOPA-R as a useful measurement tool for use with pts. with chronic low back pain
Tennen (1992)	–54 Pts. with rheumatoid arthritis	Perceived Control and Benefits, 5 items self-control, 5 items benefits from pain, 6-point Likert scale, agreement	Control	Greater perceived control was associated with less pain, but for more severe pts. more perceived control was associated with more emotional distress
De Valle (1992)	–81 Pre-operative coronary artery bypass-graft pts.	List of possible causes of coronary heart disease, 21 items, 3-point scale, yes-no, add other causes, write down main cause + Multidimensional Health Locus of Control Scale, 18 items, 6-point scale, agree–disagree	Causes, control	Causal attributions were found to be related to reported lifestyle changes. Health Locus of Control beliefs were related to the endorsement of certain causes but not to lifestyle changes

Appendix 1 *(cont.)*

First author (year)	Subjects	Assessment instrument	Assessed schema dimension	Results
Wassem (1992)	–62 Pts. with multiple sclerosis	Outcome Expectancy Scale (OES), beliefs how effective behaviours would be in influencing illness, 6 items, 5-point Likert scale, agree-disagree	Control	Outcome expectations unable to predict (social, psychological, physical) adjustment. Ceiling effect of respondent scores on the OES-scales
Weaver (1992)	–104 Pts. with chronic obstructive pulmonary disease	Attributions Interview Schedule, open-ended questions, recorded, judges coding answers into categories	Causes	Significant differences between those who did/did not ask "why me", those who had not asked were more functional
Ailinger (1993)	–59 Pts. with rheumatoid arthritis	Interview schedule based on Kleinman. Questions about causes, effects, perceived severity and expectations. Coded answers	Causes, consequences, timeline	Perceived causes: 64% none, 31% illness or physical trauma, 31% stress, 80% indicated loss of functioning in personal care, household chores, role change, work and recreation, 10% stated their hope in future cure
Bates (1993)	–372 Pts. with chronic pain: 44 Hispanics (H) 100 "Old-Americans" (OA) 28 Polish (P) 60 Irish (Ir) 50 Italians (It) 90 French Canadians (FC)	Ethnicity and Pain Questionnaire (EPQ). Subscale "Locus of Control", internal-external, 10 items, true-false	Control	Best predictors of pain intensity variation are ethnic group affiliation and locus of control style. Ethnic group identity is also a predictor of locus of control style
Flor (1993)	–213 Pts. with chronic back pain	Pain Related Control Scale (PRCS), underlying cognitive schemata of pain, 15 statements, 6-point scale, agree: not at all-very much	Control	Improvement in therapy was associated with lessening of negative cognitions. PRCS explained a significant amount of the pain severity variance

Appendix 1 (cont.)

First author (year)	Subjects	Assessment instrument	Assessed schema dimension	Results
Geisser (1993)	~60 Pts. with chronic pain	Pennebaker Inventory of Limbic Languidness (PILL), 54-symptom inventory, 5-point scales, never experienced-more than once a week	Identity	Depression related to affective and evaluative aspects of pts. pain. Somatic focus mediated relationship between depression and sensory pain experience
Kröner-Herwig (1993)	~164 Pts. with chronic pain	Kausal und Kontrollattribution Inventor (KAUKON), assessment of attributional patterns of pain pts., 4 six-point scales: perceived causes and control, both psychologically and medically oriented, 40 items, agreement	Control, causes	KAUKON tool for predicting acceptance of psychological pain therapy and its outcome. Perceived psychosocial causes and control positively associated with depression and disability
Lipchik (1993)	~96 Pts. with chronic pain, 50 receiving short-term intensive pain management program (PMU)	Pain Locus of Control (PLOC), 36 items, 3 subscales: internal, powerful others, chance, 5-point Likert scale, agree-disagree + Pain Beliefs and Perceptions Inventory, 16 items, 4-point Likert scale, agree-disagree	Control, causes, timeline	Pts. in PMU showed an increase in sense of control, decrease in pain intensity and in attribution to external factors. Pts. did not change their belief in pain endurance. Pts. who completed the PMU reduced their scores on the mystery subscale
McDonald (1993)	~65 Pts. with chronic fatigue	Interview questions about explanations and strength of beliefs for the causes of fatigue and effects on lives	Causes, conse-quences	Physical (41%), social (23%), emotional causes (15%), none 13%, family responsibility 8%. Cause had no effect on fatigue. Influence on life: none 28%, social and leisure activities 69%, sexual functioning 45%

Appendix 1 *(cont.)*

First author (year)	Subjects	Assessment instrument	Assessed schema dimension	Results
Pastor (1993)	–137 Pts. with rheumatic diseases: 32 with primary fibromyalgia syndrome 32 with rheumatoid arthritis 22 with ankylosing spondylitis 31 with osteo arthritis 20 with systemic lupus erythematosus	Multidimensional Health Locus of Control-Pain scales (MHLC-PLOC), 6 items, 6-point scale, agree-disagree	Control	Pain locus of control profile in pts. with PFS was high on "powerful others", low on "internal" and high on "fate". The locus of control profile in the other groups: high on "powerful others", high on "internal" and low on "chance". PFS pts. reported more psychological distress and pain, subjects who reported more internal control showed less disability
Pollock (1993)	–597 Pts. with various chronic illnesses: 251 with insulin-dependent diabetes mellitus 113 with hypertension 96 with rheumatoid arthritis (RA) 137 with multiple sclerosis (MS)	Perception of Illness Impact (PII), Cantril ladder with 10 divisions. Subjects rated how disabled they felt, defining their own anchoring points on the continuum, best-worst	Consequences	Perceived level of disability was related to psychosocial adaptation for all groups, but to physiological adaptation for RA and MS groups only
Rainville (1993)	–72 Pts. with chronic low back pain	Pain and Impairment Relationship Scale (PAIRS), 15 statements attributing impairment and disability to pain, 7-point Likert scale, agree-disagree	Consequences	Pain beliefs are of minimal value for predicting treatment compliance. Post-treatment PAIRS-scores correlated highly with disability measures

Appendix 1 *(cont.)*

First author (year)	Subjects	Assessment instrument	Assessed schema dimension	Results
Skevington (1993)	−44 Pts. with rheumatoid arthritis	Beliefs about Pain Control Questionnaire (BPCQ), 13 items, 3 control dimensions (internal, powerful others, chance) +	Control,	Those most depressed after two years were more likely to have believed from the outset that their pain would continue and that it would be less controllable. No differences on measures of reported pain, pain control or self-esteem
		Attributional Dimensions of Painful Symptoms, 4 ratings: stability, internality, global-specific, controllability, 7-point scales	timeline, causes, consequences, control	
Toomey (1993)	−48 Pts. with chronic pain, treated in a pain clinic −28 Pts. with chronic pain, treated in a medical clinic −22 Pts. with various illnesses without pain	Pain Locus of Control Scale (PLOC), 36 items, 6-point Likert scale, 3 scales (internality, powerful others, chance), agree-disagree	Control	Attributions of pain control varied across the treatment setting. Pain clinic pts. have significant lower scores on "powerful others". Pts. with chronic pain, regardless of treatment setting report lower "internality" scores and higher "chance" attributions than do pts. without pain
Andrykowski (1994)	−69 Pts. with leukemia	Multidimensional Health Locus of Control Scale, 18 items, 6-point Likert scale, assessing the orientation of subjects' health locus of control beliefs (Internal, Powerful Others, Chance)	Control	The relationship between control beliefs and psychological adjustment is moderated by disease severity and treatment history. Pts. with "powerful others" control belief and failure of prior cancer therapy showed the greatest distress

Appendix 1 (*cont.*)

First author (year)	Subjects	Assessment instrument	Assessed schema dimension	Results
Fowers (1994)	–71 Cardiac rehabilitation pts.	Multidimensional Health Locus of Control Scale, 18 items, 6-point Likert scale, assessing the orientation of subjects' health locus of control beliefs (Internal, Powerful Others, Chance) + Control Over Cardiac Recovery Scale (COCRS), 10 types of recovery behaviour, 6-point Likert scale, not at all-a great deal	Control, control	Appraisals of control were unrelated to psychological distress when contextual variables were statistically controlled. Interactive effect between level of life stress and perception of control significantly associated with psychological distress
Garro (1994)	–32 Pts. with malfunctioning of the temporomandibular joints of the jaw	Open-ended, semi-structured interview, sketch of illness history, start, course, diagnosis, cure, affect on life	Identity, time-line, causes, control, consequences	Analysis on an individual level. Consistent emergence of themes concerning the mind and body within and across narratives
Hampson (1994)	–61 Pts. with osteo arthritis	Personal Models of Arthritis Interview, 5 components: symptoms, seriousness, causes, control, treatment, structured interview, 60 questions, 5-point scales (not at all-extremely)	Identity, consequences, causes, control, time-line	Pts. with higher perceived seriousness reported higher levels of self-management, more utilization of medical services and experienced poorer quality of life
Heidrich (1994)	–108 Pts. with cancer	Interview question: "would you describe your cancer as acute, episodic or chronic ?"	Time-line	Perception of cancer as chronic predicted less psychological well-being, discrepancy between actual and ideal self mediated this effect

Appendix 1 *(cont.)*

First author (year)	Subjects	Assessment instrument	Assessed schema dimension	Results
Herda (1994)	–193 Pts. with chronic pain	Pain Beliefs and Perceptions Inventory, 16 items, 4-point Likert-scale, 4 subscales, agreement	Causes, timeline	Pts. blaming themselves were less frequently in pain. Belief in pain being a mystery was associated with anxiety and catastrophizing. Frequency of pain was a better predictor of psychological problems than belief in enduring pain
Ireys (1994)	–286 Pts. with various chronic illnesses	Structured interview, 1 item unpredictability (yes-no), 1 item prognosis (better, same, worse), 4 items perceived impact of illness on social interactions, 4-point scale	Timeline, consequences	Perceived impact mediated the relationship between condition characteristics (self-reported prognosis, learning disability, sensory impairment and unpredictability) and self-esteem
Jensen (1994[a])	–94 Pts. with chronic pain	Survey of Pain Attitudes (SOPA), beliefs about pain control, disability, harm, emotion, medical cure, solicitude, medication, 57 items, 5-point scale, true-untrue	Control, consequences	Changes in pts.' beliefs in control over pain and beliefs in themselves as disabled, associated with changes in depressive symptoms and physical functioning
Jensen (1994[b])	–241 Pts. with chronic pain	Survey of Pain Attitudes (SOPA), beliefs about control, disability, harm, emotion, cure, solicitude, medication, 57 items, 5-point scale (true-untrue)	Control, consequences	Belief that one is disabled by pain associated with physical disability (especially in pts. with pain of short duration), and with psychosocial dysfunction for low-to-medium pain pts. Control beliefs made no contribution to predictions of dysfunctioning

Appendix 1   *(cont.)*

First author (year)	Subjects	Assessment instrument	Assessed schema dimension	Results
Primavera (1994)	–30 Pts. with analgesic or ergotamine rebound headache	Health Attribution Test (HAT), 3 scales: internal, powerful others, chance. 22 Items, 5-point Likert scale (agree-disagree)	Control	75% of the pts. had profile representing "good" attitudes (average on "internal", low/average on "chance" and "powerful others"). No differences in length of stay between "good" and "bad" (low/average on "internal" and high/average on "powerful others" and/or "chance") profiles
Williams (1994)	study 1: –37 Pts. with chronic pain study 2: –148 Pts. with chronic pain	Pain Beliefs and Perceptions Inventory (PBPI), 5-items pain permanence, 4-items pain constancy, 4-items mystery, 3-items self-blame, Likert scale 1–4, agreement	Timeline, causes	Belief in pain constancy associated with pain and discomfort in functioning. Belief in pain permanence associated with anxiety. Belief in self causing pain associated with depression, but also with up-time. Mystery associated with distress
Yardley (1994)	–101 Pts. with vestibular disorders (vertigo)	Dizziness Beliefs Scale, 17 beliefs concerning negative consequences of attacks, 3 factors: loss of control, serious illness, severe attack, 5-point scales, agreement	Consequences	Negative beliefs about vertigo and reported autonomic symptomatology were related to handicap. Beliefs most closely related to handicap comprised concerns about incompetence and social embarrassment

Appendix 1 *(cont.)*

First author (year)	Subjects	Assessment instrument	Assessed schema dimension	Results
Kleinman (1995)	~80 Pts. with epilepsy	Semi-structured interview schedule, questions on the experience and treatment of the illness	Identity, causes, consequences	Pts. and family showed a tendency to use overwork, strong affects and a wide range of new explanations why attacks continued. Emotional, financial and family/marital burdens are reported to be extensive
Morley (1995)	~84 Pts. with chronic pain	Pain Beliefs and Perceptions Inventory (PBPI), 5-items pain permanence, 4-items pain constancy, 4-items mystery, 3-items self-blame, Likert scale 1–4, agreement	Time-line, causes	Patient groups did not differ significantly in coping strategies and beliefs. Pts. believing that pain is constant, permanent and non-mysterious were longer in pain then pts. who were neutral about its permanence and believed pain is constant and mysterious.

Pts. = patients

REFERENCES

Abramson, L.Y., Seligman, M.E.P. & Teasdale, J.D. (1978) Learned helplessness in humans: critique and reformulation. *Journal of Abnormal Psychology*, **87**, 49–74.

Adams, C.E., Power, A., Frederick, K. & Lefebvre, C. (1994) An investigation of the adequacy of MEDLINE searches for randomized controlled trials (RCTs) of the effects of mental health care. *Psychological Medicine*, **24**, 741–748.

Affleck, G., Tennen, H., Pfeiffer, C. & Fifield, J. (1987) Appraisals of control and predictability in adapting to a chronic disease. *Journal of Personality and Social Psychology*, **53**, 273–279.

Ailinger, R.L. & Schweitzer, E. (1993) Patients' explanations of rheumatoid arthritis. *Western Journal of Nursing Research*, **15**, 340–351.

Andrykowski, M.A. & Brady, M.J. (1994) Health locus of control and psychological distress in cancer patients: interactive effects of context. *Journal of Behavioral Medicine*, **17**, 439–458.

Barlow, J.H., Macey, S.J. & Struthers, G. (1992) Psychosocial factors and self-help in ankylosing spondylitis patients. *Clinical Rheumatology*, **11**, 220–225.

Bates, M.S., Edwards, W.T. & Anderson, K.O. (1993) Ethnocultural influences on variation in chronic pain perception. *Pain*, **52**, 101–112.

Baumann, L.J., Cameron, L.D., Zimmerman, R.S. & Leventhal, H. (1989) Illness representations and matching labels with symptoms. *Health Psychology*, **8**, 449–470.

Bertolotti, G., Balestroni, G., Maiani, G. & Zotti, A.M. (1989) Psychosocial responses to disease stimuli: preliminary findings. *European Respiratory Journal*, **2**, 660s–662s.

Bishop, G.D., Briede, C., Cavazos, L., Grotzinger, R. & McMahon, S. (1987) Processing illness information: The role of disease prototypes. *Basic and Applied Social Psychology*, **8**, 21–43.

Bobo, L., Miller, S.T., Smith, W.R., Elam, J.T., Rosmarin, P.C. & Lancaster, D.J. (1989) Health perceptions and medical care opinions of inner-city adults with sickle cell disease or asthma compared with those of their siblings. *Southern Medical Journal*, **82**, 9–12.

Bradley, C., Gamsu, D.S., Moses, J.L., Knight, G., Boulton, A.J.M., Drury, J. & Ward, J.D. (1987) The use of diabetes-specific perceived control and health belief measures to predict treatment choice and efficacy in a feasibility study of continuous subcutaneous insulin infusion pumps. *Psychology & Health*, **1**, 133–146.

Buckelew, S.P., Shutty Jr., M.S., Hewett, J., Landon, T., Morrow, K. & Frank, R.G. (1990) Health locus of control, gender differences and adjustment to persistent pain. *Pain*, **42**, 287–294.

Christensen, A.J., Turner, C.W., Smith, T.W., Holman, J.M. & Gregory, M.C. (1991) Health locus of control and depression in end-stage renal disease. *Journal of Consulting and Clinical Psychology*, **59**, 419–424.

Crisson, J.E. & Keefe, F.J. (1988) The relationship of locus of control to pain coping strategies and psychological distress in chronic pain patients. *Pain*, **35**, 147–154.

Dalal, A.K. & Singh, A.K. (1992) Role of causal and recovery beliefs in the psychological adjustment to a chronic disease. *Psychology & Health*, **6**, 193–203.

Deshields, T.L., Jenkins, J.O. & Tait, R.C. (1989) The experience of anger in chronic illness: a preliminary investigation. *International Journal of Psychiatry in Medicine*, **19**, 299–309.

Edwards, L.C., Pearce, S.A., Turner-Stokes, L. & Jones, A. (1992) The pain beliefs questionnaire: an investigation of beliefs in the causes and consequences of pain. *Pain*, **51**, 267–272.

Flor, H., Behle, D.J. & Birbaumer, N. (1993) Assessment of pain-related cognitions in chronic pain patients. *Behaviour Research and Therapy*, **32**, 63–73.

Flor, H. & Turk, D.C. (1988) Chronic back pain and rheumatoid arthritis: Predicting pain and disability from cognitive variables. *Journal of Behavioral Medicine*, **11**, 251–265.

Fowers, B.J. (1994) Perceived control, illness status, stress and adjustment to cardiac illness. *The Journal of Psychology*, **128**, 567–576.

Fry, R.P.W., Crisp, A.H. & Beard, R.W. (1991) Patients' illness models in chronic pelvic pain. *Psychotherapy and Psychosomatics*, **55**, 158–163.

Gallon, R.L. (1989) Perception of disability in chronic back pain patients: a long-term follow-up. *Pain*, **37**, 67–75.

Garro, L.C. (1994) Narrative representations of chronic illness experience: cultural models of illness, mind and body in stories concerning the temporomandibular joint (TMJ). *Social Science and Medicine*, **38**, 775–788.

Gaston-Johansson, F., Johansson, G., Felldin, R. & Sanne, H. (1985) A comparative study of pain description, emotional discomfort and health perception in patients with chronic pain syndrome and rheumatoid arthritis. *Scandinavian Journal of Rehabilitation Medicine*, **17**, 109–119.

Geisser, M.E., Gaskin, M.E., Robinson, M.E. & Greene, A.F. (1993) The relationship of depression and somatic focus to experimental and clinical pain in chronic pain patients. *Psychology & Health*, **8**, 405–415.

Gill, D.B.E.C. & Adams, C.E. (1995) Randomized controlled trials in the Journal of Psychosomatic Research; 1956–1993: A prevalence study. *Journal of Psychosomatic Research*, **39**, 949–956.

Gillespie, C.R. & Bradley, C. (1988) Causal attributions of doctor and patients in a diabetes clinic. *British Journal of Clinical Psychology*, **27**, 67–76.

Gilutz, H., Bar-On, D., Billing, E., Rehnquist, N. & Cristal, N. (1991) The relationship between causal attribution and rehabilitation in patients after their first myocardial infraction. A cross cultural study. *European Heart Journal*, **12**, 883–888.

Hampson, S.E., Glasgow, R.E. & Toobert, D.J. (1990) Personal models of diabetes and their relations to self-care activities. *Health Psychology*, **9**, 632–646.

Hampson, S.E., Glasgow, R.E. & Zeiss, A. (1994) Personal models of osteoarthritis and their relation to self-management activities and quality of life. *Journal of Behavioral Medicine*, **17**, 143–158.

Härkäpää, K. (1991a) Relationships of psychological distress and health locus of control beliefs with the use of cognitive and behavioral coping strategies in low back pain patients. *The Clinical Journal of Pain*, **7**, 275–282.

Härkäpää, K., Järvikoski, A., Mellin, G., Hurri, H. & Luoma, J. (1991b) Health locus of control beliefs and psychological distress as predictors for treatment outcome in low-back pain patients: results of a 3-month follow-up of a controlled intervention study. *Pain*, **46**, 35–41.

Heidrich, S.M., Forsthoff, C.A. & Ward, S.E. (1994) Psychological adjustment in adults with cancer: The self as mediator. *Health Psychology*, **13**, 346–353.

Herda, C.A., Siegeris, K. & Basler, H.D. (1994) The Pain Beliefs and Perceptions Inventory: Further evidence for a 4-factor structure. *Pain*, **57**, 85–90.

Ireys, H.T., Gross, S.S., Werthamer-Larsson, L.A. & Kolodner, K.B. (1994) Self-esteem of young adults with chronic health conditions: Appraising the effects of perceived impact. *Developmental and Behavioral Pediatrics*, **15**, 409–415.

Jensen, M.P. & Karoly, P. (1991) Control beliefs, coping efforts and adjustment to chronic pain. *Journal of Consulting and Clinical Psychology*, **59**, 431–438.

Jensen, M.P. & Karoly, P. (1992) Pain-specific beliefs, perceived symptom severity and adjustment to chronic pain. *The Clinical Journal of Pain*, **8**, 123–130.

Jensen, M.P., Karoly P. & Huger, R. (1987) The development and preliminary validation of an instrument to assess patients' attitudes toward pain. *Journal of Psychosomatic Research*, **31**, 393–400.

Jensen, M.P., Turner, J.A. & Romano, J.M. (1994a) Correlates of improvement in multidisciplinary treatment of chronic pain. *Journal of Consulting and Clinical Psychology*, **62**, 172–179.

Jensen, M.P., Turner, J.A., Romano, J.M. & Lawler, B.K. (1994b) Relationship of pain-specific beliefs to chronic pain adjustment. *Pain*, **57**, 301–309.

Jones, S.L., Jones, P.K. & Katz, J. (1991) Compliance in acute and chronic patients receiving a health belief model intervention in the emergency department. *Social Science and Medicine*, **32**, 1183–1189.

Kaplan, R.M. (1990) Behavior as the central outcome in health care. *American Psychologist*, **45**, 1211–1220.

Kerns, R.D., Finn, P. & Haythornthwaite, J. (1988a) Self-monitored pain intensity: psychometric properties and clinical utility. *Journal of Behavioral Medicine*, **11**, 71–82.

Kerns, R.D. & Haythornthwaite, J.A. (1988b) Depression among chronic pain patients: cognitive-behavioral analysis and effect on rehabilitation outcome. *Journal of Consulting and Clinical Psychology*, **56**, 870–876.

Kerns, R.D., Turk, D.C. & Rudy, T.E. (1985) The West Haven-Yale Multidimensional Pain Inventory (WHYMPI). *Pain*, **23**, 345–356.

Kleinman, A., Wang, W.Z., Li, S.C., Cheng, X.M., Dai, X.Y., Li, K.T. & Kleinman, J. (1995) The social course of epilepsy: chronic illness as social experience in interior China. *Social Science and Medicine*, **40**, 1319–1330.

Kraaimaat, F.W. & Van Schevikhoven, R.E.O. (1988) Causal attributions and coping with pain in chronic headache sufferers. *Journal of Behavioral Medicine*, **11**, 293–302.

Kröner-Herwig, B., Greis, R. & Schilkowsky, G. (1993) Kausal- und Kontrollattribution bei chronischen Schmerzpatienten: Entwicklung und Evaluation eines Inventars (KAUKON). *Diagnostica*, **39**, 120–137.

Kuckelman-Cobb, A. & Hamera, E. (1986) Illness experience in a chronic disease — ALS. *Social Science and Medicine*, **23**, 641–650.

Kutner, N.G. & Brogan, D.R. (1985) Disability labeling vs. rehabilitation rhetoric for the chronically ill: A case study in policy contradictions. *Journal of Applied Behavioral Science*, **21**, 169–183.

Laborde, J.M. & Powers, M.J. (1985) Life satisfaction, health control orientation and illness-related factors in persons with osteoarthritis. *Research in Nursing and Health*, **8**, 183–190.

Lacroix, J.M. (1991) Assessing illness schemata in patient populations. In J.A. Skelton & R.T. Croyle (Eds.), *Mental representation in health and illness* (pp. 193–219). New York: Springer-Verlag.

Lacroix, J.M., Martin, B., Avendano, M. & Goldstein, R. (1991) Symptom schemata in chronic respiratory patients. *Health Psychology*, **10**, 268–273.

Lacroix, J.M., Powell, J., Lloyd, G.J., Doxey, N.C.S., Mitson, G.L. & Aldam, C.F. (1990) Low-back pain: Factors of value in predicting outcome. *Spine*, **15**, 495–499.

Laffrey, S.C. & Crabtree, M.K. (1988) Health and health behavior of persons with chronic cardiovascular disease. *International Journal of Nursing Studies*, **25**, 41–52.

Lau, R.R. (in press) Cognitive representations of health and illness. In D. Gochman (Ed.), *Handbook of health behavior research*. New York: Plenum.

Lau, R.R., Bernard, T.M. & Hartman, K.A. (1989) Further explorations of common sense representations of common illnesses. *Health Psychology*, **8**, 195–219.

Lau, R.R. & Hartman, K.A. (1983) Common sense representations of common illnesses. *Health Psychology*, **2**, 167–185.

Leventhal, H. (1992, June) *Illness cognition: The study of the representation and coping with current and future health threats over the life span*. Paper presented at the annual Pieter de la Court readings, Leiden, The Netherlands.

Leventhal, H. & Diefenbach, M. (1991) The active side of illness cognition. In J.A. Skelton & R.T. Croyle (Eds.), *Mental Representation in Health and Illness* (pp. 247–272). New York: Springer.

Leventhal, H., Meyer, D. & Nerenz, D.R. (1980) The common sense representation of illness danger. In S. Rachman (Ed.), *Contributions to medical psychology: Vol. 2* (pp. 17–30). New York: Pergamon Press.

Leventhal, H. & Nerenz, D.R. (1985) The assessment of illness cognition. In P. Karoly (Ed.), *Measurement strategies in health psychology* (pp. 517–553). New York: Wiley.

Leventhal, H., Nerenz, D.R. & Steele, D.J. (1984) Illness representations and coping with health threats. In A. Baum, S.E. Taylor & J.E. Singer (Eds.), *Handbook of psychology and health: Vol 4* (pp. 219–252). Hillsdale, NJ: Lawrence Erlbaum Associates.

Linton, S.J., Bradley, L.A., Jensen, I., Spangfort, E. & Sundell, L. (1989) The secondary prevention of low back pain: a controlled study with follow-up. *Pain*, **36**, 197–207.

Lipchik, G.L., Milles, K. & Covington, E.C. (1993) The effects of multidisciplinary pain management treatment on locus of control and pain beliefs in chronic non-terminal pain. *The Clinical Journal of Pain*, **9**, 49–57.

Loomis, M.E. & Conco, D. (1991) Patients' perceptions of health, chronic illness and nursing diagnoses. *Nursing Diagnosis*, **2**, 162–170.

Lowery, B.J. & Jacobsen, B.S. (1985) Attributional analysis of chronic illness outcomes. *Nursing Research*, **34**, 82–88.

Lowery, B.J., Jacobsen, B.S. & McCauley, K. (1987) On the prevalence of causal search in illness situations. *Nursing Research*, **36**, 88–93.

Maes, S. & Schlösser, M. (1987) The role of cognition and coping in health behavior outcomes of asthmatic patients. *Current Psychological Research and Reviews*, **6**, 79–90.

Maes, S. & Schlösser, M. (1988) Changing health behaviour outcomes in asthmatic patients: a pilot intervention study. *Social Science and Medicine*, **26**, 359–364.

Marshall, G.N. (1991) A multidimensional analysis of internal health locus of control beliefs: separating the wheat from the chaff?. *Journal of Personality and Social Psychology*, **61**, 483–491.

McDonald, E., David, A.S., Pelosi, A.J. & Mann, A.H. (1993) Chronic fatigue in primary care attenders. *Psychological Medicine*, **23**, 987–998.

Meyer, D., Leventhal, H. & Gutmann, M. (1985) Common-sense models of illness: The example of hypertension. *Health Psychology*, **4**, 115–135.

Millard, R.W., Wells, N. & Thebarge, R.W. (1991) A comparison of models describing reports of disability associated with chronic pain. *The Clinical Journal of Pain*, **7**, 283–291.

Morley, S. & Wilkinson, L. (1995) The pain beliefs and perceptions inventory: a British replication. *Pain*, **61**, 427–433.

Moss-Morris, R., Petrie, K. & Weinman, J. (1996) Functioning in chronic fatigue syndrome: do illness perceptions and coping play a regulatory role? *British Journal of Clinical Psychology*, **1**, 15–25.

Muthny, F.A., Bechtel, M. & Spaete, M. (1992) Laienätiologien und Krankheitsverarbeitung bei schweren körperlichen Erkrankungen. *Psychotherapie Psychosomatik Medizinische Psychologie*, **42**, 41–53.

Nerenz, D.R. & Leventhal, H. (1983) Self-regulation theory in chronic illness. In T.G. Burish & L.A. Bradley (Eds.), *Coping with chronic disease* (pp. 13–37). New York: Academic Press.

Nerenz, D.R., Leventhal, H. & Love, R.R. (1982) Factors contributing to emotional distress during cancer chemotherapy. *Cancer*, **50**, 1020–1027.

Pastor, M.A., Salas, E., López, S., Rodríguez, J., Sánchez, S. & Pascual, E. (1993) Patients' beliefs about their lack of pain control in primary fibromyalgia syndrome. *British Journal of Rheumatology*, **32**, 484–489.

Pennebaker, J.W. (1982) *The psychology of physical symptoms*. New York: Springer.

Pfeiffer, C.A. & Wetstone, S.L. (1988) Health locus of control and well-being in systemic lupus erythematosus. *Arthritis Care and Research*, **1**, 131–138.

Pollock, S.E. (1993) Adaptation to chronic illness: A program of research for testing nursing theory. *Nursing Science Quarterly*, **6**, 86–92.

Powell, R., Dolan, R. & Wessely, S. (1990) Attributions and self-esteem in depression and chronic fatigue syndromes. *Journal of Psychosomatic Research*, **34**, 665–673.

Primavera, J.P. & Kaiser, R.S. (1994) The relationship between locus of control, amount of pre-admission analgesic/ergot overuse and length of stay for patients admitted for inpatient treatment of chronic headache. *Headache*, **34**, 204–208.

Rainville, J., Ahern, D.K. & Phalen, L. (1993) Altering beliefs about pain and impairment in a functionally oriented treatment program for chronic low back pain. *The Clinical Journal of Pain*, **9**, 196–201.

Raleigh, E.D.H. (1992) Sources of hope in chronic illness. *Oncology Nursing Forum*, **19**, 443–448.

Ray, C., Weir, W.R.C., Cullen, S. & Phillips, S. (1992) Illness perception and symptom components in chronic fatigue syndrome. *Journal of Psychosomatic Research*, **36**, 243–256.

Reesor, K.A. & Craig, K.D. (1988) Medically incongruent chronic back pain: Physical limitations, suffering and ineffective coping. *Pain*, **32,** 35–45.

Reinert, M. & Steurich, F. (1990) Was Weiß der Asthmatiker über seine Krankheit?. *Pneumologie*, **44**, 112–113.

Remien, R.H., Rabkin, J.G. & Williams, J.B.W. (1992) Coping strategies and health beliefs of AIDS longterm survivors. *Psychology & Health*, **6**, 335–345.

Riley, J.F., Ahern, D.K. & Follick, M.J. (1988) Chronic pain and functional impairment: assessing beliefs about their relationship. *Archives of Physical Medicine and Rehabilitation*, **69**, 579–582.

Robbins, J.M. & Kirmayer, L.J. (1991) Attributions of common somatic symptoms. *Psychological Medicine*, **21**, 1029–1045.

Rudy, T.E., Kerns, R.D. & Turk, D.C. (1988) Chronic pain and depression: toward a cognitive-behavioral mediation model. *Pain*, **35**, 129–140.

Sacks, C.R., Peterson, R.A. & Kimmel, P.L. (1990) Perception of illness and depression in chronic renal disease. *American Journal of Kidney Diseases*, **15**, 31–39.

Schiaffino, K.M. & Revenson, T.A. (1992) The role of perceived self-efficacy, perceived control and causal attributions in adaptation to rheumatoid arthritis: Distinguishing mediator from moderator effects. *Personality and Social Psychology Bulletin*, **18**, 709–718.

Schmidt, A. & Lehmkuhl, G. (1994) Krankheitskonzepte bei Kindern — Literaturübersicht. *Fortschritte der Neurologie-Psychiatrie*, **62**, 50–65.

Schober, R. & Lacroix, J.M. (1991) Lay illness models in the enlightenment and the 20th century: some historical lessons. In J.A. Skelton & R.T. Croyle (Eds.), *Mental representation in health and illness* (pp. 10–31). New York: Springer-Verlag.

Schüssler, G. (1992) Coping strategies and individual meanings of illness. *Social Science and Medicine*, **34**, 427–432.

Sharpe, M., Hawton, K., Seagroatt, V. & Pasvol, G. (1992) Follow up of patients presenting with fatigue to an infectious diseases clinic. *British Medical Journal*, **305**, 147–152.

Shutty, Jr., M.S., DeGood, D.E. & Tuttle, D.H. (1990) Chronic pain patients' beliefs about their pain and treatment outcomes. *Archives of Physical Medicine and Rehabilitation*, **71**, 128–132.

Skelton, J.A. & Croyle, R.T. (Eds.) (1991) *Mental representation in health and illness*. New York: Springer-Verlag.

Skevington, S.M. (1990) A standardised scale to measure beliefs about controlling pain (B.P.C.Q.): A preliminary study. *Psychology & Health*, **4**, 221–232.

Skevington, S.M. (1993) Depression and causal attributions in the early stages of a chronic painful disease: A longitudinal study of early synovitis. *Psychology & Health*, **8**, 51–64.

Slater, M.A., Hall, H.F., Atkinson, H. & Garfin, S.R. (1991) Pain and impairment beliefs in chronic low back pain: validation of the pain and impairment relationship scale (PAIRS). *Pain*, **44**, 51–56.

Strong, J., Ashton, R. & Chant, D. (1992) The measurement of attitudes towards and beliefs about pain. *Pain*, **48**, 227–236.

Strong, J., Ashton, R., Cramond, T. & Chant, D. (1990) Pain intensity, attitude and function in back pain patients. *The Australian Occupational Therapy Journal*, **37**, 179–183.

Tennen, H., Affleck, G., Urrows, S., Higgins, P. & Mendola, R. (1992) Perceiving control, construing benefits and daily processes in rheumatoid arthritis. *Canadian Journal of Behavioural Science*, **24**, 186–203.

Timko, C. & Janoff-Bulman, R. (1985) Attributions, vulnerability and psychological adjustment: The case of breast cancer. *Health Psychology*, **4**, 521–544.

Toomey, T.C., Mann, J.D., Abashian, S.W., Carnrike, C.L. & Hernandez, J.T. (1993) Pain locus of control scores in chronic pain patients and medical clinic patients with and without pain. *The Clinical Journal of Pain*, **9**, 242–247.

Turk, D.C. & Rudy, T.E. (1988) Toward an empirically derived taxonomy of chronic pain patients: integration of psychological assessment data. *Journal of Consulting and Clinical Psychology*, **56**, 233–238.

Turk, D.C., Rudy, T.E. & Salovey, P. (1986) Implicit models of illness. *Journal of Behavioral Medicine*, **9**, 453–474.

De Valle, M.N. & Norman, P. (1992) Causal attributions, health locus of control beliefs and lifestyle changes among pre-operative coronary patients. *Psychology & Health*, **7**, 201–211.

Vlayen, J.W.S., Geurts, S.M., Kole-Snijders, A.M.J., Schuerman, J.A., Groenman, N.H. & Van Eek, H. (1990) What do chronic pain patients think of their pain ? Towards a pain cognition questionnaire. *British Journal of Clinical Psychology*, **29**, 383–394.

Wassem, R. (1992) Self-efficacy as a predictor of adjustment to multiple sclerosis. *Journal of Neuroscience Nursing*, **24**, 224–229.

Weaver, T.E. & Narsavage, G.L. (1992) Physiological and psychological variables related to functional status in chronic obstructive pulmonary disease. *Nursing Research*, **41**, 286–291.

Weinman, J., Petrie, K., Moss-Morris, R. & Horne, R. (1996) The Illness Perception Questionnaire: A new measure for assessing the cognitive representation of illness. *Psychology & Health*, **11**, 431–445.

Westbrook, M.T., Gething, L. & Bradbury, B. (1987) Belief in ability to control chronic illness: Associated evaluations and medical experiences. *Australian Psychologist*, **22**, 203–218.

Williams, G.H. (1986) Lay beliefs about the causes of rheumatoid arthritis: their implications for rehabilitation. *International Rehabilitation Medicine*, **8**, 65–68.

Williams, D.A. & Keefe, F.J. (1991) Pain beliefs and the use of cognitive-behavioral coping strategies. *Pain*, **46**, 185–190.

Williams, D.A., Robinson, M.E. & Geisser, M.E. (1994) Pain beliefs: Assessment and utility. *Pain*, **59**, 71–78.

Williams, D.A. & Thorn, B.E. (1989) An empirical assessment of pain beliefs. *Pain*, **36**, 351–358.

Yardley, L. (1994) Contribution of symptoms and beliefs to handicap in people with vertigo: A longitudinal study. *British Journal of Clinical Psychology*, **33**, 101–113.

5

Representations of Medication and Treatment: Advances in Theory and Measurement

Robert Horne

INTRODUCTION

One of the dominant features in the development of medicine during the twentieth century has been the exponential growth in the number of effective drug treatments. The discovery of potent antibiotics during the 1940s was followed by a "therapeutic revolution" in which the burgeoning pharmaceutical industry produced a range of pharmacologically active compounds for use in a wide variety of diseases. The discovery of new drug moieties and the capability for mass production "revolutionised" the medical treatment of common conditions such as diabetes, asthma and congestive heart disease. The use of medicines has increased steadily since the 1950s and the prescription of a medicine is now one of the most common medical interventions.

Today, most patients with chronic illness are faced with the need to take regular medication. However, many fail to do this and non-adherence to medication is a major concern for health practitioners. Although generalisation is hampered by variations in the conceptualisation and measurement of adherence behaviours, it would seem that about 30–40% of medication is not taken as prescribed

(Meichenbaum & Turk, 1987). If the prescription was appropriate, then this level of non-adherence represents a lost opportunity for health gain and a wastage of health resources.

Non-adherence behaviours broadly fall into two categories. Unintentional non-adherence occurs when the patient's intentions to take the medication are thwarted by barriers such as forgetting, and inability to follow treatment instructions because of poor understanding or physical problems such as poor eyesight or impaired manual dexterity. Deliberate or intentional non-adherence, arises when the patient *decides* not to take the treatment as instructed. The latter has been called "intelligent non-compliance" in recognition of the fact that, viewed from the patient's perspective, non-adherence may be the result of a rational decision (Weintraub, 1990).

EXPLAINING INTENTIONAL NON-ADHERENCE

Why do some patients go to the trouble of visiting their doctor and then decide not to take the treatment? Theoretical developments in psychology have provided a number of social cognition models (SCMs) which attempt to explain patients' health-related decisions in terms of perceived values and expectancies and response selections based on these. Research applying these models to medication adherence provides some evidence that patients' initial decisions about treatment are influenced by their beliefs about the need for treatment and perceptions of the associated benefits and risks (e.g., Becker & Rosenstock, 1984; Cummings *et al.*, 1981; Harris & Linn, 1985; Janz & Becker, 1984; Kelly, Mamon & Scott, 1987; Newell *et al.*, 1986; Ried & Christensen, 1988).

The two models which have been most frequently applied to the issue of medication adherence are the Health Belief Model (HBM) and the Theory of Reasoned Action (TRA). Beliefs about treatment can be incorporated into both models. In most studies these have been conceptualised as general beliefs about the benefits of adherence or barriers to taking medication which are usually measured by simple items rather than by a more detailed assessment of lay beliefs about the treatment itself. However, some of these studies have demonstrated a relationship between adherence and perceived barriers, such as patients' beliefs about the degree to which the medication regimen will disrupt their normal routine (Becker *et al.*, 1978) and between general attitudes to medication — e.g., harmful versus helpful (Ried & Christensen, 1988). In other studies, patients' perceptions of the views of significant others, such as doctors or relatives, were stronger predictors of adherence (Cochran & Gitlin, 1988; Miller, Wikoff & Hiatt, 1992). The key limitations of adherence research within SCMs are that there has been little consistency across studies and the proportion of variance in adherence behaviours predicted by SCMs has generally been small (Marteau, 1995). Additionally, it is argued that health behaviour does not arise from static "one off" decisions, as implied by the SCMs, but rather that decisions are made in stages (Schwarzer, 1992; Weinstein, 1988). For a fuller discussion of SCMs and some of their limitations, see the chapter by Charles Abraham in the next section of this book.

The Self-Regulatory Model of Illness

Howard Leventhal and colleagues have developed the self regulatory model (SRM) as a framework for interpreting adherence behaviours (Leventhal & Cameron, 1987; Leventhal, Diefenbach & Leventhal, 1992). The SRM suggests that health-related behaviours or coping responses are heavily influenced by the patient's own beliefs or representations of the illness. Additionally, Leventhal asserts that people do not just think about illness in terms of perceived seriousness or susceptibility. Rather, he provides evidence that illness beliefs are structured around five themes or components: identity, time-line, cause, consequences, and cure/control. In other words, when people think about illnesses they appear to organise their thoughts around five key questions: What is it? (Identity). How long will it last? (Time-line). What caused it? (Cause). How will it/has it affected me? (Consequences). Can it be controlled or cured? (Cure/Control). An individual's representation of a particular illness is made up of their own answers to these questions (Baumann *et al.*, 1989). Evidence to support this theory is provided by research showing that, although the *structure* of illness representations seems to be constant across demographic and illness groups, the *content* varies between individuals and between patients and health practitioners (Skelton & Croyle, 1991).

Another major difference between the SRM and SCMs is that the SRM conceptualises health-related decisions as dynamic, rather than static. The selection of a coping procedure (e.g., to take medication; to smoke less) is determined by beliefs about the nature of the illness threat. This is then followed by an appraisal stage in which the patient evaluates the efficacy of their coping strategy. If the patient appraises a particular coping procedure as being ineffective, then this might result in the selection of an alternative coping strategy or even a change in the representation of the illness.

The SRM provides a useful conceptual framework for understanding intentional non-adherence. If adherence is seen as a form of coping, then the model posits that the decision to follow treatment recommendations will be influenced by the patient's representation of the illness and their subsequent view of whether the proposed treatment is appropriate. Leventhal emphasises the importance of concrete symptom experience in formulating representations and guiding appraisal of the efficacy of the coping. The dynamic interaction between representations, coping (e.g., adherence to treatment) and appraisal (was adherence to treatment beneficial?) is guided by the person's need to maintain *coherence* between these processes. In essence, the patient regulates their response to the illness threat in an attempt to achieve "common sense" coherence.

Viewed from the patient's perspective, non-adherent behaviour may be seen as the "common-sense" response to a perceived lack of coherence between the patient's ideas about the illness, their experience of symptoms and the doctor's instructions. ("Why take this medicine when I don't feel ill?", or "When I take this medicine I feel drowsy and tired. When I stop taking it I feel fine. Maybe I'm not that ill and I'll just see how I get along without the medicine."). Adherence is more likely if there is a high degree of coherence between the abstract (ideas) and concrete (symptoms) aspects of the illness representation, and if the health care provider's advice makes sense in the light of the patient's own experience and representations.

The SRM takes us from a rigid model-based view of health decisions to a more fluid framework in which beliefs and behaviour interact in a dynamic way. Leventhal conceptualises the patient as an "active problem solver" whose health-related behaviour reflects an attempt to close the perceived gap between perceived current health status and an ideal or goal state. The choice of a particular coping response (e.g., to take or not to take medication) is influenced by whether it makes sense in the light of their own ideas about the illness and personal experience of symptoms. As such, the SRM emphasises the central role of illness representations in guiding adherence decisions.

Treatment beliefs and the self-regulatory model

To date, research in this context has paid little attention to patients' beliefs about treatment. However, it is feasible that the self-regulatory patient will not just have their own ideas about the illness, but also about the treatment being offered. Thus, from Leventhal's view of the patient as an "active problem solver" it follows that, in deciding whether to adhere to a treatment schedule, the patient has to think not only about whether the illness warrants treatment but also whether the treatment is appropriate for the illness. Thus, a better understanding of the interplay between representations of illness and treatment and treatment adherence might contribute to the further development of Leventhal's SRM.

Bishop (1991) and Croyle and Williams (1991) have shown that people often hold prototypic beliefs about certain diseases which have an important role in illness cognition. It may also be true that the prominent place of medicines in health care has resulted in the formation of prototypic beliefs about medicines. People may have preconceptions or schema about *medicines in general* which might influence attitudes towards prescribed medication and personal beliefs about the most appropriate treatment for a particular disease.

The remainder of this chapter will deal with people's beliefs about medicines, beginning with an overview of the published literature and going on to describe the preliminary findings of our own research programme investigating patients' representations of medicines.

AN OVERVIEW OF EXISTING RESEARCH INTO LAY BELIEFS ABOUT MEDICINES

The published research dealing with people's beliefs about medicines falls into several broad categories. The first is essentially exploratory research into patients' knowledge of and views about medication which, although it does not appear to have been guided by psychological theory, has produced interesting insights into lay beliefs about medicines. A second type studies patients' beliefs about taking medication within the context of social cognition models. A third category comprises qualitative research eliciting patients' perspectives of illness which has identified lay representations of medication or which specifically sets out to discover the content of people's representations of medicines. Finally, a few studies have quantitatively assessed medication beliefs and systematically investigated relations between medication beliefs and other variables.

Taken collectively, this work has shown that people form beliefs about their medication and the meaning of medication taking, and suggests that such beliefs may influence adherence. Additionally, although these studies have involved a range of patients from several diagnostic groups and socio-cultural backgrounds, they seem to have uncovered common themes which will now be discussed in more detail.

Views about the General Nature of Medicines:
Healing and Harm — the Dual Nature of Medicines

An interesting insight into patients' beliefs about medicines was provided by Fallsberg (1991), who used a phenomenographic approach to analyse conceptions of medicines elicited during interviews conducted with 90 chronically ill, Swedish patients, prescribed regular medication for a range of conditions (asthma, hypertension and chronic pain). She identified several broad "conceptions" — or value judgments — about medicines in general. These included a singularly positive view of medicines derived from the beneficial effects of medicines and the idea that medicines work in unison with the body to promote health. Other patients expressed an essentially negative view which stressed the harmful effects of medication and in which medicines were seen as a form of poison which should be avoided if possible, or as a "necessary evil". A third category emphasised the dual nature of medicines which carry the potential for harm as well as benefit. In this representation, the harmful effects of medication are intrinsic, so that one cannot have the positive effects without the negative. Efficacy and toxicity somehow go hand in hand and more effective medicines implicitly have more side-effects (Lorish, Richards, & Brown, 1990). Similar categories were also identified in a more recent study of attitudes to medication in a sample of general practice patients in the UK (Britten, 1994).

These finding are analogous to those obtained in an earlier study conducted in the USA, which used the Theory of Reasoned Action to guide the development of questions to elicit rheumatoid arthritis patients' perspectives on missed dosages of their medicines (Lorish *et al.*, 1990). Patients' definitions of a "powerful" medicine were explored and questionnaire responses revealed that "powerful" was defined solely by the degree of *symptom control* (35%), solely by *potential to cause harmful side-effects* (33%), or by a *combination* of both (32%).

Leventhal's group have shown that representations of the dual nature of medicines can influence response to symptoms. In one study, a number of women with breast cancer interpreted the experience of side-effects of chemotherapy as a sign that the drugs were working. For these women, the *absence* of side-effects was a distressing indication that "chemotherapy was not having enough *beneficial* impact upon the body" (Leventhal *et al.*, 1986).

Beliefs about Efficacy

It is not surprising that some people use the perceived effects of their treatment to judge its efficacy. These judgments are usually based on symptom relief or the perceived effect of drugs in bringing back or retaining normal functioning (Arluke, 1980; Conrad, 1985). It is interesting that, although none of these studies have utilised Leventhal's SRM, they seem to support the importance of concrete symptom experience in guiding self-regulation (Leventhal *et al.*, 1986; Leventhal *et al.*, 1992).

Another representation related to efficacy has been identified in at least two studies. This is the view that if medication is taken continuously it will become less effective. The notion of becoming "immune" to the beneficial effects of the medication has been noted among rheumatology patients in the UK (Donovan & Blake, 1992) and in the USA (Lorish *et al.*, 1990), who were concerned that after regular use the medication would lose its analgesic effects.

Negative Views about Medication

Several studies have identified beliefs which were associated with a negative view of medication.

Addiction and dependence

A recurring theme, associated with negative attitudes to medicine is the notion that chronic use of medication carries the risk of dependence or addiction. It is difficult to pinpoint the precise lay meaning of these terms and they are often used interchangeably. In a medical context, "addiction" is usually defined as a state of psychological and physical dependence. Relatively few medicines are thought to have this property which is generally limited to psycho-active/ mood altering drugs. However, fear of becoming addicted or "too dependent" on medication has been cited as a key reason for intentional non-adherence by patients receiving medication for a range of diseases, including hypertension, epilepsy and asthma (Fallsberg, 1991). Conrad (1985), in his study of people with epilepsy, found that the notion of addiction or dependence was linked to the perception of having to take medication as a "threat to self reliance", and that some patients saw their medicines as symbolic of the dependence created by having epilepsy. In this context, altering the amount of medication taken could be interpreted as a means of "gaining control".

Long-term dangers

There is a belief that the *continuous* use of medication is associated with obscure long-term effects. For example, Morgan and Watkins (1988) found that several patients decided to stop taking their anti-hypertensive medication for periods of time, lasting up to a few months, in order to give the body a break from medication. People's concerns seem to arise from perceptions of danger associated with medicines in general, rather than from the personal experience of adverse effects. This is illustrated by a study conducted in the USA in which respondents who had never taken diazepam (a benzodi-azepine tranquilliser) attributed more dangers to its use than those who had taken the drug in the past (Mansbridge & Fisher, 1984).

Chemical vs natural

This representation relates to the perceived means of production of medicines. Although the term "natural" was not clearly defined, labelling of a treatment in this context was associated with a value judgment in which "natural" remedies were seen as safer than "unnatural" medicines, and that the dangerous aspects of medication were linked to their chemical/unnatural origins (Conrad, 1985). People with this view may prefer to avoid medication altogether. For example, in a study of women who had been prescribed benzodi-azepine tranquillisers for menopausal symptoms, several explained that they chose not to take them because of concerns about the potential harm which could arise from the use of these "unnatural" medicines. The symptoms of the menopause, although uncomfortable, were at least "natural" and were therefore perceived as a more favourable alternative to medication (Gabe & Thorogood, 1986). Similarly, parents who had chosen not to vaccinate their children contrasted the "unnatural" process of immunisation with the "natural" immunity possessed by the body, or the "natural" phenomena of pertussis (whooping cough) (New & Senior, 1991).

Medicine as poison

A number of Fallsberg's (1991) sample of Swedish patients expressed the belief that many medicines are poisons. This notion did not emerge as a dominant theme in other qualitative studies where the interviews were conducted in English and it may be that this representation is language specific. In this context it is interesting that the Ancient Greeks did not make a linguistic distinction between medicine and poison, but used the same word "pharmakon" to describe both types of substance (Bonuzzi, 1987).

Doctors' Overuse of Medicines

In an early UK study of general practice patients' views of medicines and prescribing, over a third of the sample thought that doctors prescribed too many medicines, but the prevalence of this view varied according to class of medicines, between antibiotics (23%), antidepressants (30%), and tranquillisers (over 50%). Also, people had clear views about the purpose of certain medicines and this seemed to influence their expectations for treatment. In a large survey of public attitudes to benzodiazepines in the USA (Clinthorne, 1986) and in a recent interview-based study conducted in the UK (Britten, 1994), patients have also expressed the view that doctors prescribe too readily and use too many medicines. However, several studies have reported that patients use the number and dosage of medications prescribed for them as an indication of severity of their illness and fluctuations in dosage as markers for improvement or deterioration (Donovan & Blake, 1992; Leventhal *et al.*, 1991; Morgan & Watkins, 1988).

Quantitative Studies Linking Medication Beliefs, Illness Beliefs and Health Behaviour

Most of the representations of medication described above have been identified from interview-based qualitative studies. Although this method provides detailed information, this type of data is time-consuming and expensive to collect and analyse, and this obviously limits the sample size. It is therefore difficult to obtain a clear insight into the prevalence of certain beliefs. Furthermore, a systematic investigation of the relationship between specific beliefs and behaviours is beyond the scope of qualitative methods. However, surprisingly few studies have attempted to quantify people's beliefs about medicine or to systematically investigate the relationship between medication beliefs and other variables.

One exception is a study of 62 German patients with asthma, in which those who emphasised the threatening aspects of corticosteroid medication were less adherent to treatment (Woller *et al.*, 1993). The sub-scale which measured the "threatening aspect" of steroids contained four items. These were responses to the statement "When I think of cortisone tablets: I'm afraid, I feel threatened, I feel despair, I think I will get addicted". This provides preliminary evidence that the representation of cortisone as potentially addictive contributed to avoidance of this medicine.

Echabe and colleagues (1992) investigated the impact of representations of health, illness and medicines on coping strategies and health promoting behaviour in 902 subjects from the Basque region. Representations of medicines were assessed using an 11 item questionnaire derived from semi-structured interviews and focus groups. Cluster analysis was used to classify respondents into groups based on their representations of health, illness, medicines and locus of control over health. Three distinct clusters were identified. The first accounted for 70% of the sample and comprised people with an "against medicine" representation. These conceptualised health as a balance between mind and body and attributed illness to stress, pollution, lack of exercise and poverty; they had an internal locus of control and held a predominantly negative view of medication. The second cluster was essentially "pro-medicine" and accounted for 12% of the sample. Here health was perceived as synonymous with being able to work and enjoy life. Control over illness focused on diet and exercise but also externally with physicians and medicines being the factors contributing to recovery. Medicines were viewed positively. The third cluster (18%) was a "half-way" position between the others. This study is one of the few to shed light on how people's beliefs about medication relate to other cognitions. Additionally, cognitions were linked to coping styles, in that people with an "against medicine" representation tended to delay going for medical check-ups, whereas those with a "pro-medicines" or "combined" representation were more likely to attend for check-ups on time. The key finding here is that views about health and illness and orientation towards medication appear to cluster together in a logical way. It is interesting that cluster analysis corroborates earlier qualitative evidence that attitudes to medication broadly fall into three groups. However, this type of distribution of views (some positive, some negative and some in-between) could probably be identified for most issues! We are still left with the question of which specific beliefs underlie these "positive", "negative" and "in-between" attitudes to medicines.

LIMITATIONS OF EXISTING RESEARCH

The research described above provides insights into the content of people's beliefs about medicines, together with a few hints as to how representations might influence attitudes and adherence to treatment. However, a number of key questions remain unanswered. Although it identifies particular beliefs, this research tells us little about the prevalence of these beliefs. We do not know the proportion of people who hold them or how strongly they are held. Furthermore, we know little about how medication beliefs are cognitively organised. For example, whether individual beliefs, such as those identified in the studies described above, are grouped together into core themes or components in the same way that illness beliefs are structured around five components (Leventhal & Nerenz, 1985). A key question here is the extent to which patients' beliefs about medicines in *general* are differentiated from their beliefs about *specific* medicines prescribed for their illness. Moreover, we need to know more about the relationship between medication beliefs and behaviours such as adherence to treatment, particularly to identify which beliefs are associated with non-adherence.

Over the past four years John Weinman at UMDS London and I have begun to address these questions in a programme of research which has been influenced by Leventhal's SRM. Although it does not set out to test the framework, the principle that patients form structured coherent beliefs about illness which influence adherence provides the theoretical basis for this work. I will now go on to describe the preliminary results of this research and to explain how this might contribute to our understanding of the patients' perspective of illness and treatment.

NEW RESEARCH INTO LAY REPRESENTATIONS OF MEDICINES

To investigate the structure and prevalence of medication beliefs in a systematic way required a method of eliciting and scoring people's beliefs about medicines. Our initial approach to this was to derive statements representing key themes identified in the literature and from our own in-depth open interviews with 35 patients receiving regular medication for chronic illness (20 haemodialysis patients and 15 patients with myocardial infarction). From this we generated 34 statements which represented common lay beliefs about medicines. The items were separated into two groups: those dealing with beliefs about *specific* medicines prescribed for a particular illness (16), and those dealing with beliefs about medicines in *general* (18). The statements were administered to over 500 patients from a range of diagnostic groups between 1991 and 1994 who were asked to rate their degree of agreement with each item on a 5-point Likert scale (strongly agree to strongly disagree). To establish whether beliefs about medicines could be assigned a simple coherent structure which was stable across different illness groups, we subjected the item responses to principal components analysis PCA with non-orthogonal (OBLIMIN) rotation, as recommended in the literature (Kline, 1994; Streiner, 1994).

Identifying Core Themes in Lay Beliefs about Medicines: The Development of the Beliefs about Medicines Questionnaire (BMQ)

The *specific* and *general* items were initially analysed separately. We reasoned that the way in which people view medication prescribed for a particular illness may, to some extent, depend on the nature of that illness and could not assume that patients with one chronic illness perceive their medication in the same way as those with another. Consequently, we began by examining specific beliefs about medicines in a single diagnostic group; hospitalised patients with chronic heart disease (n = 120), and then testing whether the factor structure obtained could be replicated in other diagnostic groups. The rationale for limiting initial exploratory factor analysis of *specific* items to a single illness group did not apply to beliefs about medicines in *general*. On the contrary, we were looking for representations of medication as a broad concept, rather than beliefs which might be unique to a particular diagnostic group. To obtain a factor structure which was representative of patients with a range of chronic illnesses, we combined data obtained from three diagnostic groups: chronic asthma (n = 78), diabetes (n = 99), and hospitalised haemodialysis patients (n = 47).

The factor structures obtained for both *specific* and *general* items by exploratory PCA were confirmed on other data sets. We also entered the combined specific and general items into a further PCA of responses from 417 patients from several diagnostic groups (asthma n = 75, diabetes n = 94, hospital haemodialyis patients n = 39, cardiac patients n = 111, psychiatric outpatients n = 88). A clear separation of general and specific items and replication of the original factor structure supported the premise that patients hold coherent complex representations of medication in which beliefs about medication prescribed for them may be distinguished from their beliefs about medicines in general. The results of PCA also indicate that certain beliefs about medicines are organised into 4 factors (or components), shown in Table 1, which were used to construct a new questionnaire measure of medication beliefs comprising the four factors as subscales. The Beliefs about Medicines Questionnaire (BMQ) is therefore split into two sections, one assessing beliefs about *specific* medication prescribed for a particular illness (BMQ-Specific), and the other assessing beliefs about medicines in *general* (BMQ-General). The development and validation of the BMQ is described elsewhere (Horne & Weinman, 1995).

As can be seen in Table 1, the factor structure obtained seems to be coherent in "common-sense" terms, and the items loading on each factor relate to each other in a logical way. The arrangement of individual beliefs to form core representations of medicines in general merits comment at this stage. Firstly, considering the *General-Harm* component it is notable that "people taking prescribed medication should stop their treatment every now and again" is linked with a representation of medication as essentially harmful, addictive poisons.

Table 1   The components of medication representation as presented in the Beliefs about Medicines Questionnaire (BMQ) (Horne & Weinman 1995)

BMQ-SPECIFIC

Specific-Necessity

Beliefs about the necessity and efficacy of medicines prescribed for specific condition.

- My health in the future will depend on medicines
- My health, at present, depends on medicines
- My life would be impossible without medicines
- Without medicines I would be very ill
- My medicines protect me from becoming worse

Specific-Concerns

Concerns about the harmful effects of medicines prescribed for specific condition

- Having to take medicines worries me
- I sometimes worry about the long-term effects of my medicines
- I sometimes worry about becoming too dependent on my medicines
- My medicines are a mystery to me
- My medicines disrupt my life

BMQ-GENERAL

General-Overuse

Beliefs that medicines in general are over-used by doctors

- If doctors had more time with patients they would prescribe fewer medicines
- Doctors use too many medicines
- Doctors place too much trust on medicines
- Natural remedies are safer than medicines

General-Harm

Beliefs that medicines in general are harmful addictive poisons

- Most medicines are addictive
- Medicines do more harm than good
- People who take medicines should stop their treatment for a while every now and again
- All medicines are poisons

The phenomenon of deliberately stopping medication was noted by Morgan and Watkins (1988) in their qualitative study of British hypertensive patients. Patients often explained this activity as being necessary to avoid becoming too dependent or addicted to the medicines. The fact that these items factor together is indicative of a coherent and complex representation of medication — the harmful effects of medication are increased if it is taken *continuously* and so one should give the body a break every now and then.

Considering the *General-Overuse* representation, it may appear surprising that the belief that "natural remedies are safer than medicines" loads on this factor, as this statement seems to relate to the intrinsic nature of medicines rather than the way in which they are used. A possible explanation is that the *General-Overuse* factor represents a concept of treatment which is essentially anti-medication and pro "natural remedies". In this representation, the belief that medication is overused by doctors is consistent with the view that natural remedies are less harmful and implicitly more favourable than medicines. This may be analogous to the first cluster obtained by Echabe and colleagues in their study of illness and medication representations, in which health was represented as a balance between body and mind, and medicines were viewed negatively (Echabe *et al.*, 1992). We are currently investigating this issue in more detail.

At first sight, the representations of medicines in general described above seem to amount to a rather negative view of medicines as harmful and overused by doctors. However, it is important to bear in mind that this does not necessarily mean that most people see medicines in this way. People can disagree with the statements on each factor and so express a view of medication as essentially safe and appropriately used. The main point here is that PCA has shown that certain beliefs link together to form coherent core representations. In other words, people seem to organise their ideas about medicines (addiction, poison, harm, regular long-term use) into coherent themes or components. Although the specific content will vary between individuals (e.g., one sees medicines as harmful and addictive, another thinks they are generally safe and non-addictive), the components are consistent.

The Distribution of Medication Representations Among Patients With Chronic Illness

Having shown that individual beliefs about general and specific medication could be grouped together in factors or "themes", it was necessary to establish the distribution of these core representations among patients with chronic illness. We did this by examining the frequency of BMQ factor scores in a pooled sample of over 500 patients from several diagnostic groups (asthma, diabetes, recipients of hospital haemodialysis, chronic heart diseases, psychiatric out-patients, and a sample of hospital in-patients).

The distribution of scores on the four BMQ factors is shown in Figure 1 and an interesting pattern emerged. Whereas beliefs about *General-Overuse*, *General-Harm* and *Specific-Concerns* were

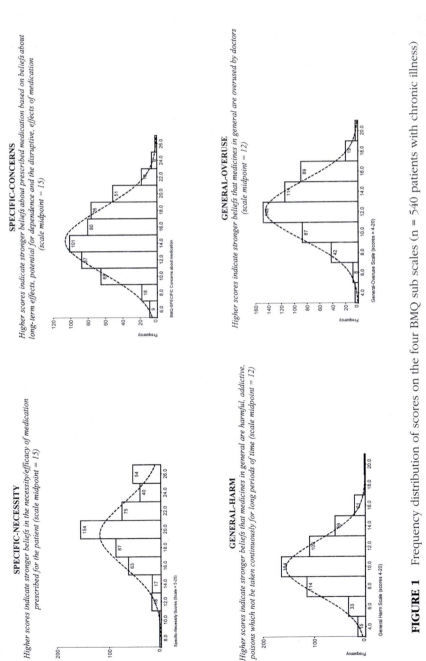

FIGURE 1   Frequency distribution of scores on the four BMQ sub scales (n = 540 patients with chronic illness)

normally distributed, *Specific-Necessity* were heavily skewed towards the positive. Over 80% had higher than mid-point scores on the *Specific-Necessity* subscale, indicating overall agreement with the view that their prescribed medicines were necessary for health. These percentages are much higher than those obtained for the *Specific-Concerns* (31%), *General-Harm* (17%), and *General-Overuse* (45%) subscales.

This gives us an interesting insight into the way patients were thinking about medication. To begin with, although the majority of patients were convinced that their prescribed medication was necessary and effective, about a third of them were clearly worried about the long term effects of prescribed medication or becoming too dependent on it. We found several things striking about this. The first was that those patients with high concerns probably had quite a different representation of their medicines than the doctors who had prescribed them. In the "medical view", none of the medicines which our patients were receiving would be considered to cause dependence or addiction and few would be expected to cause serious long term adverse effects. Secondly, it is particularly salient that concerns did not influence patients' perceptions of the necessity of their medication (over 88% of patients with strong concerns believed that their medication was necessary). Rather, these patients seemed to hold a complex representation of medicine in which firm beliefs about the *necessity* of medication were balanced against *concerns* about safety and the disruptive effects of taking medication. This provides systematic evidence that the notion of medicines as a "double-edged sword" (benefit balanced by harm) influences the way in which some chronically ill patients (about a quarter of our sample) view their medication.

What is the Relevance of Medication Representations to the Self Management of Chronic Illness?

The availability of new questionnaire-based methods for assessing patients' representations of illness (Weinman *et al.*, 1996) and both specific and general medication (Horne & Weinman, 1995), provided the basis for addressing this question. If patients' own beliefs about medication were involved in adherence decisions, then we would expect to find evidence of associations between BMQ scores and measures of adherence. Moreover, an analysis of the interrelations between sub-scales measuring representations of treatment and illness and treatment adherence, might enhance our understanding of the types of beliefs which were associated with low adherence. We began at a basic level by investigating correlations between representations of illness, specific and general representations of medication, and self-reported treatment adherence.

Adherence to medication

The correlations between BMQ sub-scales and self-reported treatment adherence were examined in a sample of 91 medical inpatients from a range of diagnostic groups (50% male; mean age = 54 years; SD = 19.8). Medication adherence was assessed using a 3-item self-report scale with a satisfactory degree of internal consistency (Cronbach's alpha = 0.72). Figure 2 provides a diagrammatic representation of the relationship between general and specific medication beliefs and adherence, based on Spearman correlations between these variables. It can be seen that those patients with stronger concerns about their prescribed medication reported that they took less of it. Moreover, these *Specific-Concerns* arose from beliefs about the potential of their prescribed medication to cause dependence and long-term effects and a representation of medication as disruptive and mysterious.

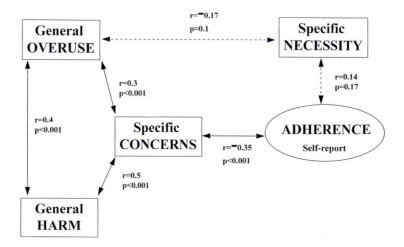

FIGURE 2   Relationship between general and specific medication beliefs and adherence

In this data set the correlation between *Specific-Necessity* beliefs and adherence was in the predicted direction, but did not reach significance. This may, in part, be attributable to the low degree of spread of responses on this sub-scale. Over 87% of the sample viewed their prescribed medication as necessary, but this was often balanced by concerns about the potential adverse effects of these medicines. Over half of those (63%) who believed that their specific medication was necessary also had strong concerns, and these concerns were associated with lower rates of adherence (rs = 0.45; n = 79; p < 0.0001). This may indicate that patients were adjusting their medication intake based on their own beliefs about the medication.

We were not surprised to obtain such high scores on the *Specific-Necessity* subscale in a sample of chronically ill patients receiving regular medication. We expect that *Specific-Necessity* beliefs will be more influential in acute conditions, or those where the relationship between medication taking and symptomatic benefit is not apparent to the patient.

This simple cross-sectional study also shows how representations of specific and general medication link together. Our patients had formed representations of medication in general which were related in a coherent way. Those with a general representation of medication as harmful, addictive poisons which should not be used continuously for long periods of time (*General-Harm*), were more likely to believe that medicines are overused by doctors who place too much trust in them (*General-Overuse*). Moreover, *General-Harm* and *General-Overuse* beliefs were associated with *Specific-Concerns* about medication prescribed for them by their doctors. It is salient that the influence of beliefs about medicines in general upon adherence to treatment seems to operate through *Specific-Concerns*, and a preliminary analysis of other data sets has shown a similar pattern of correlations. The interaction between general and specific beliefs is a key issue in health psychology and our findings corroborate other work indicating the utility of narrowing the focus of assessment to beliefs related to a specific behaviour rather than more general views.

Medication beliefs and selective treatment adherence

Identifying meaningful correlations between representations of medicines and self-reported adherence to medicines stimulated us to broaden our question to other treatment beliefs. In particular, we wondered whether *Specific-Concerns* reflected a general negativity towards treatment, or did patients distinguish between different types of treatment (e.g. medication versus diet) and moderate their behaviour accordingly? We have started to explore these issues in a sample of patients receiving hospital haemodialysis. Haemodialysis patients are required to adhere to a tripartite regimen of attendance at hospital dialysis sessions, dietary and fluid restrictions and a complex medication schedule (Will & Johnson, 1994). Although haemodialysis sessions are time-consuming and unpleasant, serial non-attendance is relatively rare, as missing only a few consecutive sessions may endanger life. However, non-adherence to medication and dietary/fluid restrictions is viewed as a major issue (Lowry & Atchison, 1980) and there is increasing interest in how patients' own beliefs influence adherence in this area (Horne & Weinman, 1994).

A study sample of 47 hospital haemodialysis patients completed the IPQ and BMQ questionnaires, in addition to a single item assessing the belief that their diet/fluid restrictions were too strict (scored from 1–5 strongly disagree to strongly agree). Patients' self-report was used as an indicator of medication adherence. Adherence to diet/fluid restrictions was assessed by recording the frequency of inter-dialysis weight gain >2kg over a 3 month period prior to administration of the questionnaires. Self-rated health was assessed using a validated subscale from the SF-36 instrument (Stewart & Ware, 1992).

The relationship between treatment beliefs and adherence indicators is shown in Figure 3. The pattern of correlations between general and specific medication beliefs and medication adherence was almost identical to that obtained in our sample of medical in-patients described above, with *Specific-Concerns* being associated with lower medication adherence. However, when we broadened our analysis to include beliefs about and adherence to diet/fluid restrictions, an interesting pattern emerged. Although *Specific-Concerns* about prescribed medication were associated with lower rates of self-reported medication adherence, they were not related to lower adherence to dietary and fluid restrictions. Similarly, patients who believed that their dietary and fluid restrictions were too strict were less likely to adhere to them, but beliefs about diet/fluid restrictions were not related to medication adherence. The fact that adherence to medication and diet/fluid restrictions

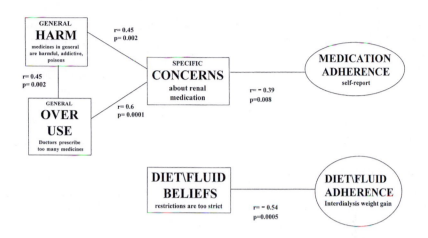

FIGURE 3   Correlations between treatment beliefs and treatment adherence in a sample of hospital haemodialysis patients (n = 47)

was not correlated is evidence that patients may adhere to some aspects of their treatment but not others. It is clearly, therefore, misleading to label a patient as generally adherent or non-adherent. Rather, it would seem that some patients were making rational decisions about whether or not to adhere to particular treatments based on their beliefs about that treatment. This finding supports Leventhal's suggestion that representations influence coping — in this case specific adherence behaviours.

Representations of Illness and Medication

The haemodialysis data set also allowed us to examine correlations between medication beliefs, illness representations and self reported medication adherence. The pattern of correlations between variables in this and other data sets (asthma; n = 78 and diabetes; n = 99) shows that medication and illness representations are both related to adherence and health status. However, although this finding was consistent across samples, the precise nature of the interaction varied across diagnostic groups. For example, in the haemodialysis data set, patients with a strong illness identity and those who perceived that their illness had more severe consequences, were *less* likely to adhere to medication. This relationship may seem counter-intuitive, as one might expect such patients to be

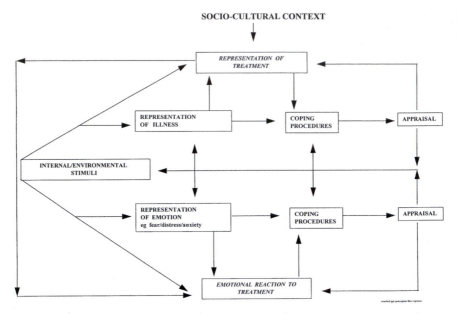

FIGURE 4 Illustration of how treatment beliefs may be incorporated into Leventhal's SRM

more inclined to take their medication. However, it may be that these patients perceived a lower sense of coherence between the medical message ("Take your medication and it will help you."), and their concrete experience ("I still feel ill even if I do."). Additionally, patients who reported lower adherence tended to rate their health status as poorer. This may, of course, be a consequence of non-adherence, but might also indicate that patients who perceived their health status as low were less inclined to follow treatment recommendation. The SRM would predict that such patients would be less motivated to adhere to their treatment.

We have also found correlations between illness representations and adherence in the asthma and diabetes samples. However, in the diabetic and asthma groups, patients with stronger time-line, Consequences and Identity beliefs were *more* likely to adhere to treatment. This may be because there is a stronger relationship between adherence and perceived symptomatic benefit in patients with asthma and diabetes than those taking medication as an adjunct to haemodialysis. In this case, taking medication makes "common-sense" as the patient perceives a greater sense of coherence between

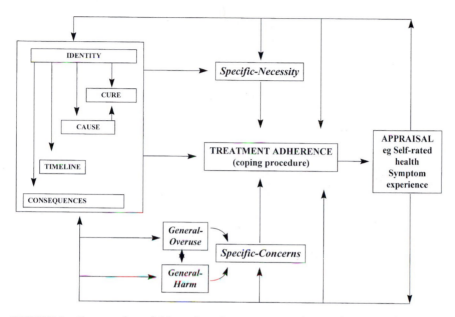

FIGURE 5 Proposed model based on Spearman correlations between illness and medication representation, coping and appraisal

representations coping and outcome. Furthermore, the value of time-line and identity beliefs in predicting adherence to treatment recommendations has been noted elsewhere (Petrie *et al.*, 1996). In summary, if adherence is viewed as a specific example of coping and self-rated health status as an example of appraisal, then our preliminary findings offer tentative support for the SRM.

Our key finding is that *medication* representations correlate with adherence, and that patients' beliefs about medicines and illness seem to be related in a logical way, even though these beliefs sometimes conflict with the medical view. For example, *Specific-Necessity* beliefs were correlated with identity and timeline representations in separate samples of patients with asthma (n = 78) and diabetes (n = 99). Typically the correlation coefficients between representations of illness and treatment and self-reported treatment adherence tend to be statistically significant but modest in size (e.g. r's = 0.3–0.5). Clearly, any conclusions based on the preliminary analysis of these data are speculative. However, the relationships between illness and medication representations and adherence suggest that the value of the SRM for explaining adherence may be enhanced by the inclusion of treatment beliefs. Figure 4 offers a diagrammatic representation of how representations of treatment might be incorporated into Leventhal's SRM. In addition, Figure 5 provides a "freeze-frame" of the dynamic interaction between illness and treatment beliefs, and adherence to treatment, based on the Spearman correlations described above.

WHAT ARE THE ORIGINS OF PATIENTS' CONCERNS ABOUT THEIR MEDICATION?

The consistent finding that *Specific-Concerns* about prescribed medication is associated with adherence has stimulated us to question where these concerns come from. Our data indicate that they are influenced by more general medicines beliefs. However, it is clear from the correlation coefficients obtained that *Specific-Concerns* do not just arise from more general beliefs that medicines are harmful (*General-Harm)* or overused by doctors (*General-Overuse).* Moreover, the direction of influence may go in both ways as concerns about specific medication may colour the patient's view of medicines in general. We have therefore begun to investigate interrelations between medication beliefs and other variables.

Beliefs about sensitivity to the adverse effects of medication

We were able to assess patients' beliefs about their sensitivity to the adverse effects of medication using the *Sensitive-Soma* Scale developed by the Leventhal group (Diefenbach, Leventhal & Leventhal, 1996). The *Sensitive-Soma* Scale was administered to the general hospital sample described above at the same time as the BMQ. It can be seen from Figure 6 that BMQ and *Sensitive-Soma* correlations suggest that patients who believed that they were more susceptible to the adverse effects of medication were more likely to believe that medicines are generally harmful, and also had stronger concerns about prescribed medication to which they were less adherent. Although we cannot be sure about the direction of influence, the interrelations are meaningful and corroborate the view that treatment beliefs are involved in self-regulation. We are currently investigating relations between BMQ factors, the Sensitive Soma Scale and current and past experience of medication side-effects.

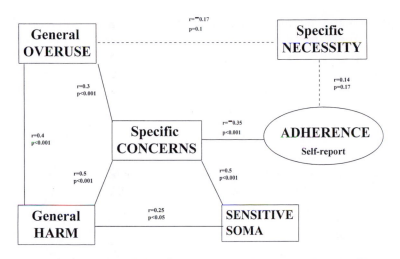

FIGURE 6   Spearman correlations between BMQ factors, the Sensitive Soma scale and treatment adherence (n = 91 medical in-patients)

Demographic factors

Our studies conducted to date indicate that medication beliefs are not overtly influenced by age and sex. We have found no relationship between sex and BMQ scale scores and the influence of age on these factors seems to be modest and limited to certain diagnostic groups. For example, in our pooled data set, age had a small but statistically significant effect on general beliefs about medicines with older patients gaining slightly higher scores on the *General-Harm* and *General-Overuse*. However, it is difficult to draw any firm conclusions from this finding since the effect of age on beliefs was very small and the relationship was not statistically significant in the smaller samples of individual diagnostic groups. The relationship between age and BMQ-Specific scores was inconsistent. We found no correlation between age and scores in the combined data set but, when we conducted the analysis in individual diagnostic groups, a mixed picture emerged. Younger cardiac patients were more concerned about the potential adverse effects of their prescribed medication as indicated by the negative correlation between age and *Specific-Concerns* (rs = –0.24; n = 116; p < 0.01) but this effect was not noted in other diagnostic groups.

Educational status was significantly related to scores on the *General-Harm* factor (p < 0.001). People educated to tertiary level were less likely to have a prototypic view of medication as harmful, whereas patients educated to secondary level or below tended to have stronger beliefs that medicines are "harmful, addictive poisons". The influence of educational status did not however, extend to representations of prescribed medication. The pattern of relationships between demographic data and beliefs about medicines in general is almost identical to that obtained by Lim, Schwarz and Lo (1980) who investigated the prevalence of "traditional" Chinese health beliefs in a sample of over 900 Hong Kong Chinese. It is interesting that those with less formal education were more likely to have stronger Chinese health beliefs. In our sample, patients with less formal education had a more negative view of medication. We might speculate that formal education leads to a more positive orientation to "western" biomedicine with its emphasis on drug treatment of disease and away from a more traditional "folk" interpretation of health and illness such as those described by Patcher (1994).

Type of illness and treatment

Further evidence that the two BMQ-General subscales (*General-Overuse* and *General-Harm*) may represent prototypic beliefs is provided by the fact that scores on these scales are independent of diagnostic group. Conversely, beliefs about prescribed medication (BMQ-Specific) were significantly influenced by the type of illness, with scores on the BMQ-Specific subscales *Specific-Necessity* and *Specific-Concerns* showing significant variation across diagnostic groups, as shown in Figure 7. These differences seem to make sense when one considers the salient features of the disease in question. For example diabetic patients, who are often aware that without treatment (insulin or oral hypoglycaemic agents) their condition may be rapidly fatal, had significantly higher *Specific-Necessity* scores than all other groups.

Leventhal has pointed out the importance of concrete symptoms experience in guiding people's representations of illness and this may also be true for representations of prescribed medication. This notion is supported by the finding that asthma patients had stronger beliefs in the necessity of their medication than psychiatric outpatients ($p < 0.005$). Each of these conditions tends to produce very different concrete symptom experiences in relation to medication. Asthma medication often produces symptom relief which the patient

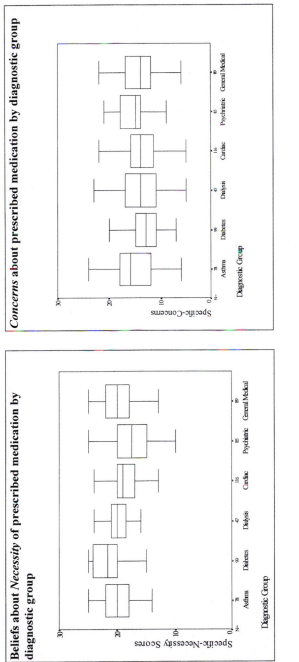

FIGURE 7   Comparison of *Specific-Concerns* and *Specific-Necessity* scores between diagnostic groups

can clearly relate to taking of the medication. Similarly, omitting medication may quickly result in adverse symptoms. Conversely, patients receiving medication for mental health-related problems may perceive a much more tenuous link between their medication and concrete benefit in terms on symptoms. Conclusions from these data are clearly tentative and more work is needed to complete our understanding of how symptom experience and medication representations are related.

Variations in scores on the *Specific-Concerns* subscale are meaningful in the light of differences between specific types of medication. Asthma patients had the highest scores on this subscale (p < 0.05), followed in close second place by psychiatric outpatients. Asthma treatment often incorporates corticosteroids. This is a large group of compounds, some of which may produce adverse side effects. Additionally, other members of this group are frequently misused in sport. In short, this class of drugs has a high "media-profile" and patients' concerns could be influenced by this, particularly if they fail to differentiate between steroids they are taking for asthma (which are generally inhaled and therefore less "dangerous") and more potent formulations upon which media attention is often focused. This idea can also be extended to help explain higher concern in the psychiatric out-patient sample, as these patients are often treated with "tranquillisers", which have received adverse media attention (Cohen, 1983).

The analysis of data, described above, has identified stable, core representations of medication and provides preliminary evidence that representations of medication are structured in a way which is analogous to the structure of illness representation identified by Leventhal and his co-workers (Leventhal & Nerenz, 1985; Leventhal *et al.*, 1991, 1992).

CONCLUSIONS AND FUTURE DIRECTIONS

The use of a questionnaire-based method for assessing beliefs about treatment (Horne & Weinman, 1995), has enabled us to augment existing qualitative research by quantifying the prevalence of specific beliefs and showing which beliefs are related to non-adherence. It is particularly interesting that medication non-adherence was not associated with the belief that medicines are unnecessary or ineffective. The majority of patients agreed that their present and future health depended on medicines. However, about a third of the patients had a complex view of medication in which beliefs about necessity and efficacy were tempered by concerns about the potential for harm, and these patients were less adherent.

Although this chapter has focused on medication beliefs, our findings emphasize the importance of patients' beliefs about treatment in general, and justify further investigation of patients' views about individual treatment options. In particular, we need to establish the extent to which representations of individual treatment options are accurate and predictive of future adjustment and adherence. Here it may be particularly salient to explore patients' perceptions of *relative* risk associated with various treatment modalities and this may have implications for the issue of informed consent and shared decision making. A further question which can be investigated with these new scales concerns the role of treatment representations in the placebo effect. The clinical importance of placebo effects is well recognised (Horwitz & Horwitz, 1993; Horwitz *et al.*, 1990), but the phenomenon is poorly understood and we are currently planning studies in this area.

So far, most of our data has been obtained from cross-sectional studies which provide a "snap-shot" of inter-relations between key variables. Further prospective studies are now needed to clarify the dynamic interaction between patients' representations of illness and treatment, and their adherence to treatment over time. Our hypothesis is that beliefs about general and specific medication will influence treatment preferences and initial orientation to prescribed medication. However, continued adherence will be determined by a dynamic interplay between abstract beliefs and concerns about medication and the degree to which the patient's concrete experience of symptoms is influenced by the medication.

The research described in this chapter has several implications for providing patients with medicines information. There is currently increasing interest in the inclusion of detailed standardised information leaflets as part of the packaging of medicines. Our research could inform this initiative in two ways. Firstly, by providing measures to assess the impact of this type of information on patients' representations of medicines, especially *Specific-Concerns*. This is necessary because, although the aim of improving patient access to medicines information is laudable, standardised information alone may not meet the needs of all patients (Weinman, 1990). Moreover, *Specific-Concerns* may arise from individual beliefs about the potential for dependence or long-term effects which might not be dealt with in the leaflet and it may therefore be appropriate to include this type of information in package inserts. Secondly, patient education about medicines is likely to be enhanced if health professionals, such as doctors and pharmacists, elicit patients' own concerns about their medication and address these issues on an individual basis rather than by relying on standardised written information alone (Horne, 1993; Webb, Bates & Horne, 1996).

In summary, our central finding that patients hold beliefs about treatment which may conflict with the medical view yet influence adherence, has implications for clinical practice. Specifically, many patients seem to have exaggerated concerns about their medication. Eliciting and alleviating these concerns may enhance the therapeutic partnership between clinician and patient and facilitate adherence to treatment.

REFERENCES

Arluke, A. (1980) Judging drugs: patients' conceptions of therapeutic efficacy in the treatment of arthritis. *Human Organization*, **39**, 84–88.

Baumann, L.J., Cameron, L.D., Zimmerman, R.S. & Leventhal, H. (1989) Illness representations and matching labels with symptoms. *Health Psychology*, **8**, 449–470.

Becker, M.H., Radius, S.M., Rosenstock, I.M., Drachman, R.H., Schubert, K.C. & Teets, K.C. (1978) Compliance with a medical regimen for asthma: a test of the health belief model. *Public Health Reports*, **93**, 268–277.

Becker, M.H. & Rosenstock, I.M. (1984). Compliance with medical advice. In A. Steptoe & A. Mathews (Eds.), *Health care and human behaviour*, London: Academic Press.

Bishop, G.D. (1991) Understanding the understanding of illness: lay disease representations. In J.A. Skelton & R.T. Croyle (Eds.), *Mental representation in health and illness* (pp. 32–60). New York: Springer-Verlag.

Bonuzzi, L. (1987) The Greek gods and the ills of man. In A. Zanca (Ed.), *Pharmacy through the ages.* Farmitalia Carlo Erba.

Britten, N. (1994) Patients' ideas about medicines: a qualitative study in a general practice population. *British Journal of General Practice*, **44**, 465–468.

Clinthorne, J.K. (1986) Changes in popular attitudes and beliefs about tranquilizers: 1970–1979. *Archives of General Psychiatry*, **43**, 527–532.

Cochran, S.D. & Gitlin, M.J. (1988) Attitudinal correlates of lithium compliance in bipolar affective disorders. *Journal of Nervous and Mental Disease*, **176**, 457–464.

Cohen, S. (1983) Current attitudes about the benzodiazepines: trial by media. *Journal of Psychoactive Drugs*, **15**, 109–113.

Conrad, P. (1985) The meaning of medications: another look at compliance. *Social Science and Medicine*, **20**, 29–37.

Croyle, R.T. & Williams, K.D. (1991). Reactions to medical diagnosis: The role of illness stereotypes. *Basic and Applied Social Psychology*, **12**, 227–241.

Cummings, K.M., Becker, M.H., Kirscht, J.P. & Levin, N.W. (1981) Intervention strategies to improve compliance with medical regimens by ambulatory haemodialysis patients. *Journal of Behavioural Medicine*, **4**, 111–127.

Diefenbach, M., Leventhal, H. & Leventhal, E. (1996) The Sensitive Soma Scale. Manuscript in preparation.

Donovan, J.L. & Blake, D.R. (1992) Patient non-compliance: Deviance or reasoned decision-making? *Social Science in Medicine*, **34**, 507–513.

Echabe, A.E., Guillen, C.S. & Ozamiz, J.A. (1992) Representations of health illness and medicines: coping strategies and health promoting behaviour. *British Journal of Clinical Psycholology*, **31**, 339–349.

Fallsberg, M. (1991) *Reflections on medicines and medication: a qualitative analysis among people on long-term drug regimens.* PhD Thesis Linkoping, Sweden: Linkoping University.

Gabe, J. & Thorogood, N. (1986) Prescribed drug use and the management of everyday life: the experiences of black and white working class women. *The Sociological Review*, **34**, 737–772.

Harris, R. & Linn, M.W. (1985) Health beliefs, compliance and control of diabetes mellitus. *Southern Medical Journal*, **78**, 162–166.

Horne, R. (1993) One to be taken as directed: reflections on non-adherence (non-compliance). *Journal of Social and Administrative Pharmacy*, **10**, 150–156.

Horne, R. & Weinman, J. (1994) Illness cognitions: implications for the treatment of renal disease. In H. McGee & C. Bradley (Eds.), Quality of life following renal failure (pp. 113–132). London: Harwood Academic.

Horne, R. & Weinman, J. (1995) The Beliefs About Medicines Questionnaire (BMQ): a new method for assessing lay beliefs about medicines. Proceedings of the Special Group in Health Psychology: *British Psychological Society.*

Horwitz, R.I. & Horwitz, S.M. (1993) Adherence Treatment and Health Outcomes. *Archives of Internal Medicine,* **153**, 1863–1868.

Horwitz, R.I., Viscoli, C.M., Berkman, L., Murray, C.J., Ransohoff, D.F. & Sindelar, J. (1990) Treatment adherence and the risk of death after a myocardial infarction. *Lancet,* **336**, 542–545.

Janz, N.K. & Becker, M.H. (1984) The health belief model: a decade later. *Health Education Quarterly,* **11**, 1–47.

Kelly, G.R., Mamon, J.A. & Scott, J.E. (1987) Utility of the health belief model in examining medication compliance among psychiatric outpatients. *Social Science and Medicine,* **25**, 1205–1211.

Kline, P. (1994) *An easy guide to factor analysis,* London: Routledge.

Leventhal, H. & Cameron, L. (1987) Behavioral theories and the problem of compliance. *Patient Education and Counselling,* **10**, 117–138.

Leventhal, H. & Diefenback, M. (1991) The Active Side of Illness Cognition. In: J.A. Skelton & R.T Croyle (Eds.), *Mental representation in health and illness* (pp. 245–271). New York: Springer Verlag.

Leventhal, H., Diefenbach, M. & Leventhal, E.A. (1992) Illness cognition: using common sense to understand treatment adherence and affect cognition interactions. *Cognitive Therapy and Research,* **16**, 143–163.

Leventhal, H., Easterling, D.V., Coons, H.L., Luchterhand, C.M. & Love, R.R. (1986) Adaption to chemotherapy treatments. In B.L. Andersen (Ed.), *Women with cancer: psychological perspectives* (pp. 172–203). New York: Springer Verlag.

Leventhal, H. & Nerenz, D. (1985) The assessment of illness cognition. In P. Karoly (Ed.), *Measurement strategies in health psychology* (pp. 517–555). New York: Wiley and Sons.

Leventhal, H., Nerenz, D.R., Leventhal, E.A., Love, R.R. & Bendena, L.M. (1991). The behavioral dynamics of clinical trials. *Preventative Medicine*, **20**, 132–146.

Lim, L.P., Schwarz, E. & Lo, E.C.M. (1994) Chinese health beliefs and oral health practices among the middle-aged and elderly in Hong Kong. *Community Dentistry and Oral Epidemiology*, **22**, 364–368.

Lorish, C.D., Richards, B. & Brown, S. (1990) Perspective of the patient with rheumatoid arthritis on issues related to missed medication. *Arthritis Care and Research*, **3**, 78–84.

Lowry, L. R. & Atchison, E. (1980) Home dialysis dropouts. *Journal of Psychosomatic Research*, **24**, 173–178.

Mansbridge, B. & Fisher, S. (1984) Public knowledge and attitudes about diazepam. *Psychopharmacology*, **82**, 225–228.

Marteau, T.M. (1995) Health beliefs and attributions. In A. Broome & S. Llewellyn (Eds.), *Health psychology: processes and applications* (2nd ed.) (pp. 3–20). London: Chapman & Hall.

Meichenbaum, D. & Turk, D.C. (1987) *Facilitating treatment adherence: A practitioner's handbook*, New York: Plenum Press.

Miller, P., Wikoff, R. & Hiatt, A. (1992) Fishbein's model of reasoned action and compliance behaviour of hypertensive patients. *Nursing Research*, **41**, 104–109.

Morgan, M. & Watkins, C.J. (1988) Managing hypertension: beliefs and responses to medication among cultural groups. *Sociology of Health and Illness*, **10**, 561–578.

New, S.J. & Senior, M.L. (1991) "I don't believe in needles": qualitative aspects of a study into the uptake of immunisation in two English health authorities. *Social Science and Medicine*, **33**, 509–518.

Newell, S.M., Price, J.H., Roberts, S.M. & Baumann, R.R. (1986) Utility of the modified Health Belief Model in predicting compliance with treatment by adult patients with advanced cancer. *Psychological Reports*, **59**, 783–791.

Pachter, L.M. (1994) Culture and clinical care. Folk illness beliefs and behaviors and their implications for health care delivery. *Journal of the American Medical Association*, **271**, 690–694.

Petrie, K.J., Weinman, J., Sharpe, N. & Buckley, J. (1996) Predicting return to work and functioning following myocardial infarction: the role of the patient's view of their illness. *British Medical Journal*, **312**, 1191–94.

Ried, L.D. & Christensen, D.B. (1988) A psychosocial perspective in the explanation of patients' drug-taking behavior. *Social Science and Medicine*, **27**, 277–285.

Schwarzer, R. (1992) Self-efficacy in the adoption and maintenance of health behaviours: theoretical approaches and a new model. In R. Schwarzer (Ed.), *Self-efficacy: Thought control of action* (pp. 217–243). Washington: Hemisphere Publishing Corporation.

Skelton, J.A. & Croyle, R.T. (1991) *Mental representation in health and illness*, New York: Springer-Verlag.

Stewart, A.L. & Ware, J.E. (1992) *Measuring functioning and well-being: The medical outcomes study approach*. Chapel Hill, NC: Duke University Press.

Streiner, D.L. (1994) Figuring out factors: the use and misuse of factor analysis. *Canadian Journal of Psychiatry*, **39**, 135–140.

Webb, D., Bates, I. & Horne, R. (1996) The "New Luddites". *Pharmaceutical Journal*, **256**, 367.

Weinman, J. (1990) Providing written information for patients: psychological considerations. *Journal of the Royal Society of Medicine*, **83**, 303–305.

Weinman, J., Petrie, K.J., Moss-Morris, R. & Horne, R. (1996) The Illness Perception Questionniare: a new method for assessing cognitive representations of illness. *Psychology and Health*, **11**, 431–445.

Weinstein, N.D. (1988) The precaution adoption process. *Health Psychology*, **7**, 355–386.

Weintraub, M. (1990) Compliance in the elderly. *Clinics in Geriatriatric Medicine*, **6**, 445–452.

Will, E.J. & Johnson, J.P. (1994) Options in the medical management of end-stage renal failure. In H. McGee & C. Bradley (Eds.), *Quality of life following renal failure* (pp. 15–32). London: Harwood Academic.

Woller, W., Kruse, J., Winter, P. & Mans, E.J. (1993) Cortisone image and emotional support by key figures in patients with bronchial asthma: An empirical study. *Psychotherapy and Psychosomatics*, **59**, 190–196.

6

Representations of Disability

Marie Johnston

INTRODUCTION

Disability is a commonly used, frequently undefined and diversely measured construct. It is a term in common discourse as well as belonging in many academic and applied disciplines including sociology, psychology, medicine, physiotherapy, occupational therapy, social policy, health economics and health services research. The use of the construct suggests varying underlying representations of disability in terms of its content and cause, but these are not always reflected in the theoretical models proposed nor in the measurement approaches adopted. These representations have influenced the research in the field, but have not influenced the development of models of disability.

Mental representations are involved in two kinds of model of disability: models which *explain the consequences* of disability and models which *explain disability* itself. Psychological models of the consequences treat disability as an "illness", life-event or stressor and examine the impact on mood and quality of life. These models typically identify critical mental representations (e.g. attributions for the disability, seriousness of the disability) which determine the impact of the event and which can be applied to disability as to any other threat, stressor, life-event or illness-event. Hence, in this context, disability can be conceptualised and investigated in the same manner and the findings obtained are similar to those for any other illness-related threat and needs no special consideration. For example, Earll, Johnston and Mitchell (1993) explored the impact on patients' adjustment of motor neurone disease, including the disabling aspects of the disease. Using Leventhal, Nerenz and Steele's (1984) Self-Regulation Model, five components of mental representations (identity, time-line, cause, consequences and cure) as well as coping and the evaluation of coping were investigated as predictors of mood and well-being. Similarly, Schulz and Decker (1987) found that social support, high perceived control and self-blame were associated with adjustment in people with spinal cord injuries.

By contrast, models that explain disability are more intimately concerned with the nature and definition of disability itself. It can be conceptualised within a predominantly biological framework, in which case the explanations are largely biological. Alternatively, it can be conceptualised primarily as a behavioural construct, which encourages more psychological explanations. Unlike disease outcomes such as survival, immune function, blood pressure or lung function, where biological end-points are likely to have more variance explained by biological parameters, it is likely that psychological factors can play an important role in the explanations of disability.

This chapter deals with models that *explain disability*. It examines the biological explanations and explores additional psychological explanatory variables. The dominant model explaining disability is the WHO (1980) model, which defines disability in behavioural terms but considers it in a biological framework as a consequence of disease. The model conflicts with much research evidence and the assumptions underlying the delivery of health care. Psychological models tend to be presented as alternatives although the research undertaken suggests that they have more potential as modifications to the basic model. In this chapter, the models of disability used in research are considered, examining definitions and measurement approaches, before considering the explanatory value of the WHO model. Since this model only explains a limited amount of the findings on disability, psychological factors that might serve to explain additional variance are explored. Three psychological domains offer some *a priori* expectation of explanatory power: control cognitions, coping and emotional factors. Current evidence gives clearest support to the role of control cognitions and the final section examines how they might be incorporated in the WHO model. It is argued that it is not necessary to invent a new model of behaviour, but rather to identify appropriate psychological models which incorporate control cognitions as a critical predictor of behaviour and therefore of disability. By combining such a psychological model with the WHO model, a more satisfactory model of disability is proposed.

REPRESENTATIONS OF DISABILITY IN RESEARCH

Definitions

Disability is defined in a variety of ways with resulting problems in measurement and communication of results. The working definition used for this chapter is the WHO (1980) definition:

> *Disability: Any restriction or lack (resulting from impairment) of ability to perform an activity in the manner or within the range considered normal for a human being.*

which contrasts disability with impairment and handicap defined as:

> *Impairment: Any loss or abnormality of psychological, physiological or anatomical structure or function. ...*

> *Handicap: A disadvantage for a given individual, resulting from an impairment or disability, that limits or prevents the fulfilment of a role (depending on age, sex and social and cultural factors) for the individual.*

Other authors use the word disability differently, even when adopting quite similar models of the process of consequences of disease. For example, Johnson and Wolinsky (1993) define disability as "physical limitations ... that may be caused by the underlying disease burden" (p. 108) and postulate separate dimensions for upper and lower body limitations. They propose that functional limitations, indicated by performance of activities of daily living, are the result of disability. Thus their concept of disability is closer to the WHO concept of impairment and their functional limitations closer to the WHO concept of disability. Patrick and Peach (1989), in developing a UK version of the Sickness Impact Profile (SIP) called the Functional Limitations Profile (FLP), made no attempt to separate disability and handicap, preferring to use a combined concept of "disablement". In some countries the term disability may even refer to the conditions that attract welfare support.

In part, the confusion arises from the use of the term *activity* by some authors to refer to a motivated performance and by others to define an anatomically and/or physiologically limited performance. In addition, the WHO model includes the notion of *normal* performance with resultant ambiguity regarding whether normality is a statistical or a value-laden construct.

Orbell (in press) has proposed that three main models or representations of disability are used. The Biological Model represents disability as the result of failing body parts or systems as in the WHO model. The second, Environmental Constraints Model, sees disability as "not directly related to severity of impairment, but ... moderated by the extent to which the environment facilitates or impedes performance of an activity" (manuscript p. 5). Orbell's third model, the Psychological Model, proposes that the observed performance is the result of a motivational process and that measures of both behaviour and motivational constructs are necessary to adequately represent disability.

Measurement

As Orbell indicates, measurement approaches reflect the authors' representations of the core construct. She proposes that the Biological Model is represented by measures such as those developed by Partridge, Johnston and Edwards (1987), or the OPCS (Martin, Meltzer & Elliot, 1988) where the individual can be requested to illustrate "normal" performance of activities. Measurements within the Environmental Constraints Model depend on performance of everyday activities with little regard to the "normality" of the performance, for example, the Barthel Index (Mahoney & Barthel, 1965) or Katz *et al.*'s (1963) ADL scale.

Differences in representations occur both in the items included and in the scaling adopted. Measures with items which elicit performance of movements assume that the disability is a constant, inherent aspect of the individual which can reliably be produced on demand. By contrast, measures of activities of daily living or ADL use reports or performance under ordinary, rather than assessment, conditions. A large number of ADL measures have been developed, often motivated by the need to assess the assistance required in everyday life. When used as more general research tools they reflect a situational and, possibly, motivational construct of disability. Smith and Clark (1995) have proposed scales which separate competence from performance of ADL and demonstrate validity of scaling designed to separate these constructs in stroke patients. Thus there continues to be debate over the type of items that constitute disability.

Most measures use additive scaling, indicating a concept of equivalence of items or activities. In these measures, failure on feeding, self-care or mobility would contribute in a similar manner to the overall score. Other measures such as the Sickness Impact Profile (SIP) (Bergner *et al.*, 1981) or Functional Limitations Profile (FLP) (Patrick & Peach, 1989) use weighted additive scores, where failure on some items counts for more than failure on other items; for example, difficulties in walking a long distance count for less than difficulties in walking a short distance. Williams *et al.* (1976) proposed that a cumulative hierarchical model was appropriate and used scaling methods that represented this model and others have adopted this approach (e.g. Whiting & Lincoln, 1980). Using this approach, the underlying theoretical model proposes that disabilities are acquired or lost in a systematic, ordered way; failure on an "easy" item then reflects both more disability and more severe disability.

In developing the OPCS scales, Martin *et al.* (1988) have used a Thurstone scaling approach to create a set of hierarchical scales for each area of disability, e.g. locomotion, dexterity, personal care. For each scale, the value of each item was determined by judges' ratings. The method of *combining* disabilities was also empirically derived to reflect the judgements of expert raters. It is heavily weighted by the individual's most severe disabilities, the score being derived from the formula:

$$worst + 0.4 \ (second \ worst) + 0.3 \ (third \ worst)$$

This contrasts with averaging or additive models which carry the implication that many mild disabilities, e.g. walking more slowly, being unable to walk half a mile and being unable to climb stairs, may be equivalent to one severe disability, e.g. being unable to walk at all.

Further questions arise over the dimensional structure of disability and whether a single dimension of disablement or multiple dimensions such as impairment, disability and functional limitations, are represented (e.g. Johnson & Wolinsky, 1993). Recent developments of measures of health status or of health related quality of life often include items that have traditionally been incorporated in measures of disability, along with other items assessing symptoms, mood, handicap, etc. This suggests that disability does not even represent a dimension but is only a component of the more global variable. As I have argued elsewhere (Johnston, 1995), such global measures may have some value as outcome measures but have little value in understanding the processes involved. If disability is postulated to result in handicap, global measures will not permit that relationship to be evaluated.

Conclusion

Definitions and measurement of disability indicate a wide diversity of views about what the word "disability" represents. On the other hand, there is some agreement about the phenomena that need to be investigated. The WHO definition of disability will be adopted for the remainder of this chapter. Measures which assess limitations in activities due to impairment or disease will be accepted as measures of disability. Clearly the issues raised in consideration of measurement indicate the lack of a satisfactory model of disability and will be addressed in examining explanations of disability.

THE BIOLOGICAL OR "MEDICAL" MODEL

The WHO model proposes that disability is due to physical impairment which is in turn due to disease or disorder (Figure 1). One might expect different patterns of disability to be associated with different patterns of impairments as suggested by Martin *et al.* (1988) and Orgogozo (1994) and therefore with different diseases. However this is not always observed; for example we have found a single pattern of disability for a community based group of old people, rather than a series of patterns which differentiated the main disease groups such as arthritis, stroke, respiratory disease or

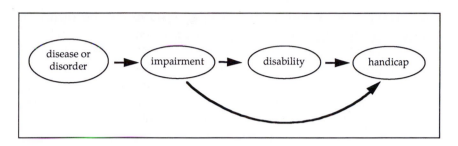

FIGURE 1   WHO model of Disability (WHO, 1980)

coronary heart disease (Williams *et al.*, 1976) and this has been replicated in subsequent studies.

Johnson and Wolinsky (1993) propose that disease affects "functional limitation" (equivalent to WHO disability) both directly and indirectly via functional impairment of upper and lower body separately. However using structural equation modelling, they demonstrate that impairments, rather than diseases, are the major determinants of disability (functional limitation). Their model does not investigate the influence of other factors, but clearly there is unexplained variance in the relationship between impairment and disability in their data.

Neither the WHO nor the Johnson and Wolinsky (1993) models seek further explanatory mechanisms, but other authors do. For example, Orgogozo (1994) suggests that the factors which influence the relationship between impairment and disability following stroke are "neural connectivity and plasticity ..., drive and strategies of compensation". A fundamental premise of rehabilitation therapies is that disabilities are not completely determined by impairment and that interventions can result in the impaired individual being less disabled. The finding that rehabilitation therapists report less disability than nurses do for the same patients (Johnston *et al.*, 1987) may be due to their greater success in intervening to reduce the disabling effects of impairments.

Disability may be further explained using variables that relate to the physical environment, social policy and the social environment, but the focus here is on psychological factors. It is conceivable that the effects of more macro level variables are mediated by psychological factors.

PSYCHOLOGICAL FACTORS INTERVENING BETWEEN IMPAIRMENT AND DISABILITY

A wide range of psychological variables has been found to be related to and to predict disability. However without further control for impairment level, it is possible that these psychological variables are predictive only because of their relationship with impairment. If so, then they may simply function as proxy measures for impairment and these findings would only serve to further confirm the basic tenet of the WHO model. More convincing are studies where the effects of impairment have been controlled statistically or where a randomised controlled trial has shown effects of a psychological intervention on disability, when one can assume that impairment was equally distributed in the control and intervention groups.

Numerous psychological interventions have resulted in reduced disability. For example, the self-management programme designed by Lorig and her colleagues (1989) has shown evidence of reducing disability for people with rheumatoid arthritis using the HAQ as the outcome measure. Kaplan, Atkins and Reinsch (1984) showed improvements in disability for patients with chronic obstructive pulmonary disease following cognitive and behavioural exercise programmes.

As with all psychological interventions, it can be difficult to identify the explanatory mechanism. In both the above studies, the authors suggest that these effects are due to changes in self-efficacy as a result of the programme. Kaplan *et al.* (1984) found that changes in self-efficacy were correlated with performance following their programme.

Control Cognitions

Control cognitions have been defined, described and related to health in a number of ways. Wallston *et al.* (1989) differentiate theoretical constructs of locus of control, self-efficacy and attributions, each referring to some aspect of control but deriving from the different theoretical conceptualisations of social learning theory, social cognitive theory and attribution theory respectively. The different theoretical approaches focus on different time perspectives (past, present, future) and apply control to different functions (behaviour, processes, outcomes).

Working within social cognitive theory, O'Leary *et al.* (1988) hypothesised that self-efficacy would mediate disease management. They found that an intervention to increase self-efficacy in 15 patients with rheumatoid arthritis resulted in reduced joint impairment compared with a control group and that end of treatment self-efficacy predicted follow up disability.

Control cognitions occur as spontaneous mental representations of patients with disabling conditions. Partridge (1984) found that patients in rehabilitation settings, in response to semi-structured interview questions, frequently commented on perceptions of control. Using statements by patients who had experienced stroke and wrist fracture, she went on to develop the Recovery Locus of Control (RLOC) scale which satisfied basic psychometric requirements (Partridge & Johnston, 1989). In a longitudinal prospective study of patients entering a rehabilitation programme, initial RLOC assessments predicted recovery from disability allowing for initial levels of disability in patients following stroke and wrist fracture (Partridge & Johnston, 1989). These findings were replicated in a larger group of stroke patients followed up from one month following discharge from hospital to 6 months after discharge (Johnston *et al.*, 1996). Support for the predictive value of the RLOC, controlling for initial levels of disability, was found for both self-report and observer-assessed measures of disability. These results allow the possibility that perceptions of control are not only predictive, but may play a causal role in determining recovery from disability. It was hypothesised that coping mediated this relationship and this is examined below in the section on coping.

A further study demonstrated that control cognitions as assessed by the RLOC were amenable to change (Johnston *et al.*, 1992). Patients entering a rehabilitation programme were randomly allocated to receive either the standard appointment letter or an experimental letter designed to enhance control beliefs. After one week in the programme, the experimental group had higher RLOC scores. Having demonstrated that control cognitions could be altered, it was possible to test the causal hypothesis that altering control cognitions would influence disability.

Patients with chronic pain were randomly allocated to manipulations designed to either enhance or diminish control cognitions (Fisher & Johnston, in press). Perception of control was increased by recalling occasions when the individual had achieved control, and decreased by recalling occasions when they had failed to retain control. The results showed that the manipulation was successful in influencing control cognitions as assessed by a visual analogue scale. It also influenced disability, assessed by the observed performance of a lifting task; patients having the increased control manipulation showed greater lifting tolerance (less disability) after the manipulation than before and those having the decrease control cognition had greater disability levels.

These results indicate the potential value of control cognitions in explaining some of the variance in the relationship between impairment and disability. Clearly impairment had not changed in the above study, but disability had and the results are therefore not explicable by the simple medical or WHO model. However, the result raises a further question: why should mental representations of disability affect disability?

Coping

Psychological factors such as perceived control may influence disability by altering coping. Working with Leventhal *et al.*'s (1984) Self-Regulation Model, the individual may develop mental representations of their impairments which would in turn determine their coping and, extending the model, one can postulate that coping would influence the final pattern of disability observed as proposed in Figure 2.

Moore and Stambrook (1995) have proposed a similar model for traumatic brain injury. They propose that: "How the person explains what has happened, why and to what extent it has changed his/her life situation and how it will affect the future … affects choice of coping strategies and motivation. These choices subsequently influence many of the other moderating and outcome factors." They found that locus of control beliefs accounted for more variance in disablement (SIP) than an index of impairment (the Glasgow Coma Scale). Using cluster analyses they found that a cluster of patients characterised by both coping strategies and control beliefs had lowest disabilities. These findings are compatible with a model proposing that coping mediates the relationship between cognitions and disability, but the authors did not examine the causal pathways between the three variables.

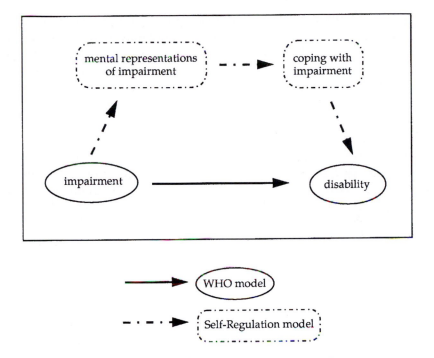

FIGURE 2   Integration of Self-Regulation and WHO models of disability

However, their analysis does not rule out the possibility that the control cognitions, rather than coping, determine the disability observed, which would conflict with the proposed model. Further, as the authors point out, this cross-sectional design allows the possibility that control cognitions and coping strategies are the result, rather than the cause of disability. Other cross-sectional studies showing correlations between coping and disability (e.g., Roberto, 1992) for women with hip fractures, also give no indication of the direction of causality and it is plausible that observed coping is a result of disability. Where longitudinal studies have been undertaken, coping has been found to be a *result* rather than a cause of health outcomes. For example, in longitudinal analyses over one year of 100 patients following myocardial infarction, Gudmundsdottir (1995) found that coping (assessed using the COPE, Carver, Scheier & Weintraub, 1989) was predicted by distress, rather than being predictive of distress, and Revenson and Felton (1989) found that change in disability was correlated with changes in coping (Ways of Coping Scale) in a prospective study of 25 patients with rheumatoid arthritis.

Appealing as the model presented in Figure 2 is in explaining disability, there is little evidence to support this model in longitudinal studies. In the study of stroke patients where control cognitions predicted disability, mental representations did not predict coping and coping did not predict disability 6 months after discharge from hospital (Johnston *et al.*, 1996). Coping was measured in two ways. First, it was proposed that the critical coping response was coping by engagement in exercise and a series of indices of engagement in exercise was developed. Despite some evidence of the validity of these measures, there was no evidence of this form of coping mediating disability. Second, we examined the fifteen coping scales of the COPE (Carver *et al.*, 1989). While there were some significant correlations, there was no evidence that coping strategies mediated the relationship between mental representations of impairment and disability. Control cognitions continued to predict recovery from disability when coping scales were included in the analyses and the latter did not explain any additional variance.

Revenson and Felton (1989) found that changes in the coping strategy of acceptance were negatively related to changes in disability in their group of individuals with rheumatoid arthritis, but do not present data on the simple prediction from coping, rather than changes in coping. The results are therefore compatible with a model of coping being influenced by disability and changes in disability. Other studies by Earll (1994) on people with MS, Petrie and Moss-Morris (1994) on people with chronic fatigue, and P. Kennedy (personal communication) on people with spinal injuries, have also found that coping did not predict and therefore did not influence disability. Earll (1994) used in-depth interviews to explore mental representations and coping in three groups of people who had had multiple sclerosis for less than 6 months, 2 years and 7 years respectively. Illness representations of identity and consequences as conceptualised in Leventhal *et al.*'s (1984) model predicted later disability (assessed using standard OPCS measures, Martin *et al.*, 1988). Coping was investigated using open questions addressing commonly reported modes of coping for these patients concerning action taken to keep healthy, to manage specific problems or difficulties, to increase understanding or actions other than those advised by the doctor. By contrast with illness representations, coping was not predictive of disability outcomes, even when coded using a simple binary classification of taking action or not.

It may be that these findings are specific to this group of clinical conditions. In each of these conditions, little can be done by the individual patient that affects the outcome and coping may be a more critical variable where clear action by the individual can affect outcomes. However these results are incompatible with the simple model proposed in Figure 2. Further, results of the studies by Johnston *et al.* (1996) and Earll (1994) have indicated that mental representations are more successful than coping in predicting disability.

Emotional Factors

A further possibility is that mental representations affect emotional state which in turn influences disability. Cognitive theories of emotional disorder assert that certain dysfunctional cognitions cause the emotions and that the emotional disorder can be treated by interventions which alter these cognitions. It is possible that the emotions rather than the cognitions are the main mediating variables between impairment and disability.

A key feature of Leventhal *et al.*'s self-regulation theory is that coping with emotions is seen as a parallel process to coping with objective problems and most modern approaches to coping separate emotion-focused coping from problem-focused coping. Complex feedback loops within the model allow emotions and coping with emotions to influence the process of coping with the objective problem (the impairments in Figure 2), but the latter process can occur independently of emotional processing. It is therefore difficult to derive a testable hypothesis of the role of emotions from this model. Moore and Stambrook's (1995) modified model incorporates emotional states. Based on their clinical observations and their reading of the literature on cognitive models of depression, Moore and Stambrook (1995) proposed that emotions influence outcomes by partially mediating the effects of perceptions of control on coping. However, the failure of coping to predict disability in the above studies makes this an implausible mechanism.

Emotion might function by some means other than coping. However, there was no support for emotional state as a mediator of the relationship between control cognitions and subsequent disability in our study of stroke patients (Johnston *et al.*, 1996). On the other hand, an experimental mood manipulation resulted in changes in disability in patients with chronic pain. In a study parallel to the control manipulation study described above, Fisher and Johnston (1996) used standard mood manipulation techniques and found that those in the anxiety reduction group had reduced disability while those in the anxiety increase group had more disability than before. In addition, changes in mood were correlated with change in disability, whereas changes in perceived control were not correlated with change in disability in the Fisher and Johnston (in press) study. These results would suggest that the critical factor in both manipulation studies might be emotional state. However, in the stroke study emotional state did not mediate the effects of perceived control on disability, nor did it explain any additional variance. There would appear to be a complex relationship between control cognitions and emotional state in determining disability. It is not clear whether the cognitions act directly or are mediated by their effect on mood.

MODELS OF MENTAL REPRESENTATIONS AND DISABILITY

Given the limitations of the WHO model and the evidence on psychological factors intervening between impairment and disability, an explanatory model which incorporates psychological factors is clearly required, but the model presented in Figure 2 is inadequate. In explaining disability, numerous psychological constructs have been investigated including coping and emotional states, as well as representational factors. While there is support for the explanatory power of mental representations, the mediating role of coping inherent in some models has not been empirically supported. It is suggested that other psychological models, those that give a major role to social cognitions, may have more explanatory power. It is proposed that psychological models are not alternatives to the WHO model, but that the models can be combined to offer a better explanation of the behaviours that are defined as disability.

A more satisfactory model should continue to include mental representations, specifically control cognitions, but need not incorporate coping. The explanation should be capable of incorporating the essential elements of the WHO model and offer some explanation of disability in addition to the explanation provided by impairment. The WHO definition of disability clearly defines disability as a behaviour and therefore any model which predicts behaviour from cognitions is potentially viable. In health psychology, the main models fulfilling this role are social cognition models, especially the Theory of Planned Behaviour (TPB) (Azjen, 1988) and Social Cognitive Theory (Bandura, 1986; 1989), which have been applied successfully to health behaviour, e.g. in explaining uptake of screening, participation in exercise, modification of diet. Both models include control cognitions as predictors of behaviour and are therefore compatible with the findings reported above.

The TPB would predict that behaviour, including behaviours defined here as disability, are determined by a combination of behavioural intention and perceived behavioural control. Applying this model to disability, one would predict that the lifting tolerance in the patients in the studies of chronic pain (Fisher & Johnston, in press, 1996) was determined by their intention to hold the weight for longer and their perception that they could hold it for longer. The intention is determined by three factors: 1) attitude to the behaviour (e.g. "when I hold the weight for any length of time it is painful, I dislike pain and I am therefore not in favour of holding it for long"); 2) subjective norm for the behaviour (e.g. "the psychologist wishes me to hold the weight for as long as possible, I wish to please her and I shall therefore hold it as long as I possibly can") and perceived behavioural control over the behaviour (e.g. "I am confident that I am able to hold the weight for a long time").

This model satisfactorily incorporates the causal role of perceived control. It makes the unusual prediction that disability is to some extent determined by intention and this is worth considering in more detail. While at first glance, one might expect everyone to have the intention of performing everyday tasks, one can see that the individual experiencing repeated failures due to impairment would develop negative attitudes toward the task, might be surrounded by family who do not expect the individual to perform the task and would have low expectations of being able to perform the behaviour; they might therefore have little intention of performing the behaviour. This is illustrated by an anecdotal observation. A woman recovering from a stroke reported that she had not tried a

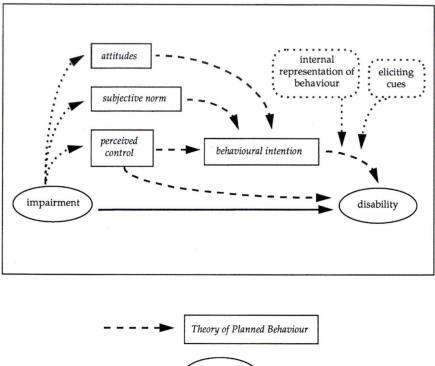

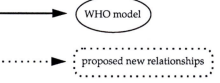

FIGURE 3   Theory of Planned Behaviour and WHO Model: An integrated model of disability

particular task until the morning of the research interview when she found she could do it. Her success in overcoming this disability occurred because she tried it (intention) and she did this because she knew the interviewer would ask her to do it (subjective norm) and not because she had overcome the underlying impairment.

By incorporating the TPB in the WHO model (Johnston, 1996) it is possible to integrate the causal influences of control cognitions and impairments as in Figure 3. Impairment is proposed to have a direct effect on disability and an indirect effect mediated by mental representations including perceived control and intention.

This model also brings other cognitions into play. Both the attitude and subjective norm component introduce value systems. Attitudes toward performing the activity incorporate the value held for the outcomes of the behaviour and implies balancing negative and positive outcomes. Activities which result in pain or failure are obviously likely to attract a negative value. But if the same activity results in positive outcomes such as retaining personal independence or dignity, then the balance may be positive and will increase the intention to perform the task. If there are culturally shared values for tasks, then one might expect patterns of disability that do not precisely mirror underlying patterns of impairment or disease. For example, a shared high value for privacy when toileting would result in this activity being retained in diverse disease conditions with resultant impairments in energy, mobility, breathing etc., while apparently easier activities but of lower value were lost. Then the model would predict the shared hierarchical patterns of disability found across diverse diseases by Williams *et al.* (1976). It would also predict that one would find idiosyncratic patterns for individuals or groups with specific values and might therefore predict different patterns of disability, given the same impairments, for men compared with women, for people of different social or educational groups, for people with different hobbies and so on.

Similarly, the value system built into subjective norm implies that different patterns of disability may be observed depending on the critical social influences. One would therefore expect to find different patterns of disability in individuals with the same impairments cared for at home, in a nursing home or in a rehabilitation setting. This prediction is consistent with the finding that nurses and rehabilitation therapists report different levels of disability (Johnston *et al.*, 1987). Different professions have different treatment goals (Dekker, in press) and it seems plausible that nurses assist the individual in achieving the goal, whereas rehabilitation therapists help the person to perform the activities which achieve the goal. It is not surprising then that nurses find the patients more disabled than the therapists. Similarly, the model predicts that patients will perform in a more disabled manner in social environments which have lower expectations and demands, a prediction that is confirmed by clinical observation in institutional and home settings.

The TPB offers a new approach to modelling disability but has recognised limits. Many authors have noted that the model is more successful in predicting intention than in predicting behaviour and refer to this as the "intention-behaviour gap". In applying the model to disability, one can see that someone with both the intention to perform a task and perceived control over the performance might fail to perform the task if their expectations were unrealistic or they forgot at the critical time. Thus a patient with visual neglect following a stroke might be unable to negotiate a doorway despite having the intention and the belief that they could do it. A patient with memory impairments might fail to perform self-care tasks even though they intended to and believed they could do the task, simply because they forgot. Thus some additional elements are required in the model to enhance the explanation of the action, as against the motivational stage of the performance.

Social cognition researchers are currently investigating various possible additional elements to the TPB (e.g. Gollwitzer, 1993; Schwarzer, 1992). All of these address the action phase of the model. In the proposed model for disability, two variables have been added: Internal Representations of the Behaviour and Eliciting Cues. Internal Representations of the Behaviour refer to the availability of the components of the behaviour at some level within the individual. This might be information and knowledge about the behaviour, the necessary skill to perform, or the required physical attributes. If the individual does not know how to undo new garments provided by the hospital, has not been taught how to use a wheelchair or is currently catheterised, they may fail to toilet successfully regardless of their intentions and control cognitions. The person may have representations of the performance in some situations which do not apply in others; environmental factors may demand alternative modes of performance or skills which the individual has not practised.

Eliciting Cues are external cues or triggers to action which remind the individual to perform the behaviour and have been incorporated into other social cognition models. They are akin to the antecedents as specified in behavioural accounts of performance and may serve to explain why the individual may be more disabled in some situations than in others.

It is possible that conceptualisation of disability has been restricted by the medical domain in which it has arisen and been used. The model proposed applies equally well to any limitations in performance resulting from anatomical or physiological limitation. Thus the terms "Impairment" and "Disability" could readily be replaced by the terms "Limitations of anatomy or physiology" and "Limitations of performance of activities". A model of limitations in performance readily incorporates the concept of disability, highlights the range of explanatory variables available and avoids the evaluative/pejorative overtones of the word disability.

The model does not include emotional state and the evidence presented in a previous section suggests that emotions may also influence disability, although their effect is likely to be closely linked to the effects of mental representations of control. Current theorising on cognition and emotion suggests that cognitions both determine and are determined by emotional states (Mathews & Macleod, 1994). For example, depression is caused by dysfunctional cognitions and, by selectively influencing recall processes, affects cognition. Thus a model which incorporates cognition may subsequently be adaptable to account for emotional processes too.

SUMMARY AND CONCLUSIONS

The dominant WHO model of disability used in medical and rehabilitation settings proposes that disability is determined by impairment resulting from disease or disorder. As it stands, this model is incapable of explaining many of the findings in the field, including observed shared cumulative patterns of disability and systematic discrepancies between the ratings of disability made by different health professions. Some of the problems can be overcome if disability is examined as a behaviour (rather than as the result of a disease/disorder or as a cause of emotional distress) and psychological models of behaviour can be integrated with the WHO model of disability.

Leventhal's self-regulation model proposes that mental representations influence coping. If coping in turn affects behaviour, including disability, then, integrating this model with the WHO model introduces factors which might moderate the impact of impairment on disability. However this approach did not satisfactorily explain the results of studies where coping did not predict disability but mental representations did.

A new approach is proposed based on social cognition models of behaviour. While a variety of models is available, examination of the Theory of Planned Behaviour suggests that this model might be useful in studying disability. Integrating it with the WHO model leads to predictions that impairment influences attitudes, social norms and perceived behavioural control over the behaviours characterised as disability and that these cognitions determine the individual's intention to perform the behaviour. This intention is proposed as the main proximal determinant of the performance, with other factors, including perceived behavioural control, internal representations of the behaviour and external eliciting cues, also influencing the observed disability. This model can account for current empirical observations which challenged the simple WHO model and makes predictions relevant to impairments and disabilities which have not as yet been tested.

REFERENCES

Azjen, I. (1988) *Attitudes, personality and behaviour.* Milton Keynes: Open University Press.

Bandura, A. (1986) *Social foundations of thought and action: A social cognitive theory.* Englewood Cliffs, NJ: Prentice-Hall.

Bandura, A. (1989) Human agency in social cognitive theory. *American Psychologist,* **44**, 1175–1184.

Bergner, M., Bobbitt, R.A., Carter, W.B. & Gibson, B.S. (1981) The Sickness Impact Profile: development and final revision of a health status measure. *Medical Care,* **19**, 789–805.

Carver, C.S., Scheier, M.F. & Weintraub, J.K. (1989) Assessing coping strategies: a theoretically based approach. *Journal of Personality and Social Psychology,* **56**, 267–283.

Dekker, J. (in press). Application of the ICIDH in survey research on rehabilitation: The emergence of functional diagnosis. *Disability and Rehabilitation.*

Earll, L. (1994) *Coping with chronic neurological illness: An analysis using self-regulation theory.* PhD thesis: University of London.

Earll, L. & Johnston, M. (1994) *Illness representations and coping in multiple sclerosis.* Paper presented at the British Psychological

Society Special Group in Health Psychology Annual Conference, Sheffield.

Earll, L., Johnston, M. & Mitchell, E. (1993) Coping with motor neurone disease: an analysis using self-regulation theory. *Palliative Medicine*, **7**, 21–30.

Evans, R.L., Kiolet, C.L. & Smith, K.M. (1985) Treatment outcome as a function of expectations and prior adjustment. *Journal of Social Behavior and Personality*, **1**, 133–136.

Fisher, K. & Johnston, M. (in press). Experimental manipulation of perceived control and its effect on disability. *Psychology and Health*.

Fisher, K. & Johnston, M. (1996). Emotional distress as a mediator of the relationship between pain and disability: an experimental study. *British Journal of Health Psychology*, **1**, 207–218.

Gollwitzer, P.M. (1993) Goal achievement: the role of intentions. In W. Stroebe & M. Hewstone (Eds.), *European review of social psychology* (Vol. 4). Chichester: Wiley.

Gudmundsdottir, H. (1995) *Coping strategies and causal attributions following myocardial infarction: a longitudinal study*. PhD thesis, University of St Andrews.

Johnson, R.J. & Wolinsky, F.D. (1993) The structure of health status among older adults: disease, disability, functional limitation and perceived health. *Journal of Health and Social Behaviour*, **34**, 105–121.

Johnston, M. (1995) The quality of health. In J. Rodriguez-Marin (Ed.), *Quality of life*. Alicante University.

Johnston, M. (1996). Models of disability. *The Psychologist*, **9**, 205–210.

Johnston, M., Bromley, I., Boothroyd-Brooks, M., Dobbs, W., Ilson, A. & Ridout, K. (1987) Behavioural assessment of physically disabled patients: agreement between rehabilitation therapists and nurses. *International Journal of Research in Rehabilitation*, **10(Suppl.)**, 205–213.

Johnston, M., Gilbert, P., Partridge, C. & Collins, J. (1992) Changing perceived control in patients with physical disabilities: an intervention study with patients receiving rehabilitation. *British Journal of Clinical Psychology*, **31**, 89–94.

Johnston, M., Morrison, V., MacWalter, R.S. & Partridge, C.J. (1996) *Perceived control, coping and recovery from disability following stroke*. Manuscript submitted for publication.

Kaplan, R.M., Atkins, C.J. & Reinsch, S. (1984) Specific efficacy expectations mediate exercise compliance in patients with COPD. *Health Psychology*, **3**, 223–242.

Katz, S., Ford, A., Moskowitz, R., Jackson, B. & Jaffe, M. (1963) Studies of illness in the aged. *Journal of the American Medical Association*, **185**, 914–919.

Leventhal, H., Nerenz, D. & Steele, D.J. (1984) Illness representations and coping with health threats. In A. Baum, S.E. Taylor & J.E. Singer (Eds.), *Handbook of psychology and health: social psychological aspects of health* (Vol. 4). Hillsdale, NJ: Lawrence Erlbaum.

Lorig, K., Seleznick, M., Lubeck, D., Ung, E., Chastain, R.L. & Holman, H.R. (1989) The beneficial outcomes of the arthritis self-management course are not adequately explained by behavior change. *Arthritis and Rheumatism*, **32**, 91–43.

Mahoney, F.I. & Barthel, D.W. (1965) Functional evaluation: the Barthel Index. *Maryland State Medical Journal*, **14**, 61–65. [also in Johnston, M., Wright, S. & Weinman, J. (1995) *Measures in health psychology: A user's portfolio*. Windsor: NFER-Nelson].

Martin, J., Meltzer, H. & Elliot, D. (1988) *The prevalence of disability among adults*. London: HMSO.

Mathews, A. & Macleod, C. (1994) Cognitive approaches to emotion and emotional disorders. *Annual Review of Psychology*, **45**, 25–50.

Moore, A.D. & Stambrook, M. (1995) Cognitive moderators of outcome following traumatic brain injury: a conceptual model and implications for rehabilitation. *Brain Injury*, **9**, 109–130.

O'Leary, A., Shoor, S., Lorig, K. & Holman, H.R. (1988) A cognitive-behavioral treatment for rheumatoid arthritis. *Health Psychology*, **7**, 527–544.

Orbell, S. (in press). Concepts of disability. In V. Aitken, G. Jordan & H. Jellicoe (Eds.), *Behavioural sciences for health care professionals*.

Orgogozo, J.M. (1994) The concepts of impairment, disability and handicap. *Cerebrovascular Disorder*, **4(Suppl.)**, 2–6.

Patrick, D.L. & Peach, H. (1989) *Disablement in the community*. Oxford: Oxford University Press.

Partridge, C.J. (1984) *Cognitions and emotions as predictors of recovery in conditions involving physical disability*. PhD thesis, University of London.

Partridge, C.J. & Johnston, M. (1989) Perceived control and recovery from physical disability. *British Journal of Clinical Psychology,* **28**, 53–60.

Partridge, C.J., Johnston, M. & Edwards, S. (1987) Recovery from disability after stroke: normal patterns as a basis for evaluation. *Lancet,* **1**, 373–375.

Petrie, K. & Moss-Morris, R. (1994, July) *The impact of illness perceptions on disability in chronic fatigue syndrome.* Paper presented at the International Society of Behavioural Medicine, Amsterdam.

Revenson, T.A. & Felton, B.J. (1989) Disability and coping as predictors of psychological adjustment in rheumatoid arthritis. *Journal of Consulting and Clinical Psychology,* **57**, 344–348.

Roberto, K.A. (1992) Coping strategies of older women with hip fractures: Resources and outcomes. *Journal of Gerontology: Psychological Sciences,* **47**, 21–26.

Schulz, R. & Decker, S. (1987) Long-term adjustment to physical disability: the role of social support, perceived control and self-blame. *Journal of Personality and Social Psychology,* **48**, 1162–1172.

Schwarzer, R. (1992) Self-efficacy in the adoption and maintenance of health behaviour. Theoretical approaches and a new model. In R. Schwarzer (Ed.), *Self-efficacy: thought control of action.* Hemisphere: London.

Smith, D.S. & Clark, M.S. (1995) Competence and performance in activities of daily living of patients following rehabilitation from stroke. *Disability and Rehabilitation,* **17**, 15–23.

Wallston, K., Wallston, B.S., Smith, S. & Dobbins, C.J. (1989) Perceived control and health. In M. Johnston & T.M. Marteau (Eds.), *Applications in health psychology.* New Brunswick: Transaction Press.

Whiting, S. & Lincoln, N. (1980) An ADL assessment for stroke patients. *Occupational Therapy,* Feb., 44–47.

Williams, D.A., Nicholas, M.K., Richardson, P.H., Pither, C.E., Justins, D.M., Chamberlain, J.H., Harding, V.R., Ralphs, J.A., Jones, S.C., Dieudonne, I., Featherstone, J.D., Hodgson, D.R., Ridout, K.L. & Shannon, E.M. (1993) Evaluation of a cognitive behaviour programme for rehabilitating patients with chronic pain. *British Journal of General Practice,* **43**, 513–518.

Williams, R.G.A., Johnston, M., Willis, L. & Bennett, A.E. (1976) Disability: a model and a measurement technique. *British Journal of Preventive and Social Medicine*, **30**, 71–78.

World Health Organisation. (1980) *International classification of impairments, disabilities and handicaps.* Geneva: WHO.

Section 2
Illness Perspectives in Prevention and Health Screening

7
Cognitive Representations and Preventive Health Behaviour: A Review

Charles Abraham & Paschal Sheeran

ASSUMPTIONS, CAUTIONS AND OPTIMISM

Social representations (Moscovici, 1981) refer to widely shared beliefs about a phenomenon which are established and maintained through interpersonal communication. Herzlich (1973) explored social representations of health and illness. She found that her French participants viewed health as something which was taken for granted until illness struck and that they understood illness both in terms of; (i) a loss of equilibrium in individuals' lifestyles and (ii) a limited reserve of health derived partly from inherited constitutions. Such broad characterisations of social understanding help to map out the meaningful background, or 'common sense', against which individuals construct representations of their own health and illness (see also Farr, 1977). They do not, however, help to identify who will become ill (see Adler & Matthews, 1994) or take preventive health action.

Available evidence suggests that self-report measures based on models of individual cognition can contribute to the prediction of future health and health behaviour. Peterson, Seligmann and Vaillant (1988) have shown that people who explain negative events in terms of stable and pervasive aspects of themselves (that is, those who have a "pessimistic explanatory style") are more likely to have poorer doctor-assessed health 20–30 years later. King (1982), study-ing hypertension screening, found that self-reported intentions and health beliefs could correctly distinguish between those who did and did not attend in 82% of cases. Explanatory style, intentions and health beliefs are descriptions of individual cognitions derived from a group of theoretical models known as "social cognition models" (see Conner & Norman, 1996). The self-reports used to measure such constructs are viewed as markers of intrapersonal processes involved in the regulation of individual decision-making and behaviour control. They can be used to characterise individual cognition patterns and their predictive value can be assessed in relation to particular outcome measures. This chapter will review the application of social cognition models to preventive health behaviour.

Preventive health behaviour has been linked to life expectancy (e.g. Breslow & Enstrom, 1980) and it is possible that a better under-standing of the cognitive prerequisites of such behaviour could lead to more effective health promotion activities. Modifiable self-reported cognitions, such as perceived confidence in one's ability to perform a specified behaviour (e.g. Bandura, 1989; Cervone, 1989) may be used to enhance the effectiveness of health interventions by high-lighting intrapersonal changes most likely to result in behaviour modification (e.g. Schaalma *et al.*, in press; Wiedenfeld *et al.*, 1990). However, the impact of health promotion activities should not be overestimated (Carroll, Bennett & Davey Smith, 1993). There is con-siderable evidence suggesting that one's socio-economic status is a major determinant of life expectancy (Wilkinson, 1990). For example, Hein, Suadicani and Gyntelberg (1992) demonstrated that social class had a much greater impact on heart disease than smoking behaviour. Such findings imply that health promotion cannot, in itself, provide a basis for public health policy-making. Nevertheless, the promotion of preventive health behaviour remains important to public health policy and cognition measures may partially account for the effect of socio-economic position on individual health (Adler *et al.*, 1994).

The application of social cognitive models is based on a series of assumptions. Central amongst these is the idea that individuals' rep-resentations of illness and health behaviour can be compared and contrasted. For example, researchers might assume that a person who agrees strongly that they are susceptible to HIV infection means the same by "susceptible" as the person who strongly disagrees. The validity of such assumptions depends upon the degree of cultural homogeneity amongst those studied. For example, someone who believes that HIV-related illness is the result of witch-craft may have a very different idea of susceptibility to someone who accepts current medical explanations of HIV transmission and its effects on immunological functioning. However, even within "Western" cultures the social construction of illnesses may create sub-cultural differences. Sontag (1988), for example, argues that our understanding of HIV infection has become imbued with moral values and social identities so that it is understood;

> *"as a disease incurred by people both as individuals and as members of a 'risk group' — that neutral-sounding bureaucratic category which also revives the archaic idea of a tainted community that illness has judged" (p. 46).*

Social representations of this kind shape individual understandings and may result in differences in cognitive structures or differences in the relationship between cognitions and health behaviours across cultural sub-groups. For example, van der Velde and van der Pligt (1991) report that higher perceived susceptibility was positively related to intentions to use condoms amongst their sample of het-erosexuals with multiple partners but negatively related to intentions amongst their sample of gay men, suggesting that further emphasis on personal susceptibility could be counter-productive for the latter group. Similarly, Abraham *et al.* (1996) found that while young men's intentions to use condoms were positively related to subse-quent reports of condom use, young women's intentions were not, suggesting a gender difference in the ability to translate condom-use intentions into action.

These examples underline the need to empirically determine the generalisability of relationships specified by cognitive models. Careful piloting of research instruments, the use of both qualitative and quantitative methods and replications of studies across sub-samples can be used to check the ecological validity of these models (Carey, 1992; Sheeran & Abraham, 1996; Steckler *et al.*, 1992). There is, however, reason to be cautiously optimistic since measures specified by social cognition models have been found to be associated with health behaviour across a wide variety of European and North American samples (e.g., Oettingen, 1995) and some have been found to operate successfully with individuals from individualist and collectivist cultures (Earley, 1993).

Social cognitive modelling is implicitly or explicitly based on assumptions about how experience is stored in memory, how retrieval from memory affects subsequent behaviour (including reporting behaviour) and how social contexts influence what is reported. There has been some debate about self-presentational bias in the reporting of health-related cognitions and behaviours (see Abraham & Hampson, 1996) and it is clear that researchers must pay close attention to participants' motivation, especially when collecting reports of socially approved or disapproved behaviours (Davis & Best, 1995). Nevertheless, self-report measures of behaviour have been found to be reliable when objective tests are available. For example, Glasgow *et al.* (1993) observed disconfirmation rates of only 4% when biochemical measures were used to validate self-reported smoking. Moreover, when such measures can successfully distinguish between groups in terms of prospective health outcomes (e.g. Peterson, Seligman & Vaillant, 1988), there is reason to believe that they express important health-related individual differences. Therefore, while appropriate methodological sophistication is essential in assessing the reliability of self-reports (e.g., Davis & Best, 1995; Sheeran & Abraham, 1996) the evidence does not suggest that self-report measures are inherently unreliable.

BELIEFS ABOUT HEALTH AND ILLNESS

During the 1950s US public health researchers began to identify psychological targets for health education programmes (Rosenstock, 1974). Early research suggested that health beliefs concerning susceptibility and illness severity could differentiate between those who did and did not participate in tuberculosis X-ray screening and by the early 1970s a series of studies had confirmed the relationship between these beliefs and various health behaviours. The model which emerged from this research became known as the health belief model (HBM) (Becker & Maiman, 1975). It focuses on two aspects of individual representation of health and health behaviour; threat perception and behavioural evaluation. Each consists of two distinct sets of beliefs. Threat perception includes perceived susceptibility to illness and anticipated severity of the consequences of the illness. Behavioural evaluation depends upon beliefs concerning the benefits or efficacy of a recommended health behaviour and those concerning the costs of, or barriers to, enacting the behaviour. In addition, the model proposed that cues to action may trigger health behaviour when appropriate beliefs are held. These "cues" included a diverse range of triggers such as individual perceptions of symptoms, social influence and health education campaigns. Finally, an individual's general health motivation was included in later versions of the model.

The HBM has been applied to a variety of preventive health behaviours, including smoking, dieting, exercising, breast self-examination and condom use (see Sheeran & Abraham, 1996 for a review). In their 1984 review Janz and Becker (1984) identified 46 studies using the HBM and counted the number of studies which found each of the HBM constructs to be significantly associated with health behaviours. Eighteen of these studies used a prospective design and in these studies, perceived susceptibility was found to be a significant predictor in 82%, perceived severity in 61%, perceived benefits in 81% and perceived barriers in 100%. These results suggested a causal role for the four main HBM beliefs across a range of health-related behaviours, but did not assess the size of the observed relationships. Harrison, Mullen and Green (1992) used meta-analysis to address this issue. They located 234 published empirical tests of the HBM but found only 16 which measured each of the four major components and included reliability checks. Only six of these used prospective designs and four of these had been included in the Janz and Becker review. These findings suggest that the model has rarely been subjected to the most rigorous empirical tests. Considering only the six prospective studies and using Pearson's r to represent the relationship between HBM components and health behaviours, Harrison *et al.* (1992) found average weighted effect sizes of 0.19, 0.13, 0.10 and –0.16 for perceived susceptibility, severity, benefits and barriers, respectively. These correlations are statistically significant ($p < 0.01$) but small in substantive terms, with each variable accounting for between 1.0% and 3.6% of the variance in behaviour measures. However, effect sizes for individual variables do not assess the predictive power of the combined HBM variables. In a more recent meta-analytic review of 30 studies relating HBM to preventive health behaviour, Zimmerman and Vernberg (1994) found that, on average, 24% of the variance in behaviour was accounted for by combined HBM variables. This leaves 76% of the variance in preventive behaviour unexplained and indicates that further cognitive prerequisites could be identified. It also suggests that promoting HBM-specified beliefs could make a substantial contribution to the effectiveness of health education interventions. Rosenthal and Rubin (1982) have used a "binomial effect size display" to translate percentages of variance explained into increases in outcome or success rates. They calculate that explaining 25% of variance corresponds to a potential success-rate increase from 25% to 75%. This suggests that if 25% of a target population currently engage in preventive action and a 100% successful health promotion campaign persuaded the remaining 75% of the beliefs specified by the HBM, then 75% of that population might be expected to take preventive action after the intervention.

Overall, the evidence suggests that the beliefs specified by the HBM are prerequisites for preventive health behaviours, but that other cognitions are likely to be involved in prompting such behaviour. In the next sections we consider how other models and theories have elaborated our understanding of the individual determinants of preventive health behaviour. However, it is worth noting here that the HBM has focused researchers' and health care professionals' attention on modifiable psychological prerequisites of behaviour and provided a basis for practical interventions across a range of behaviours. For example, Haefner and Kirscht (1970) demonstrated that an educational intervention designed to increase participants' perceived susceptibility, perceived severity and anticipated benefits resulted in a greater number of medical check-up visits amongst participants compared with controls over the subsequent eight months. Jones, Jones and Katz (1987) used the model to develop and evaluate an educational intervention for patients attending an accident and emergency department with asthma symptoms. Patients were provided with information tailored to alter beliefs specified by the HBM and then advised to make an appointment to see their doctor. Results showed that 75% complied with this advice compared to only 10% in a control group. Similarly, in a review of the determinants of compliance Ley (1988) concluded that HBM-specified beliefs and, in particular perceived susceptibility, are correlated with patient compliance with medical advice, suggesting that health care professionals could enhance the effectiveness of their services by assessing and promoting these beliefs.

FROM ILLNESS REPRESENTATION TO ACTION-RELATED REPRESENTATIONS

The cost-benefit analysis inherent in the HBM is intuitively plausible, but the model does not propose any cognitive mechanism by which beliefs about the threat of illness and preventive behaviour are translated into action. Such a mechanism is central to the theory of reasoned action (TRA) (Fishbein & Ajzen, 1975) which developed out of research into the relationship between people's attitudes and their behaviour (Eagly & Chaiken, 1993). The theory suggests that intention formation precedes and predicts behaviour and that intentions are themselves determined by beliefs constituting a person's attitude and subjective norm regarding particular behaviours.

Attitudes are defined as the product of beliefs about the likely consequences of a particular behaviour and evaluations of those consequences. For example, a smoker might believe that s/he is more likely to feel positive and relaxed when smoking and may highly value such mood control. S/he may accept that smoking increases the chances of lung cancer and may acknowledge that this outcome would be disastrous, but may also believe that the increased risk is small for the number of cigarettes s/he smokes. The TRA proposes that people hold a series of such beliefs about any particular behaviour and that these partially determine the extent to which they intend to undertake it. The perceived likelihood of anticipated consequences multiplied by the degree to which they are positively or negatively evaluated is taken to represent the way in which such beliefs influence intention formation.

The TRA acknowledges that other people's views affect our intentions and behaviour and this is represented in the subjective norm measure. A person's subjective norm combines two sets of beliefs. First, their perceptions of the extent to which other people approve of a behaviour (e.g. do my friends think I should not smoke? or does my partner think we should use a condom during intercourse?). These are injunctive social norms in that they refer to perceptions of what others think we should do, rather than perceptions of what others themselves do, which are referred to as descriptive social norms (Cialdini, Kallgren & Reno, 1991). Secondly, their desire to conform to these people's wishes (e.g. I very much want to do what my friends/partner thinks I should). The degree to which a series of relevant others are perceived to think that a specified behaviour should/should not be undertaken is multiplied by the person's motivation to comply with each of these people's wishes and the products summed to provide an overall subjective norm measure for any particular behaviour.

Fishbein and Ajzen (1975) and Ajzen (1988) point out that attitude measures are most likely to be correlated with intention and behaviour measures when all three define the behaviour at the same level of specificity. For example, measures of attitudes towards eating chocolate cake with afternoon coffee is much more likely to be associated with this behaviour than measures of general attitudes towards healthy eating. Attitudes towards particular behaviours and intentions to undertake them may depend upon the context, the time or occasion. For example, while someone may hold a positive attitude towards using condoms with new partners, they may think that the benefits are outweighed by the costs of using them with their present regular sexual partner. Even if they intend to use a condom with a new partner, the perceived consequences of raising the issue of condom use (when their partner does not) may be enough to undermine this intention. Therefore, attitudinal and intention measures which specify the behaviour as precisely as possible (for example, buying condoms in the next month, carrying them when going out in the evenings during the next month and raising the issue of condom use with one's next new sexual partner) are likely to be most closely related to behaviour. This means that we should not expect general illness representations to be good predictors of specific preventive actions. Action-specific cognitions are likely to be more important proximal prerequisites of behaviour. This may partially explain why perceptions of illness severity, which are not linked to a particular behavioural response, are relatively weak correlates of preventive health behaviour (Abraham *et al.,* 1994; Wurtele & Maddux, 1987).

The TRA has received empirical support across a range of behaviours including smoking, exercise and diet. Even in the case of condom use, which is a complex, joint action dependent on a series of preparatory actions (Abraham & Sheeran, 1994), intentions have been shown to be significantly associated with future condom use reported three and four months subsequently (Boyd & Wandersman, 1991; van der Velde, Hookyaas & van der Pligt, 1992). Sheppard, Hartwick and Warshaw (1988) conducted a meta-analysis of 87 studies applying the TRA and Eagly and Chaiken (1993) report the results of a more extensive but unpublished meta-analysis by van den Putte (1991) based on 113 articles. These analyses found mean correlations of 0.68 (Sheppard *et al.*, 1988) and 0.68 (van den Putte, 1991) for the relationship between attitudes and subjective norm and intention and correlations of 0.53 (Sheppard *et al.*) and 0.62 (van den Putte) for the relationship between intentions and behavioural measures. Although the strength of the intention-behaviour relationship varies considerably across behaviours (Eagly & Chaiken, 1993), these results identify intention formation as an important predictor of future action.

There have been few studies comparing the degree to which the HBM and the TRA can explain health behaviour. Mullen, Hersey and Iverson (1987), for example, compared the accuracy with which the two models predicted five reported behaviours eight to nine months after initial cognition assessment. Unfortunately the intention measure was only correctly specified for one of the five behaviours. In this case TRA accounted for 25% of the variance in reported attempts to quit smoking, while the HBM accounted for 8%. In a review of 15 studies Zimmerman and Vernberg (1994) found that the mean variance in preventive health behaviour explained by the TRA was 34% compared to only 24% explained by the HBM (across 30 studies).

Mullen *et al.* (1987), Zimmerman and Venberg (1994) and others have concluded that intention measures should be included in research attempting to identify the cognitive precursors of health behaviours and this has been supported by empirical studies. King (1982), for example, found that intention was the best predictor of hypertension screening using an extended HBM, and Warwick, Terry and Gallois (1993) reported that the effects of health beliefs on a subsequent measure of condom use at last intercourse were entirely mediated by an intention measure.

The TRA has three theoretical advantages over the HBM. First, the empirically-supported proposal that intentions mediate the effects of beliefs on behaviour provides a parsimonious model of how (frequently contradictory) beliefs culminate in a decision (that is, an intention) to act. Secondly, the focus on action-specific cognitive measures shifts attention from general representations of illness to representations of particular behaviours and enhances behavioural prediction. Thirdly, the theory acknowledges the impact of social influence on individual behaviour through the subjective norm measure. The TRA also allows a number of key HBM beliefs, in particular, perceived benefits, perceived barriers and perceived severity to be included as components of the attitude measure. Each of these beliefs refer to the perceived likelihood of the consequences of taking or not taking action. Perceived personal susceptibility to illness may not be as easily translated into a component of attitude measures and may, therefore, need to be added to TRA conceptions of the prerequisites of health behaviours (e.g. Vallie *et al.*, 1993).

PERCEPTIONS OF CONTROL

The importance of perceived control to preventive health behaviour has been highlighted in research into "health locus of control" (HLOC) based on the work of Rotter (1966) and Wallston and Wallston (1978). Rotter distinguished between two types of causal understandings; internal attributions in which an event is perceived as being caused by the person themselves, and external attributions when the cause is perceived to be outside the person's control. He also proposed that people tended to favour one of these explanation types and could be categorised as "internals" or "externals". Internals believe their own actions shape their experience, while externals see events as beyond their personal control. Applying this to health behaviour, it was proposed that internals were more likely to take responsibility for their health and so be more likely to take preventive action. Early work suggested that patients also distinguish between having personal control over their health and feeling that powerful others such as doctors can control their health (Wallston & Wallston, 1978). Wallston, Wallston and DeVellis (1978) then developed the multidimensional health locus of control (MHLC) scales which measure the extent to which people attribute their health to internal factors such as their own action, to the actions of powerful others or to chance.

Although a number of studies have shown that those with higher internal scores on the MHLC scales are more likely to take preventive behaviour, the overall pattern of evidence is inconsistent (see Norman & Bennett, 1996 for a review; Wallston & Wallston, 1982). Attempts to improve the utility of locus of control measures have included the development of behaviour-specific scales. For example, Kelly *et al.* (1990) found that gay men who explained HIV infection in terms of luck, on an AIDS-specific health locus of control scale, were more likely to engage in unprotected anal intercourse. The development of behaviour-specific locus of control scales can be seen as analogous to the employment of action-specific cognition measures in the TRA (Fishbein & Ajzen, 1975). Unlike the TRA, however, locus of control measures are not based on a cognitive theory of action regulation which links attributions directly to behaviour. Therefore, even when such attributional patterns convincingly predict health outcomes, the means by which they do so remain speculative (see Peterson *et al.*, 1988).

Bandura's (1989, 1992) articulation of self-efficacy mechanisms offers theoretical clarification of the potential links between perceived control and health behaviour. Bandura has argued that perceived self-efficacy, the belief that one can successfully perform a specified behaviour, affects motivation and behavioural control during performance. Those who believe they will succeed are more likely to; formulate intentions to act, set themselves higher goals, exert greater effort, regard errors and failures as learning experiences and persevere for longer. They are also less likely to be distracted by high anxiety and self-doubt during performance.

It has been proposed that beliefs about the causes of events may affect preventive health behaviour through their impact on perceived self-efficacy (Bandura, 1992). For example, those attributing previous failure to a lack of ability or previous success to luck may have reduced confidence in their ability to succeed in future. This view is supported by studies which show that the effects of attributions on behaviour are mediated by perceived self-efficacy scores (Bandura, 1992; Hospers, Kok & Stecher, 1990; Kok *et al.*, 1992). However, attributions may also affect other cognitions. For example, a person who attributes infection to bad luck or understands disease in terms of genetic inheritance may have little faith in the effectiveness of suggested precautions. Such perceived response-efficacy can be measured as a part of the attitudinal component of the TRA and might be expected to affect intention formation (King, 1982).

Self-efficacy beliefs have been found to be associated with the successful performance of a range of preventive health behaviours including exercise, condom use and smoking (Bandura, 1992; Schwarzer, 1992; Schwarzer & Fuchs, 1996). Their importance has been acknowledged by their inclusion in a reformulation of the HBM (Rosenstock, Strecher & Becker, 1988) and the addition of a very similar concept to the TRA. Ajzen and Madden (1986) tested a revised TRA (the theory of planned behaviour), which included a measure of "perceived behavioural control" which was found to have direct effects on behaviour as well as indirect effects through intention formation. Perceived self-efficacy has been distinguished from perceived behavioural control by the use of references to the self in measures of the former. In other words, measures of perceived self-efficacy explicitly refer the individual's action-specific confidence, that is, the ease or difficulty with which they think they could accomplish a task, while measures of perceived behavioural control may refer to beliefs about the general ease or difficulty of a task (Schwarzer, 1992). In practice, however, many researchers regard the two constructs as identical and tend to favour explicitly self-referencing measures of the kind used to assess perceived self-efficacy.

Combining perceived self-efficacy with TRA results in a sophisticated cognition model of how intention-formation and performance appraisal direct behaviour. Studies using this combined model have found that both intention and perceived self-efficacy have powerful effects on future behaviour. For example, in a study of smoking onset, De Vries, Backbier, Kok and Dijkstra (1995) found that intention measures were able to account for 39% of variance in reported smoking (with biochemical validation) twelve months later while perceived self-efficacy measures did not add to the variance explained. By contrast, Schwarzer and Fuchs (1996) found that intention and perceived self-efficacy were equally strong predictors of reported healthy eating measured six months later, with approximately 20% of the variance being explained by measures of intention, perceived self-efficacy, beliefs about the health consequences of healthy eating and perceived susceptibility to heart attack and stroke.

Perceived self-efficacy can be modified in laboratory settings and such changes affect subsequent behaviour (Cervone, 1989). This suggests that enhancing perceived self-efficacy would be an effective health promotion strategy. Ewart (1992) has shown that self-efficacy scores can be increased amongst post myocardial infarction patients using follow-up consultations involving treadmill exercising, interpretation of results by a cardiologist and counselling by a doctor and nurse. Perceived self-efficacy scores assessed immediately after treadmill exercising were also found to be better predictors of subsequent exercise adherence than heart rate measures during treadmill exercising. Such results suggest that perceived self-efficacy can be enhanced and is predictive of preventive health behaviour. It is worth noting, however, that mistaken beliefs about the effectiveness of precautions combined with high perceived self-efficacy could have negative effects by encouraging ineffective preventive action. For example, perceived self-efficacy in relation to assessment of partner HIV-risk-status through questioning has been found to be associated with higher levels of unprotected intercourse amongst students (O'Leary *et al.*, 1992).

REPRESENTATIONS OF ANTICIPATED EMOTION

An important anticipated consequence of undertaking any preventive health action is how one will feel during it, after completing it or after failing to complete it. Cognitive representations of affect can have important effects on planning, emotion felt during action and action control (Bagozzi, 1992; Fiske, 1981). Some researchers have, therefore, developed measures of anticipated affect which particularly highlight these effects. For example, socially learned emotional responses to sexuality have been related to condom use. Higher sex guilt has been found to be associated with unprotected sex (Gerrard, 1982) and greater acceptance and comfort with sexuality, as measured by "erotophilia-erotophobia" scales, has been shown to be associated with greater condom use even when the effects of intention are accounted for (Fisher, 1984). However, the most impressive findings have been reported in relation to measures of anticipated regret (Janis & Mann, 1977). Richard, van der Pligt and De Vries (1995) have shown that adding anticipated regret measures to those specified by the theory of planned behaviour increases the variance explained in condom use expectations (which can be regarded as a measure of intention — see Sheppard *et al.* 1988). They have also found that reported anticipated regret is related to subsequent condom use. Students received a questionnaire asking how they would expect to feel after sexual intercourse with an attractive partner if they (i) had used a condom and (ii) had not used a condom. Respondents were more likely to report anticipated negative affect when asked to focus on how they would feel after intercourse without a condom. Moreover, respondents expressing higher anticipated regret were more likely to expect to use condoms in subsequent sexual encounters and more likely to report having used a condom with new partners during the five months following initial data collection (Richard, van der Pligt & De Vries, 1996). Successful replications of interventions using anticipated regret prompts could confirm the potential of this approach for health promotion campaigns.

REPRESENTATIONS OF ACTION PROMPTS AND CONTEXTS

Self-report measures of attitude, subjective norm, intention, perceived self-efficacy and anticipated regret have all proved useful in distinguishing between those who do and do not engage in preventive health behaviour. These measures do not, however, capture the detail of our experience of action planning, particularly in the case of new action sequences. Cognitive modelling influenced by artificial intelligence (e.g. Miller, Galanter & Pribram, 1960) and clinical practice (e.g. Meichenbaum, 1977) has emphasised the hierarchical nature of goal-directed behaviour and the need to translate goals and intentions into context-related sub-routines to ensure successful performance. The importance of planning and cognitive rehearsal of action sequences, as well as self-instruction during action have been recognised as prerequisites of behaviour change by cognitive-behaviour therapists (e.g. Meichenbaum, 1977).

Recent theoretical and empirical work in social cognition has emphasized the importance of assessing individual differences in planning and rehearsal in relation to specified behaviours. Schwarzer (1992), for example, has outlined a new model based on perceived self-efficacy and the theory of planned behaviour; the Health Action Process Approach. The model suggests that measures of perceived susceptibility and perceived severity should be explicitly added to the TRA framework and distinguishes between measures which assess the progress towards intention formation and those relating to processes involved in the translation of intentions into action. These latter "action phase" processes include the formulation of action plans, specific action control perceptions and perceptions of contextual factors which may constrain or facilitate action (including social support in the action context). No guidelines for operationalising these action phase measures have been provided and further empirical work will be required to assess whether the Health Action Process Approach provides a better framework for the prediction of preventive health behaviour than the theory of planned behaviour.

Bagozzi (1992) also addresses the translation of intentions into action in his Volitional Model of Goal-Directed Behaviours. This model highlights the means, behavioural sub-routines or "instrumental acts" which constitute the enactment of intentions. Planning and control of such instrumental acts and investing the commitment and effort necessary to ensure their completion are viewed as prerequisites of goal achievement. Bagozzi proposes that cognitions included in the theory of planned behaviour should be measured in relation to specific instrumental acts, in particular; (i) the perceived effectiveness of identified means (for example, how effective a smoking-cessation strategy is planning not to buy cigarettes and/or resolving to ask one's smoking friends not to give one cigarettes?), (ii) perceived self-efficacy in relation to specific means (for example, how difficult does the respondent think it will be to resist buying cigarettes and/or insist that his/her friends do not share their cigarettes in social settings?) and (iii) anticipated affective reactions to the means themselves (for example, anticipated anxiety, embarrassment or rejection). It is possible to see these proposals as an extension of Fishbein and Ajzen's (1975) recommendations regarding the specificity of attitude and intention measures. Viewed in this way, Bagozzi's proposals serve to remind us that many preventive health behaviours are actually complex sequences of instrumental acts about which people may hold inconsistent views. Therefore, cognition measures should refer specifically to these instrumental acts. For example, the cognition measures which are most closely related to intentions to carry and use condoms may differ and these relationships may be different for men and women (Abraham *et al.*, 1992).

Bagozzi (1992) argues that the likelihood of performing a particular instrumental act (such as asking one's friends not to share their cigarettes) depends upon the individual's commitment to that act. He defines commitment as emotional attachment to and ego preoccupation with the specific intention and suggests that it could be measured by self-report statements such as "I cannot imagine changing my intention to do X" and "My intention is well thought through". Commitment, then, appears to be a strength of intention measure and can be usefully compared to previous work on attitude strength measures. Measures such as self-reported confidence in an attitude have been found to correlate with the speed of response to inquiries concerning that particular attitude (Eagly & Chaiken, 1993). Moreover, those given multiple opportunities to rehearse their attitudes and those whose attitudes are based on direct experience with the attitudinal object respond more quickly to attitudinal enquiries (Fazio *et al.*, 1982). The time taken to respond to an attitudinal enquiry appears to be a marker of attitudinal strength or attitude accessibility in working memory and people with more accessible attitudes are more likely to act in an attitude-congruent manner when the opportunity presents itself (Fazio & Williams, 1986). Fazio and colleagues conclude that rehearsal and direct experience strengthen attitudes by making them more accessible in memory and, therefore, more likely to be automatically retrieved (without deliberation) in response to relevant contextual cues such as inquiries or opportunities to act in an attitude-relevant manner. Eagly and Chaiken (1993) suggest that Fazio's work can be regarded as supplementary to the theory of planned behaviour, explaining why some attitudes have priority over others in the intention formation process. However, it also offers insights into the plausible mechanisms by which one intention may be prioritised over another in the generation of action.

Gollwitzer (1993) has conducted further work on the way in which action planning and rehearsal may affect the relationship between intention and behaviour. He proposes that before intentions are enacted they are translated into "implementation intentions" specifying when and where a particular act is to be undertaken. The idea of act-specific intentions is similar to Bagozzi's (1992) concept of instrumental acts but also incorporates Schwarzer's (1992) suggestion that the representation of context is important in the translation of intentions into action. In a similar fashion to Fazio and colleagues, Gollwitzer (1993) proposes that those who have elaborated their intentions by formulating implementation intentions are more likely to retrieve their intentions once the context specified in their implementation intentions is encountered. It also seems possible that the formation of implementation intentions is itself a marker for commitment or intention strength. Gollwitzer has shown that those who have formed implementation intentions are better able to recall presented descriptions of the means to carry out an action, more likely to identify environmental cues relevant to their planned action and faster to initiate action in response to situational prompts. Applying this idea to health promotion, Orbell, Hodgekins and Sheeran (1996) found that women who completed a questionnaire inviting them to say when and where they would perform breast self-examination during the subsequent month (i.e. inviting them to form implementation intentions) were considerably more likely, than those who completed a questionnaire without these items, to report having undertaken breast self examination at follow up.

Gollwitzer (1993) notes that the differences in speed of response between those who have and have not formed implementation intentions is similar in some respects to observed differences between people who have had direct experience of the behaviour in question and those who have not. This suggests that rehearsal which prompts elaboration of intentions into context-related implementation intentions referring to specific instrumental acts may promote action by enhancing the accessibility of these context-related instrumental intentions. Indeed Orbell *et al.* (1996) suggest that, in certain cases, simple questions prompting further context-specific planning may increase the likelihood preventive health action. These are encouraging findings but further work on the capacity of self-assessed planning and rehearsal measures to predict the translation of intentions into behaviour and on the use of planning prompts to stimulate behaviour change is required to ascertain the power of these techniques.

DECIDING AND ACTING: COGNITIVE STAGES OR INTER-RELATED PROCESSES?

Recent work on conceptualising the elaboration of goal-related intentions (such as quitting smoking) into context-related act-specific intention sequences (such as not buying cigarettes with the morning paper tomorrow) has led some researchers to view intention formation as cognitively distinct from the translation of intentions into action (Schwarzer, 1992; Weinstein, 1988). The Health Action Approach Model, for example, explicitly distinguishes between the cognitive processes culminating in intention formation (which are the focus of the theory of planned behaviour) and action phase cognitions which account for the translation of intentions into behaviour. This parallels the growing use of stage models of behaviour change in addiction research (e.g. Prochaska, DiClemente & Norcross, 1992) and has already resulted in the development of behaviour-specific stage models such as the AIDS Risk Reduction Model (Catania, Kegeles & Coates, 1990).

Despite the popularity of the stages of change concept, there appears to be little empirical evidence suggesting that people progress towards action or behaviour change through distinct cognitive stages. Sutton (1996), for example, has questioned the empirical support for Prochaska and DiClemente's transtheoretical model (Prochaska *et al.*, 1992) which is one of the most widely cited stage models. He points out that smokers' self reports, collected every six months over two years (Prochaska *et al.*, 1992) reveal that only 16% progressed, without regression, from one stage to the next and that none progressed, without regression, through more than two stages. He also notes that self-help smoking cessation manuals matched to the individual's self-reported stage of change were no more successful in promoting prolonged cessation than standardised manuals (Prochaska, DiClemente & Rossi, 1993). It may, therefore, be premature to view behaviour change as a series of cognitive plateaux linked by distinctive psychological pathways.

Viewed from an information processing perspective, it seems implausible that rehearsal or observational learning which strengthens attitudes towards a behaviour will not also affect the elaboration of intentions. There is also evidence that counter-attitudinal behaviour promotes attitude change (e.g., Fazio, Zanna & Cooper, 1977), suggesting that 'action-phase' change may prompt changes in 'motivational-stage' cognitions. Therefore, although we can identify distinct self-report measures (such as attitudes and implementation intentions) and describe their separate associations with specific health behaviours, it is unlikely that they map onto discrete cognitive sequences which follow one another in a progressive manner. Self-report measures are more likely to be broad indicators of an individual's overall cognitive preparedness to undertake specified behaviours in particular contexts.

This does not mean that health promotion work should not be based on cognitive assessments of target audiences. It is useful to identify target audiences who are already persuaded of the need to take preventive action when this action is perceived as having few costs and is easy to manage. In such cases health promotion initiatives or legislation (e.g. Robertson, 1986) may facilitate widespread adoption by enhancing access or providing incentives. There is also considerable evidence that particular cognitive measures are predictive of health behaviour so that self-reports can be used to reveal the extent of attitudinal, normative or action-facilitating change which may be required to generate behaviour change within a particular target population. However, it seems unlikely that these measures will be able to differentiate between individuals in discrete cognitive states which can be predictably altered using stage-specific interventions.

CONCLUSIONS

The social cognition models reviewed here define a set of self-report cognition measures which can be used to identify those most in need of educational interventions and to specify psychological characteristics demonstrably associated with preventive health behaviour which should be targeted by educational initiatives. The theory of reasoned action suggests that attitudes towards specific behaviours (operationalised as the perceived likelihood and value of expected outcomes) and subjective norm measures (operationalised as the perceived views of others whose approval is valued) will be related to behaviour through intention. Intention can be measured using self-reports of how much one intends to act and how strong one's certainty or commitment is to this intention. It has also been suggested that particular outcome expectancies be added to the theory; perceived severity, perceived susceptibility and the extent to which regret is anticipated if preventive action is not taken. Perceived self-efficacy has also been found to be associated with intention formation and behavioural performance. Finally, planning and cognitive rehearsal may facilitate action. In particular, the formulation of implementation intentions which link performance to specific contextual cues may render action more likely. Collectively these constructs provide a model of the cognitive prerequisites of specific context-related action. The model highlights the kind of information which might be persuasive and identifies some of the psychological components of skilled performance.

Ideally, health promotion should proceed by identifying which cognition measures are most closely associated with the target behaviour amongst particular populations. Different preventive behaviours may be related in different ways to cognition measures. For example, Bagozzi and Kimmel (1995) point out that dieting is typically 'event-initiated' because external events determine when one should implement one's dieting intentions and action follows more or less immediately. Exercising, by contrast, is 'self-initiated' and requires planning and preparation. Similarly, some preventive behaviour may involve eradicating or replacing old routines (such as smoking cessation or dieting), while others (such as dental flossing) may only involve making time to set up new behavioural routines. Such differences in the target behaviour may alter the predictive power of particular cognitions for particular behaviours. Differences in the relationships between cognition measures and preventive behaviour patterns may also be observed between different groups, so that group-specific educational campaigns may be most effective.

This complexity suggests that effective health educational interventions may require substantial planning and preparatory research (Mullen, Green & Persinger, 1985). Unfortunately, however, many interventions are not theoretically-based and not grounded in research into the preparedness of target audiences (e.g., Fisher & Fisher, 1992). They may, therefore, employ general educational strategies (such as information provision, fear appeals or the promotion of general self-esteem) which do not target the most important prerequisites of preventive action (Kok, 1993). Further co-operation between social cognition researchers and health promotion practitioners could enhance the effectiveness of many health promotion campaigns.

REFERENCES

Abraham, C. & Hampson, S.E. (1996) A social cognition approach to health psychology, *Psychology and Health*, **11**, 233–241.

Abraham, C. & Sheeran P. (1994). Modelling and modifying young heterosexuals' HIV-preventive behaviour; a review of theories, findings and educational implications. *Patient Education and Counselling*, **23**, 173–186.

Abraham, C., Sheeran, P., Spears, R. & Abrams, D. (1992) Health beliefs and the adoption of HIV-preventive intentions among teenagers; a Scottish perspective. *Health Psychology*, **11**, 363–370.

Abraham, C., Sheeran, P., Abrams, D. & Spears, R. (1994) Exploring teenagers' adaptive and maladaptive thinking in relation to the threat of HIV infection. *Psychology and Health*, **9**, 247–266.

Abraham, C., Sheeran, P., Abrams, D. & Spears, R. (1996) Health beliefs and teenage condom use; a prospective study. *Psychology and Health*, **11**.

Adler, N.E., Boyce, T., Chesney M.A., Cohen S., Folkman, S., Kahn, R.L. & Syme, S.L. (1994) Socio-economic status and health: The challenge of the gradient, *American Psychologist*, **49**, 15–24.

Adler, N. & Matthews, K. (1994) Health Psychology: Why do some people get sick and some stay well. *Annual Review of Psychology*, **45**, 229–259.

Ajzen, I. (1988) *Attitudes, personality and behaviour*. Milton Keynes, Open University Press.

Ajzen, I. & Madden, T.J. (1986) Prediction of goal-directed behaviour: attitudes, intentions and perceived behavioural control. *Journal of Experimental Social Psychology*, **22**, 453–474.

Bagozzi, R.P. (1992) The self-regulation of attitudes, intentions and behaviour. *Social Psychology Quarterly*, **55**, 178–204.

Bagozzi, R.P. & Kimmel, S.K. (1995) A comparison of leading theories for the prediction of goal-directed behaviours. *British Journal of Social Psychology*, **34**, 437–461.

Bandura, A. (1989) Perceived self-efficacy in the exercise of personal agency. *The Psychologist*, **2**, 411–424.

Bandura, A. (1992) Exercise of personal agency through the self-efficacy mechanism. In R. Schwarzer (Ed.), *Self-efficacy: thought control of action* (pp. 3–38). Washington: Hemisphere Publishing Corporation.

Becker, M.H. & Maiman, L.A. (1975) Sociobehavioural determinants of compliance with health and medical care recommendations. *Medical Care*, **13**, 10–24.

Boyd, B. & Wandersman, A. (1991) Predicting undergraduate condom use with the Fishbein and Ajzen and the Triandis attitude-behaviour models: implications for public health interventions. *Journal of Applied Social Psychology*, **21**, 1810–1830.

Breslow, L. & Enstrom, J.E. (1980) Persistence of health habits and their relationship to mortality. *Preventive Medicine*, **9**, 469–483.

Carey, J.W. (1992) Linking qualitative and quantitative methods; integrating cultural factors into public health. *Qualitative Health Research*, **3**, 298–318.

Carroll, D., Bennett, P. & Davey Smith, G. (1993) Socio-economic health inequalities: their origins and implications. *Psychology and Health*, **8**, 295–316.

Catania, J.A., Kegeles, S.M. & Coates, T.J. (1990) Towards an understanding of risk behaviour: An AIDS Risk Reduction Model (ARRM). *Health Education Quarterly*, **17**, 247–261.

Cervone, D. (1989) Effects of envisioning future activities on self-efficacy judgements and motivation: an availability heuristic interpretation. *Cognitive Therapy and Research*, **13**, 247–261.

Cialdini, R.B., Kallgren, C.A. & Reno, R.R. (1991) A focus theory of normative conduct; a theoretical refinement and re-evaluation of the role of norms in human behaviour. *Advances in Experimental Social Psychology*, **24**, 201–234.

Conner, M. & Norman, P. (1996) *Predicting health behaviour: research and practice with social cognition models*. Buckingham: Open University Press.

De Vries, H., Backbier, E., Kok H. & Dijkstra, M. (1995) The impact of social influences in the context of attitude, self-efficacy, intention and previous behaviour as predictors of smoking onset. *Journal of Applied Social Psychology*, **25**, 237–257.

Davis, J.B. & Best, D.W. (1995) Demand characteristics and research into drug use, *Psychology and Health*, **10**, 291–299.

Earley, P.C. (1993) East meets west meets mideast: Further explorations of collectivistic and individualistic work groups. *Academy of Management Journal*, **36**, 319–348.

Eagly, A.H. & Chaiken, S. (1993) *The psychology of attitudes*. Fort Worth: Harcourt Brace Jovanovich.

Ewart, C.K. (1992) Role of physical self-efficacy in recovery from heart attack. In R. Schwarzer (Ed.), *Self-efficacy: thought control of action* (pp. 217–243). Washington: Hemisphere Publishing Corporation.

Farr, R.M. (1977) Heider, Harré and Herzlich on health and illness. Some observations on the structure of 'représentations collectives'. *European Journal of European Social Psychology*, **7**, 491–504.

Fazio, R.H., Chen, J., McDonel, E.C. & Sherman S.J. (1982) Attitude accessibility, attitude-behaviour consistency and the strength of object-evaluation association. *Journal of Experimental Social Psychology*, **18**, 339–357.

Fazio, R.H. & Williams C.J. (1986) Attitude accessibility as a moderator of attitude-perception and attitude-behaviour relations: an investigation of the 1984 presidential election. *Journal of Personality and Social Psychology*, **51**, 505–514.

Fazio, R.H., Zanna, M.P. & Cooper, J. (1977) Dissonance versus self-perception: an integrative view of each theory's proper domain of application. *Journal of Experimental Social Psychology*, **13**, 464–479.

Fishbein, M. & Ajzen, I. (1975) *Belief, attitude, intention and behaviour: an introduction to theory and research*. Reading MA: Addison-Wesley.

Fisher, W.A. (1984) Predicting contraceptive behaviour among university men: the role of emotions and behavioural intentions. *Journal of Applied Social Psychology*, **14**, 104–123.

Fisher, J.D. & Fisher W.A. (1992) Changing AIDS risk behaviour. *Psychological Bulletin*, **111**, 455–474.

Fiske, S.T. (1981) Social cognition and affect. In J. Harvey (Ed.), *Cognition, social behaviour and the environment*. Hillsdale, New Jersey: Lawrence Erlbaum.

Gerrard, M. (1982) Sex, sex guilt and contraceptive use. *Journal of Personality and Social Psychology*, **42**, 153–158.

Glasgow, R.E., Mullooly, J.P., Vogt, T.M., Stevens, V.J., Lichtenstein, E., Hollis, J.F., Lando, H.A., Severson, H.H., Pearson, K.A. & Vogt, M.R. (1993) Biochemical validation of smoking status: Pros, cons and data from four low intensity intervention trials. *Addictive Behaviors*, **18**, 511–527.

Gollwitzer, P.M. (1993) Goal achievement: the role of intentions. *European Review of Social Psychology*, **4**, 142–185.

Harrison, J.A., Mullen, P.D. & Green, L.W. (1992) A meta-analysis of studies of the health belief model with adults. *Health Education Research*, **7**, 107–116.

Haefner, D.P. & Kirscht, J.P. (1970) Motivational and behavioural effects of modifying health beliefs. *Public Health Reports*, **85**, 478–484.

Herzlich, C. (1973) *Health and illness; a social psychological analysis* (trans. D. Graham). London: Academic Press.

Hein, H.O., Suadicani, P. & Gyntelberg, F. (1992) Ischaemic heart disease incidence by social class and form of smoking: the

Copenhagen Male Study — 17 years follow-up. *Journal of Internal Medicine*, **231**, 477–483.

Hospers, H.J., Kok, G.J. & Stecher, V.J. (1990) Attributions for previous failures and subsequent outcomes in a weight reduction program. *Health Education Quarterly*, **17**, 409–415.

Janis, I.L. & Mann, L. (1977) *Decision making: A psychological analysis of conflict, choice and commitment.* New York: Free Press.

Janz, N. & Becker, M.H. (1984) The health belief mode: A decade later. *Health Education Quarterly*, **11**, 1–47.

Jones, P.K., Jones, S.L. & Katz, J. (1987) Improving compliance for asthma patients visiting the emergency department using a health belief model intervention. *Journal of Asthma*, **24**, 199–206.

Kelly, J.A., St. Lawrence, J.S., Brasfield, T.L., Lemke, A., Amidei, T., Roffman, R.E., Hood, H.V., Kilgore, H., Smith, J.E. & McNeill Jr., C. (1990) Psychological factors that predict AIDS high-risk versus AIDS precautionary behaviour. *Journal of Consulting and Clinical Psychology*, **58**, 117–120.

King, J.B. (1982) The impact of patients' perceptions of high blood pressure on attendance at screening: an attributional extension of the health belief Model. *Social Science Medicine,* **16**, 1079–1091.

Kok, G. (1993) Why are so many health promotion programs ineffective? *Health Promotion Journal of Australia*, **3**, 12–17.

Kok, H., Dan Boer, D., De Vries H., Gerards, F., Hospers H.J. & Mudde A.N. (1992) Self-efficacy and attribution theory in health education. In R. Schwarzer (Ed.), *Self-efficacy: thought control of action* (pp. 246–262). Washington: Hemisphere Publishing Corporation.

Ley, P. (1988) *Communicating with patients: improving communication, satisfaction and compliance.* London: Croom Helm.

Marmot, M.G., Smith, G.D., Stansfield, S., Patel, C., North, F., Head, J. White, I. Brunner, E. & Feeney, A. (1991) Health inequalities among British civil servants: the Whitehall II study. *Lancet*, **337**, 1387–1393.

Meichenbaum, D. (1977) *Cognitive, behaviour modification: An integrative approach.* New York: Plenum Press.

Miller, G.A., Galanter, E. & Pribram, K.H. (1960) *Plans and the structure of behaviour.* New York: Holt.

Moscovici, S. (1981) On social representations. In J.P. Forgas (Ed.), *Social cognition: Perspectives on everyday understanding* (pp. 181–209). London: Academic Press.

Mullen, P.D., Green, L.W. & Persinger, G. (1985) Clinical trials for patient education for chronic conditions: a comparative meta-analysis of intervention types. *Preventive Medicine,* **14**, 753–781.

Mullen, P.D. Hersey, J.C. & Iverson, D.C. (1987) Health behaviour models compared. *Social Science and Medicine,* **24**, 973–983.

Norman, P. & Bennett, P. (1996) Health locus of control. In M. Conner & P. Norman (Eds.), *Predicting health behaviour: research and practice with social cognition models* (pp. 62–94). Buckingham, UK: Open University Press.

Oettingen, G. (1995) Cross-cultural perspectives on self-efficacy. In A. Bandura (Ed.), *Self-efficacy in changing societies* (pp. 149–176). Cambridge: Cambridge University Press.

O'Leary, A., Goodhart, F., Jemmott, L.S. & Boccher-Lattimore, D. (1992) Predictors of safer sexual behaviour on the college campus; a social cognitive theory analysis. *Journal of American College Health,* **40**, 254–263.

Orbell, S., Hodgekins, S. & Sheeran P. (1996) Implementation intentions and the theory of planned behaviour. Manuscript submitted for publication.

Peterson, C., Seligman, M.E.P. & Vaillant, G.E. (1988) Pessimistic explanatory style is a risk factor for physical illness: A thirty-five-year longitudinal study. *Journal of Personality and Social Psychology,* **55**, 23–27.

Prochaska, J.O., DiClemente, C.C. & Norcross, J.C. (1992) In search of how people change, applications to addictive behaviours. *American Psychologist,* **47**, 1102–1114.

Prochaska, J.O., DiClemente, C.C. & Rossi, J.S. (1993) Standardised, individualized, interactive and personalized self-help programs for smoking cessation. *Health Psychology,* **12**, 399–405.

Prochaska, J.O., Velicer, W., Guadagnoli, E., Rossi, J.S. & DiClemente, C.C. (1991) Patterns of change: dynamic topology applied to smoking cessation. *Multivariate Behavioural Research,* **26**, 83–107.

Richard, R. & van der Pligt, J. (1991) Factors affecting condom use among adolescents. *Journal of Community and Applied Social Psychology,* **1**, 105–116.

Richard, R., van der Pligt, J. & De Vries, N. (1995) Anticipated affective reactions and prevention of AIDS. *British Journal of Social Psychology,* **34**, 9–21.

Richard, R., van der Pligt, J. & De Vries, N. (1996) Affective reactions and time perspective; Changing sexual risk-taking behaviour. Manuscript submitted for publication.

Robertson, L.S. (1986) Behavioural and environmental interventions for reducing motor vehicle trauma. *Annual Review of Public Health*, **7**, 13–34.

Rosenstock, I.M. (1974) Historical origins of the health belief model. *Health Education Monographs*, **2**, 1–8.

Rosenstock, I.M., Strecher, V.J. & Becker, M.H. (1988) Social learning theory and the health belief model. *Health Education Quarterly*, **15**, 175–183.

Rosenthal, R. & Rubin D.B. (1982) A simple general purpose display of magnitude of experimental effect. *Journal of Educational Psychology*, **74**, 166–169.

Rotter, J.B. (1966) Generalized expectancies for internal versus external control of reinforcement. *Psychological Monographs*, **80**, (1, Whole No 609).

Schaalma, H., Kok, G., Bosker, R., Parcel, G., Peters, L., Poelman, J. & Reinders, J. (in press). Short-term effects of a systematically developed school-based AIDS/STD education for secondary school students in the Netherlands. *Health Education Quarterly*.

Schwarzer, R. (1992) Self-efficacy in the adoption and maintenance of health behaviours: theoretical approaches and a new model. In R. Schwarzer (Ed.), *Self-efficacy: thought control of action* (pp. 217–243). Washington: Hemisphere Publishing Corporation.

Schwarzer, R. & Fuchs, R. (1996) Self-efficacy and health behaviours: theoretical approaches and a new model. In M. Conner & P. Norman (Eds.), *Predicting health behaviour: research and practice with social cognition models* (pp. 163–196). Buckingham UK: Open University Press.

Sheeran, P. & Abraham, C. (1995) Measurement of condom use in 72 studies of HIV-preventive behaviour: a critical review. *Patient Education and Counselling*, **24**, 199–216.

Sheeran, P. & Abraham, C. (1996) The health belief model. In M. Conner & P. Norman (Eds.), *Predicting health behaviour; research and practice with social cognition models* (pp. 23–61). Buckingham UK: Open University Press.

Sheppard, B.H., Hartwick, J. & Warshaw, P.R. (1988) The theory of reasoned action: a meta-analysis of past research with recommendations for modifications and future research. *Journal of Consumer Research*, **15**, 325–343

Sontag, S. (1988) *AIDS and its metaphors*. Penguin Books, London.

Steckler, A., McLeroy, K.R., Goodman, R.M., Bird, S.T. & McCormick, L. (1992) Towards integrating qualitative and quantitative methods; an introduction. *Health Education Quarterly*, **19**, 1–8.

Sutton, S. (1996) Can 'stages of change' provide guidance in the treatment of addictions? A critical examination of Prochaska and DiClemente's model. In G. Edwards & C. Dare (Eds.), *Psychotherapy, psychological treatments and the addictions* (189–205). Cambridge: Cambridge University Press.

Vallie, M.S.B., Calnam, M., Rutter, D.R. & Wall, B. (1993) Breast cancer screening services in three areas: uptake and satisfaction. *Journal of Public Health Medicine*, **15**, 37–45.

van den Putte, B. (1991) 20 years of the theory of reasoned action of Fishbein and Ajzen: a meta analysis. Unpublished manuscript, University of Amsterdam, The Netherlands.

van der Velde, F.W., Hookyaas, C. & van der Pligt, J. (1992) Risk perception and behaviour: pessimism, realism and optimism about AIDS-related health behaviour. *Psychology and Health*, **6**, 23–38.

van der Velde, F.W. & van der Pligt, J. (1991) AIDS-related health behaviour: coping, protection motivation and previous behaviour. *Journal of Behavioural Medicine*, **14**, 429–451.

Wallston, B.S. & Wallston, K.A. (1978) Locus of control and health: a review of the literature. *Health Education Monographs*, **6**, 107–117.

Wallston, K.A., Wallston, B.S. & DeVellis, R. (1978) Development of the control (MHLC) scales. *Health Education Monographs*, **6**, 160–170.

Wallston, K.A. & Wallston, B.S. (1982) Who is responsible for your health? The construct of locus of control. In G. S. Saunders & J. Suls (Eds.), *Social psychology of health and illness* (pp. 65–95). Hillsdale: Lawerence Erlbaum Associates.

Warwick, P., Terry, D. & Gallois, C. (1993). Extending the theory of reasoned action: the role of health beliefs. In D.J. Terry, C. Gallois & M. McCamish (Eds.), *The theory of reasoned action: its application to AIDS-preventive behaviour*. Oxford: Pergamon Press.

Weinstein, N.D. (1988) The precaution adoption process. *Health Psychology*, **7**, 355–386.

Wiedenfeld, S.A., O'Leary, A., Bandura, A., Brown, S., Levine, S. & Raska, K. (1990) The impact of perceived self-efficacy in coping with stressors on components of the immune system. *Journal of Personality and Social Psychology*, **59**, 1082–1094.

Wilkinson, R.G. (1990) Income distribution and life expectancy. *British Medical Journal*, **304**, 165–168.

Wurtele, S.K. & Maddux, J.E. (1987) Relative contributions of protection motivation theory components in predicting exercise intentions and behaviour. *Health Psychology*, **6**, 453–466.

Zimmerman, R.S. & Vernberg, D. (1994) Models of preventive health behaviour: Comparison, critique and meta-analysis. *Advances in Medical Sociology*, **4**, 45–67.

8

Illness Representations After The Human Genome Project: The Perceived Role of Genes in Causing Illness

Theresa M. Marteau & Vicky Senior*

Rapid developments in genetics have resulted in the identification of genes that predispose to many common conditions, including heart disease, breast cancer, multiple sclerosis, Alzheimer's and arthritis (Department of Health, 1995). Such information could be used to screen populations to identify those at increased risk of developing these conditions and in some instances offer medical treatments or behavioural advice.

Little is known about the psychological impact of these developments. How will greater knowledge of the genetic contribution to illness affect perceptions of that illness? How will people respond to screening programmes in which they will receive personalised risks based upon genetic testing for conditions that are not wholly determined by genes? Addressing these and other questions requires an understanding of how people conceptualise genetic, alongside other influences upon health and illness. While new information about

*Theresa Marteau is supported by the Wellcome Trust, Vicky Senior is supported by a studentship from the Medical Research Council, United Kingdom.

genetic predispositions to illness may influence many aspects of illness representations, it is likely to have most influence upon people's causal beliefs about illness, given that genetic information is specifically about causes. The focus of this chapter is therefore upon causal beliefs about illness.

The chapter is divided into two main sections. The first describes the content and structure of causal beliefs, focusing upon beliefs about inheritance and genetics. The second considers how these beliefs might change as a result of new information about the genetic determinants of multifactorial diseases. The consequences of perceiving genes to have a role in causing illness and recovery for what people do to reduce threats to their own health or to help others, are also considered. This chapter is written at a time when there has been relatively little research that directly addresses these issues. We therefore draw largely upon research in other areas to consider the research questions and methods that seem most promising for developing understanding of illness representations in the 21st century when the Human Genome Project will be complete. The Human Genome Project is the largest ever international scientific endeavour, the purpose of which is to map and sequence the entire human genome.

CAUSAL BELIEFS

People's beliefs about the causes of illness have been the focus of study in two psychological paradigms: attribution theory and the study of illness cognition. Attribution theory is concerned with the ways in which people formulate causal explanations for phenomena. Attributions about the causes of disease have been found to be associated with coping strategies and adjustments to health threats (Michela & Wood, 1986; Turnquist, Harvey & Anderson, 1988). Illness representations have been found in many studies to have five core components: beliefs about the cause of diseases, as well as identity, time-line, consequences and cure (Leventhal & Diefenbach, 1991).

The frequency of seeking causal explanations for threats, including health threats, varies with the severity of the threat: the more serious the outcome is perceived to be, the more likely people are to make causal attributions (Affleck *et al.*, 1987; Tennen, Affleck &

Gershman, 1986). The extent to which an event is unexpected also influences the extent to which people seek causal explanations (Wong & Weiner, 1981), as does the time since diagnosis (Turnquist, Harvey & Anderson, 1988) and the nature of the condition. For example, in a study of lay conceptions of genetic disorders, Shiloh and Berkenstadt (1992) found that causal beliefs did not figure prominently in lay representations. This may be because the cause of the condition is explicit in the label of the disease: genetic.

In summary, there is a large body of research documenting that, when people think about an illness, some of these thoughts will concern the causes of that illness. Such cognitions form part of the organised and stable cognitive representations of diseases which guide how people respond, behaviourally and emotionally to illness information (Bishop, 1991).

Causal beliefs have been conceptualised as reflecting core dimensions, such as the attributional dimensions of controllability, stability and internality (Weiner, 1971), or dimensions of internality, powerful others and chance, as assessed by the Mulitidimensional Health Locus of Control scale (Wallston, Wallston & DeVellis, 1978) and as particular causal agents (e.g., germs, pollution, genes: de Valle & Norman, 1992; Weinman *et al.,* 1996). Some investigators have attempted to look at the relationship between causal agents and dimensions, using factor analysis (e.g., Landrine & Klonoff, 1994; Lau & Hartman, 1983). The next two sections consider the content and the structure of causal beliefs, with particular reference to genetic influences.

Content of Causal Beliefs about Illness

Beliefs that some illnesses can "run in families" and that aspects of constitution can be inherited are well rooted in both medical and lay cultures in the West (Blaxter & Paterson, 1982; Davison, Frankel & Davey Smith, 1989). In a series of interviews with a sample of the general population in France, heredity was seen as the major determinant of health (Herzlich, 1973). In a UK study, heredity was seen as the third major cause of illness, after germs and lifestyle (Pill & Stott, 1986). There are, however, major differences in causal beliefs held by people in different parts of the world and within different cultural groups in the Western world. This is discussed in the section under social and cultural differences, later in this section. Much of the research by psychologists has been conducted on the dominant cultural group in the West, as reflected in this chapter.

The public see most illnesses as multifactorial in origin, encompassing environmental as well as genetic causes. This is the case both for what are traditionally thought of as purely genetic diseases and for diseases not traditionally associated with genes. In a study of families affected by a dominantly inherited condition that leads to bowel cancer, familial adenomatous polyposis, the great majority of those interviewed considered onset of the condition to be multifactorially determined (Michie, McDonald & Marteau, 1996). While inheriting a gene was seen as important, it was not considered sufficient for onset of the condition. This was expressed in various ways by participants in this study when asked what caused familial adenomatous polyposis:

> *I think the gene's already in you. I think you're born with it. I think everybody's got like cancerous cells, haven't they and I think maybe stress brings it out.*

> *I don't know. It could be born in your genes and it passes through generation to generation but you catch it I suppose ... I relate the catch it with the way that you live and your lifestyle and that I suppose ... I still seem to think it's, you know, keeping fit and the exercises, but I'm not too sure.*

One of the themes to emerge from this study was the reluctance of those who received low risk results from genetic testing to abandon regular bowel screening. In addition to the many cognitive, emotional and behavioural explanations already put forward for this (Michie *et al.*, 1996), a further explanation is that, given the multifactorial representation of this condition, a negative result on genetic testing may not be seen as sufficient to remove the threat of developing the condition. It may be difficult for patients to see how a blood test for a genetic marker provides credible evidence about a bowel condition. That is, the identity of the test and the condition may not match. Heart disease, until more recently, has been a condition presented in health education campaigns as largely behavioural in origin. Yet lay representations of the condition encompass strongly inheritance and lifestyle in the notion of a "coronary candi-

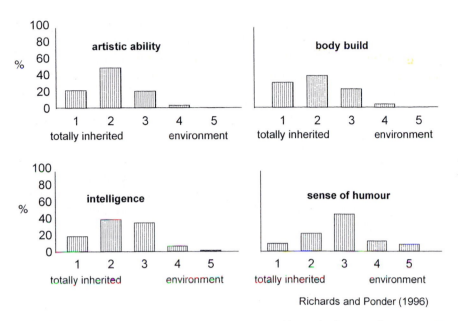

FIGURE 1   Perceived heritability and environmental basis for human characteristics

date" (Davison *et al.*, 1991). Most traits and human characteristics, such as artistic ability and a sense of humour, are also seen as multi-factorial in origin (Richards & Ponder, 1996: see Figure 1).

Caution, however, is needed in interpreting the results from this and other studies that have used similar measures to that used by Richards and Ponder (personal communication), such as those used in a recent public opinion survey (Gallup, 1995). Causal beliefs were assessed using a closed, as opposed to an open-ended, question to explore how people think about causes. A single scale was used to measure two dimensions: genetic and environmental influences. Placing these at each end of a scale provides an explicit model of causality: the more genes are influential in cause, the less important will be environmental influences. The issue here is not to do with scientific plausibility, but with how people conceptualise the interplay between genes and environment. People may well have an antagonistic representation of the interplay between genes and environment, as is implicit in the scale used. But we do not know if this is the case. Research is needed to determine how people conceptualise relationships between causes and from this, develop the appropriate methodologies for assessing these cognitions. As a beginning, it may be useful to distinguish between representations of inheritance, genes and genetic causes of illness. Possible methods for approaching this are discussed in the section on Methodological Issues, later in this chapter.

Representations of inheritance

Most people are familiar with the idea of inheriting character-istics from both parents. These beliefs diverge from a scientific Mendelian model in several important ways (Richards, 1996). For example, there is a widespread view amongst children that off-spring are more likely to take after the same sex parent (Clough & Wood-Robinson, 1985; Kargbo, Hobbs & Erickson, 1980). Implicit in many descriptions of inheritance is a belief that genes are inherited en masse so that an individual who is held to resemble in character or appearance those who had a disease, are also thought likely to develop the disease (Davison, Frankel & Davey Smith, 1989; Kessler, 1988). A further phenomenon described by Richards (1996) is that people overestimate shared inheritance with children and parents and underestimate shared inheritance with siblings, aunts or uncles. Richards provides some data to support the idea that the degree of perceived genetic connection is more a function of the closeness of the kin tie rather than the genetic closeness.

Representations of genes

While there are some good descriptions of how people represent inheritance, it would appear that many people do not have a concept of a process that links genes with the development of par-ticular characteristics (Richards, 1996). Even when people know that a disease in their family is inherited through a dominant gene, their conceptualisation of a gene may be less clear. When asked what genes do, members of families at risk for familial adenoma-tous polyposis were quite unclear (Michie *et al.*, 1996):

> ... *I don't understand genes.*

> ... *it's hard to think — because I never thought that much about it. I know it was a hereditary disease so I never really tried to analyse what it was and how it started.*

*To be honest, I don't know. All I know is, it is hereditary
and it's passed on like that. Why, I don't know.*

Cultural and Social Differences

While there are clearly documented differences in causal beliefs
across conditions, individuals vary in how they perceive causes for
the same condition. The sources of such individual differences have
been little studied. Gender differences may be one source. In a
recent survey, respondents were asked to state which of a list of illnesses they thought were hereditary, defined as "running in families" (Gallup, 1995). The perceived contribution of inheritance to the
cause of disease varied across conditions. Women, however, were
significantly more likely than men to perceive five of the six conditions shown as inherited, there being no difference between women
and men in their perceptions of the heritability of diabetes.

   In another study women were also found to be significantly
more likely than men to invoke heredity as a cause of illness
(Landrine & Klonoff, 1994). Such gender differences may reflect

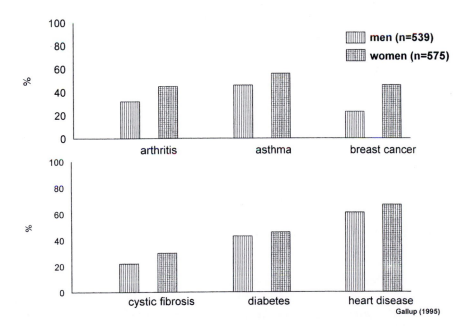

Gallup (1995)

FIGURE 2   Gender differences in perceptions of a genetic cause in six chronic
illnesses

greater knowledge amongst women, who have been described as the "genetic housekeepers" for families (Richards, 1996). Women often take the primary role within families in giving information about a genetic condition, even if they themselves are not at risk (e.g., Shakespeare, 1992). Another explanation is that men may perceive themselves as having more control than women and hence perceive the origins of disease to be more controllable, i.e., not genetic. These and other possible mediators or moderators of causal models of illness require study.

A further source of variation in causal beliefs is cultural background. Anthropological and sociological research suggests that there is considerable cultural diversity in beliefs about the causes of illness (Landrine & Klonoff, 1992, 1994). Much research in health psychology on causal beliefs has been informed by a Western cultural tradition in which illness is viewed as an "… episodic, intrapersonal deviation caused by microlevel, natural etiological agents such as genes, viruses, bacteria and stress" (Landrine & Klonoff, 1992). By contrast, non-Western cultural groups are more likely to view illnesses as entailing "… macrolevel, interpersonal and supernatural etiological agents" (Landrine & Klonoff, 1992). Thus, in Western groups illness is frequently attributed to diet, heredity, weight, smoking, alcohol use, stress and lack of exercise and other intrapersonal variables. Amongst non-Western groups, Landrine & Klonoff report five major etiological agents of illness: violations of interpersonal norms; violations of the demands and expectations of social roles; the emotions entailed in such transgressions (such as envy or jealousy, which are assumed to be illness provoking); violations of moral and religious taboos; and, quasi-natural agents such as types of food, the weather and various states of one's blood. Landrine and Klonoff suggest that the failure to consider non-Western causal beliefs in studies in the multicultural Western world accounts for the poor predictive power of scales such as the Multidimensional Health Locus of Control scale (Wallston *et al.*, 1978) and the Attributional Style Questionnaire (Peterson *et al.*, 1982). The extent to which the five etiological agents of disease emerge as distinct categories of causal beliefs remains to be determined. Research is also needed to test the hypothesis that the predictive power of the Multidimensional Health Locus of Control scale is increased if it is used to predict behaviour in the cultural group in which the scale was developed.

Structure of Causal Beliefs Concerning Genetic Causes of Illness

Turnquist, Harvey and Anderson (1988) observed that researchers have categorised attributions to inheritance and genes in all possible ways including coding it as "external" (e.g., DuCette & Keane, 1984), "internal" (e.g., Lowery, Jacobsen & Murphy, 1993), "other" (e.g., Abrams & Finesinger, 1953) or "chance" (e.g., Koslowsky, Croog & LaVoie, 1978). Such inconsistencies in conceptualising inheritance are likely to have obscured any consistencies across studies. Determining how people conceptualise the means by which individuals inherit characteristics and how genes cause illness within individuals, is a first step towards understanding how people will respond to information concerning genetic predisposition to disease. As yet, there has been little work on this. Two studies that begin to address this issue are described below.

Mothers' beliefs about the causes of their children's genetic disorders have been studied using Q-sort methodology (Weil, 1991). Two categories of causal beliefs were identified. In one, the beliefs were based upon an impersonal scientific view, in which cause was attributed to chromosomes, pollution, egg or sperm problems. The other category was more personal with the cause being more likely to be attributed to the mother being specially selected to care for a child with problems. Mothers with the two belief patterns were equally knowledgeable about genetics.

Preliminary evidence from an analogue study suggests that conceptualisations of inheritance are, to some extent, situationally dependant (Senior, Marteau & Weinman, 1996). Participants were asked to imagine that they had been tested by their general practitioners and found to have an increased risk of heart disease. They were randomly allocated to one of two conditions, varying in the type of test used to determine susceptibility to heart disease. In one condition, participants were told that they had been tested using a new genetic test, the results showing whether or not they had inherited a gene that predisposed them to heart disease. In the other condition, the type of test was not disclosed and the increased risk of heart disease was not attributed to inheritance of a particular gene. While the types of causal beliefs and the factor structure of those beliefs were similar in the two experimental conditions, the loading of "genes" and "chance" on the same factor differed. Genes loaded negatively with chance when the type of test was genetic and loaded positively with chance when the test was not specified. One possible explanation for this finding is that the term gene invokes the notion of chance or uncertainty when the gene is not linked to the person; when told one has a gene, genetic becomes the very opposite of chance, to mean fate or certainty.

This explanation for a difference in perception according to whether the representation assessed is for an illness that a person has, or is vulnerable to, or for an illness which has no particular personal relevance, is supported by the results of a study by Bishop (1991). Participants rated 22 diseases on a series of 18 bipolar scales (Bishop, 1991). The scales comprised a number of potentially relevant characteristics including causal beliefs (e.g., contagious, inherited, caused by the environment), beliefs about seriousness (life threatening, serious) and beliefs about cure (easily cured, controllable). Using multidimensional scaling and cluster analysis, the results showed that lay people organise diseases into two categories based upon perceptions of contagiousness and the degree to which diseases are life threatening. Thus some causal beliefs form a critical part of general, as well as specific disease representations. This result suggests that illness representations differ according to whether an individual is rating their own illness or the illness of others: people use fewer concepts or dimensions when considering diseases more generally, or when considering an illness that they do not have. The two categories identified by Bishop reflect two core components of risk perception: a lack of controllability (inherent in the term contagious) over events that are adverse (such as life-threatening illness) (Brun, 1994), suggesting a commonality in prototypes used to appraise threats. These two dimensions also reflect primary appraisal (how threatening is the event?) and secondary appraisal (how controllable is it?) (Lazarus & Folkman, 1984).

In summary, causal beliefs about illnesses frequently encompass beliefs concerning inheritance. Further work is needed to determine the content of these beliefs and how people conceptualise inheritance and genes. This may lead to a more elaborate classification of these causal beliefs. Such work needs to consider cultural diversity and other individual differences as well as situational influences upon the content and structure of causal beliefs about illness.

IMPACT OF GENETIC INFORMATION UPON CAUSAL BELIEFS

In addition to understanding how causal beliefs are organised, it is also important to understand their relationship to beliefs about treatment or cure and hence their links with emotional and behavioural responses to risk information. People's beliefs about the causes of an illness affect not only how they respond to that illness in themselves, but also how they respond to others with that illness. Knowing the genetic basis of illnesses raises the questions of how such information will affect causal beliefs and in turn health-related behaviour and emotional adjustment, as well as attitudes and behaviour towards those at risk for, or with, conditions that have an identified genetic cause.

Causal Beliefs, Health-related Behaviour and Emotional Adjustment

The impact of causal beliefs upon behaviour has mainly been studied within the illness representation paradigm referred to at the beginning of this chapter. By contrast the role of causal beliefs in the emotional adjustment to illness has mainly been studied from an attributional theory perspective.

Illness cognitions affect the likelihood that someone will follow health advice. In a study of representations of common illnesses such as colds and 'flu, Lau and Hartman (1983) hypothesised that "illness schemas frequently include a one-to-one relationship between the cause of the disease and the cause of recovery" (p. 169). They found some support for this hypothesis: 41.5% of reported causal and cure beliefs matched on a one-to-one basis. Examples of these matched cause and cure beliefs are: getting sick because of too little sleep — getting better because of more sleep or rest; getting sick because of germs — getting better because of doctors or medicine. In a study of men awaiting coronary artery by-pass grafts, significant associations were found between making changes to diet, smoking and exercise and beliefs about the causes of their heart disease (de Valle & Norman, 1992). Whether these findings translate to situations where people possess a genetic risk for illness remains to be determined. In part, this will depend upon how controllable people perceive an illness with a genetic risk to be.

Information about the cause of a condition may affect emotional adjustment through causal beliefs and beliefs about the cure or treatment for a condition. In a review of studies using attributions to predict adjustment to illness, Turnquist, Harvey and Anderson (1988) found that overall, emotional adjustment to illness was better when the person affected had made a causal attribution but that the nature of the attribution was not predictive. They concluded that one of the most consistent findings in this literature was that ...” with few exceptions ... investigators have found that patients who report an explicit attribution are better adjusted in a variety of domains than patients who fail to report any type” (p. 58). Although the majority of this research is cross-sectional in design, most investigators appear to have an implicit causal model of attributional processes. In this model attributions play a causal role in predicting emotional responses to a threat. One possible mechanism for this relationship is that making an attribution provides an explanation and thereby makes the event seem more controllable and hence easier to adjust to. There are however other explanations for why reporting attributions is associated with better outcomes. According to the emotion-driven model, emotional responses to a threatening event have a causal impact upon attributional processes and hence subsequent outcomes. One mechanism through which this might work is that those who are better adjusted emotionally are more likely to have “spare” cognitive capacity and hence more likely to try to explain the causes of events. A further explanation for the relationship between making attributions and adjustment is that they have a correlational, not a causal relationship. Thus both attributions and emotions form only part of a larger process and it is some other, unknown variable that is predictive of outcome.

Whereas the type of explanation does not predict adjustment, whether or not blame is attributed does. Emotional adjustment is poorer when those affected blame others for the cause of an illness or adverse event (Tennen & Affleck, 1990). This finding may reflect the greater difficulty in adjusting to events that are perceived as personally uncontrollable. Alternatively it may stem from poorer emotional adjustment leading to more blame. Data from prospective or experimental studies are lacking on the causal nature of associations between attributions and emotional outcomes (Downey, Cohen Silver & Wortman, 1990).

Given that causal beliefs may affect both emotional adjustment and behaviour, it is apposite to consider how causal beliefs may be affected by information about a genetic influence upon the cause of a disease. Preliminary results from an analogue study of ours suggest that causal beliefs are affected by such information (Senior, Marteau & Weinman, 1996). Students (n = 212) were asked to imagine that they had received a positive screening test result showing that they were at increased risk for (a) heart disease and (b) arthritis. These two conditions were chosen as ones that differed in the threat they posed: in a pilot study of another group of students the mean perceived seriousness for heart disease was 7.67 (SD:1.39) and for arthritis it was 4.80 (SD:1.80), using a ten-point rating scale. For half the participants the screening test was described as a new genetic test which had detected a dominant gene for the condition. For the other half, the screening test was described only as a new test which had detected an increased risk for developing the condition. Causal beliefs were assessed using ten-point rating scales requiring respondents to state how important they perceived each of seven factors to be in causing the condition for which they were asked to imagine they had just been given a positive test result.

When risk to either disease was determined by a genetic as opposed to an unspecified test, the cause of the condition was more likely to be attributed to genes and less likely to be attributed to lifestyle. The condition was seen as less preventable when a genetic cause was emphasized. The results of this analogue study suggest that personalised genetic information is likely to affect causal and cure beliefs. The generalisability of these findings to clinical settings needs to be established.

Causal Beliefs and Helping Behaviour

Perceptions of others' problems can determine the kind of help offered. This applies to people in all possible helping roles such as relatives, friends, strangers, doctors, nurses or policy makers. One of the main perceptions that has been studied is causal beliefs or explanations for a behaviour. Attributions for the cause of an illness or problem are associated with different attitudes towards the affected person. For example, college students rated an obese girl more positively if they were told that the obesity was due to a thyroid complaint than if they were told it was due to overeating (De Jong, 1980). That the attributions of health professionals may influence their attitudes towards patients was evident in a study of nurses' and doctors' attitudes towards patients with the same conditions but with different behavioural histories (Marteau & Riordan, 1992). Across five conditions, patients who had engaged in a relevant preventive behaviour, such as not smoking in those with lung cancer, were seen as more compliant, more likely to be concerned about their condition and more enjoyable to work with than those with the same condition but who had not engaged in a relevant preventive behaviour. Brewin (1984) found that attributions made by medical students influenced their willingness to prescribe psychotropic medication: if patients' depression was attributed to uncontrollable rather than controllable life events, the students were more likely to consider psychotropic medication an appropriate form of treatment.

Two of the conceptual frameworks that have been used to predict helping behaviour are the attributional theory of helping behaviour (Weiner 1979, 1986) and a cost-benefit perspective (Dovidio, 1984). The attributional theory of helping behaviour has two central components. First, helping behaviour is caused primarily by the emotional reactions of sympathy and anger which respectively facilitate or inhibit the tendency to help (Batson *et al.*, 1981). Second, attributions of controllability are regarded as the primary determinants of such emotional reactions as sympathy and anger. Cost-benefit appraisals predict that helping behaviour is associated with higher expectations that help will be successful (Sharrock *et al.*, 1990). This model has two central components. First, helping behaviour is caused primarily by the expectation that help will be successful. Second, attributing a problem to unstable, but controllable causes, is the primary determinant of the expectation that help will be successful. There is evidence to support each of these models of helping behaviour, suggesting that both cognitive and emotional variables mediate helping, although the circumstances in which they may be more or less important remain to be determined.

How might a genetic emphasis upon the causes of illness or behaviour affect helping? If the effect is to make an outcome appear less controllable, it would be predicted from attribution theory that people would be less likely to attribute blame for the outcome. So, for example, presentation of homosexuality as genetic in origin has been greeted by some gay rights activists as heralding the end of blame for such a sexual orientation. If, on the other hand, the effect of a genetic technology causes an adverse outcome to be perceived as more controllable, then less help and more blame may be attributed to those experiencing such an outcome. Evidence for this was obtained in an analogue study of attributions for the birth of a child with Down's syndrome (Marteau & Drake, 1995). The birth of a child with Down's syndrome to a mother who had declined testing was perceived as more controllable than the birth of a child to a mother who had not been offered the test. While a certain amount of blame was attributed to mothers for giving birth to children with Down's syndrome with either screening history, significantly more blame was attributed when the mother declined testing than when she was not offered it.

If the likelihood of successful interventions is deemed lower following an emphasis upon the genetic basis to a condition, then it would be predicted from the cost-benefit model that there would be less willingness to help. So, for example, if intelligence is seen to be an inherited more than a socially determined characteristic, there may be less willingness to invest in education (Duster, 1990; Lewontin, 1991; Rose, Lewontin & Kamin, 1984). In health contexts, there may be less willingness to invest in health education programmes if some of the major causes of mortality and morbidity become attributed largely to inheritance. Conversely, if interventions were deemed more likely to succeed if targeted at a group more likely to benefit, such as those at known genetic risk for heart disease being offered life-style advice, then there might be more willingness to provide help in the form of such programmes.

In addition to effects upon causal beliefs, other illness beliefs may be affected by information about genetic causes of illnesses, which in turn may affect attitudes towards those with such conditions. For example, willingness to interact with someone with one of a range of illnesses has been found to be largely dependant upon the extent to which the illness was perceived to be contagious (Bishop, 1991). The more a condition was seen as inherited, the more willing participants were to interact with people with the condition, an effect mediated by a lower perceived contagiousness for such conditions. If the effect of emphasizing the genetic contribution to an illness is to reduce the extent to which it is perceived to be contagious, then such an emphasis would make people more willing to interact with those with the condition.

All these hypotheses require testing in the context of screening for genetic susceptibility to multifactorial disease.

METHODOLOGIES FOR STUDYING CAUSAL BELIEFS

The key methodological issue in this area concerns how best to determine and analyse the content and structure of causal beliefs.

Determining and Measuring Salient Beliefs

Open-ended questions are most often used to determine causal beliefs for an illness, sometimes using questionnaires (e.g., Landrine & Klonoff, 1994; Lau & Hartman, 1983), but most often as part of an unstructured or semi-structured interview. Such an approach was used by Davison and colleagues in a study of lay representations of heart disease. Much of the early data on illness representations were collected during interviews in which patients were invited to speak openly about their illnesses (Leventhal & Nerenz, 1985; Meyer, Leventhal & Gutmann, 1985). Those working within an attributional framework have also used this approach to elicit spontaneous attributions (e.g., Stratton *et al.,* 1988)). Different methods have been used to analyse the material produced from open-ended questions. Davison and colleagues used a grounded theory approach to analyse their data, in which beliefs are inductively inferred from the narrative of the interview. Stratton and colleagues used a standardised rating scale to measure the beliefs elicited during their interviews: the Leeds Attributional Coding Scheme (LACS: Stratton *et al.,* 1988). Bishop and colleagues (Bishop *et al.,* 1987) conducted a content analysis of open-ended responses concerning disease prototypes.

Other methods of assessing causal beliefs include the use of checklists, rating scales and rank ordering. The widely held assumption that eliciting beliefs using open-ended formats is the most valid way of determining people's beliefs about illness is challenged by the results of several studies. Elig and Frieze (1979) used the multitrait-multimethod approach to test the reliability of three main attributional measures: open-ended responses, scale ratings and ipsative percentage judgements (i.e., those in which the score of one attribution must influence the score of other attributions, as when the "total cause" of an event (100%) must be accounted for from the given number of particular causes). Open-ended measures of causal attribution had poorer inter-test reliability than structured response measures. The rating scale method was preferred over the percentage method by respondents. Landrine and Klonoff (1994) found differences in causal beliefs elicited according to whether responses were to open-ended questions or to experimenter-provided dimensions. Respondents were more likely to attribute illness to supernatural causes when responding to experimenter-provided items than when responding to open-ended questions. The authors suggest that these differences are a function of social desirability, with most people not wanting to reveal supernatural beliefs. These results point to the importance of comparing results obtained using different methods. It is likely that the value of open-ended methods is higher at the pilot stage of research (Maruyama, 1982).

Turnquist *et al.* (1988), writing about attributions, describe the different ways that concepts are assessed, in particular the use of different terms and different response options. Studies using more than one method have found low convergence between methods (e.g., Bulman & Wortman, 1977; de Valle & Norman, 1992; Landrine & Klonoff, 1994; Taylor, Lictman & Wood, 1984). Croyle and Barger (1993) point out that slightly different analysis techniques can produce quite different results. However, they conclude from a review of the literature that the results of several studies are consistent, implying that these methodological problems have not compromised the validity of the studies. Weinman *et al.* (1996) report that the use of a self-administered questionnaire measuring illness representations produces similar responses to those obtained during an interview. A more robust investigation of this critical issue requires a systematic literature review (Chalmers & Altman, 1995) to determine outcomes of different methods of assessing and analysing causal beliefs.

The causal beliefs used in different studies vary widely in their specificity. For example, some studies have assessed causes of heart disease using specific factors such as eating fatty foods and not taking exercise (e.g., Norman, 1992). In others, more general factors are used, such as "something about my own behaviour" or "something to do with someone else" (e.g., Weinman *et al.*, 1996). The consequences of assessing these different levels of specificity are unknown. Comparisons of responses obtained using different methods should be used to assess convergent and predictive validity.

The extent to which measuring presence or absence of beliefs or belief strength in different ways needs to be determined in moving towards more reliable and valid measures in this area. The use of the multitrait-multimethod matrix to determine convergent and discriminant validity (Campbell & Fiske, 1959; Schmitt & Stults, 1986; Williams, Cote & Buckley, 1989) would seem particularly important in an area that has spawned numerous measures offering little more than face validity.

Determining and Measuring the Structure of Beliefs

The relationship between beliefs have most often been assessed using statistical techniques including factor analysis, cluster analysis and multidimensional scaling. Factor analytic methods have been the most frequently used. One of the first standardised measures of illness cognitions to be produced was the 45-item Implicit Models of Illness Questionnaire (IMIQ: Turk, Rudy & Salovey, 1986). Occasionally the structure of beliefs has been determined using judgments by raters (e.g., Landrine & Klonoff, 1994).

The validity of any proposed structure of beliefs depends critically upon the sample of stimuli chosen by the researcher and the type of people studied. Researchers' assumptions about the structural dimensions can influence their choice of beliefs, thus leading to structures that perhaps reflect more the initial choice of items rather than the structural dimensions along which people's beliefs are organised. The original factor analysis of the IMIQ has been criticised for being based on pooled responses of diverse groups, namely: patients with diabetes, diabetes educators and college students (Lau, 1988). A similar problematic approach was taken in a study which failed to replicate the original IMIQ in which pooled responses were taken from students and patients with rheumatoid arthritis, multiple sclerosis and human immunodeficiency virus (Schiaffino & Cea, 1995). Such analyses are based upon an unfounded assumption that the factor structures of illness cognitions will be similar across diverse groups. Evidence that this is not a valid assumption comes from studies that show differences in beliefs between those with and those without a particular illness, as discussed above.

Data Analysis

In addition to variations in determining the structure of causal beliefs, there is variation in the way that factor or cluster scores are used. The way that factor scores are most often used in data analysis jeopardises their predictive power. Usually, data are analysed using group means derived either from factor scores or single causal items (e.g., Lau & Hartman, 1993; Weinman *et al.*, 1996). This may not, however, be the most sensitive or valid way of analysing such data. A complementary method is to use patterns of scores across factors as a way of describing causal models that people hold about an illness. Such a method was advocated by Wallston and Wallston (1982) for the analysis of scores on the multidimensional health locus of control scale. The usefulness of this method of analysis has yet to be demonstrated, although theoretically it has much to recommend it.

Future Directions for Assessing the Structure of Causal Beliefs

Most research on causal beliefs has focused upon assessing these beliefs in isolation, as reflected in the dominant approaches to analysis discussed above. For example, while most people perceive diet, inheritance and exercise to each play a role in the development of heart disease, how do they see the relationship between these causes? Two models that have been considered in the structure of people's beliefs about causal processes in nature are linear hierarchical patterns (White, 1992): first, an Aristotelian unidirectional hierarchy and second, a two-way systems hierarchy. In the former there is a seat of power at the top of the hierarchy and causal influence proceeds down through the levels of the hierarchy to the bottom but not upwards. In a two-way hierarchy any given level receives inputs from and gives outputs to any adjacent level, so that no level has control of the hierarchy as a whole and no level is immune to influence from other levels.

Various methods can be used to examine relationships between causes. One method is network analysis (Antaki, 1988; Knopke & Kuklinski, 1982), which has been used successfully to describe the structure of causal beliefs for such phenomena as student political action (Antaki, 1989), loneliness (Lunt, 1991), examination failure (Lunt, 1988), poverty (Heaven, 1994) and coronary heart disease (de Valle & Norman, 1992; Green & McManus, 1995). One approach to using this method is to start by deriving a list of putative causes for a phenomenon, such as the onset of an illness. Using these, people are asked to consider whether each cause could be considered to affect each of the other causes. From this, a network of causes is generated to determine whether generalisable causal links exist between them. For each pair of causes, a link can be absent or present in one or both directions. Causes can be classified as distal, proximal or mediating. The strength of this technique is that it facilitates complex understanding of the perceived relationships between putative causes, based upon large numbers of people. The predictive validity of the resulting causal schema has yet to be determined.

Other methods that may prove useful in assessing causal links are experimental studies in which the presence of different possible causes is manipulated to determine the impact upon perceived likelihood of developing the illness.

CONCLUDING COMMENT

There is growing evidence for the importance of causal beliefs in influencing both cognitions about the controllability of an illness and behaviour to reduce risks or enhance recovery. There is now a need to develop reliable and valid methods of determining causal beliefs and their structure. Understanding how people conceptualise genes in causing multifactorial diseases will provide the foundation for determining how to communicate effectively about the results of any tests undergone and provide one of the surest ways of addressing some key questions raised by the Human Genome Project (HGP):

> *"The HGP will generate tools to help us learn much about human biology, to understand unique new connections between the genome and morphological as well as behavioral expression. What is the relationship between the human genome and the human organism that geneticists should, as experts, promote to the public? Can that relationship be modeled in a way that is accessible to the public, accurately reflects scientific progress and does not suggest a loss of personal freedom and integrity?"*

> *Fogle (1995) p. 537.*

As this chapter has hopefully shown, psychology has the theories and methods to answer these questions.

REFERENCES

Abrams, R.D. & Finesinger, J.E. (1953) Guilt reactions in patients with cancer. *Cancer*, **6**, 474–482.

Affleck, G., Pfeiffer, C., Tennen, H. & Fifield, J. (1987) Appraisals of control and predictability in adapting to chronic disease. *Journal of Personal Social Psychology*, **53**, 273–279.

Antaki, C. (1988) Structures of belief and justification. In C. Antaki (Ed.), *Analysing everyday explanations: A casebook of methods* (pp. 60–73). New York: Sage.

Antaki, C. (1989) Structured causal beliefs and their defence in accounts of student political action. *Journal of Language and Social Psychology*, **8**, 39–48.

Batson, C.D., Duncan, B.D., Ackerman, P., Buckley, T. & Birch, K. (1981) Is emphatic emotion a source of altruistic motivation? *Journal of Personality and Social Psychology*, **40**, 290–302.

Bishop, G.D. (1991) Lay disease representations and responses to victims of disease. *Basic and Applied Social Psychology*, **12**, 115–132.

Bishop, G. D., Briede, C., Cavazos, L., Grotzinger, R. & McMahon, S. (1987) Processing illness information: The role of disease prototypes. *Basic and Applied Social Psychology*, **8**, 21–44.

Blaxter, M. & Paterson, E. (1982) *Mothers and daughters: a three generational study of health attitudes and behaviour.* London: Heinemann Educational Books.

Brewin, C.R. (1984) Perceived controllability of life-events and willingness to prescribe psychotropic drugs. *British Journal of Social Psychology*, **23**, 285–287.

Brun, W. (1994) Risk perception: Main issues, approaches and findings. In G. Wright & P. Ayton (Eds.), *Subjective probability* (pp. 163–184). Chichester: John Wiley & Sons Ltd.

Bulman, R.J. & Wortman, C.B. (1977) Attributions of blame and coping in the 'real world': Severe accident victims react to their lot. *Journal of Personality & Social Psychology*, **35**, 351–363.

Campbell, D.T. & Fiske, D.W. (1959) Convergent and discriminant validation of the multitrait-multimethod matrix. *Psychological Bulletin*, **56**, 81–105.

Chalmers, I. & Altman, D.G. (1995) *Systematic reviews.* London: BMJ Publishing Group.

Clough, E.E. & Wood-Robinson, C. (1985) Children's understanding of inheritance. *Journal of Biological Education,* **19**, 304–310.

Croyle, R.T. & Barger, S.D. (1993) Illness cognition. In S. Maes, H. Leventhal & M. Johnston (Eds.), *International review of health psychology* (pp. 29–47). Chichester: John Wiley & Sons Ltd.

Davison, C., Frankel, S. & Davey Smith, G. (1989) Inheriting heart trouble: the relevance of common-sense ideas to preventive measures. *Health Education Research,* **4**, 329–340.

De Jong, W. (1980) The stigma of obesity: The consequences of naive assumptions concerning the causes of physical deviance. *Journal of Health and Social Behaviour,* **21**, 75–87.

Department of Health (1995) The genetics of common diseases: A second report to the NHS Central Research and Development Committee on the new genetics. Leeds, England: Department of Health, Research and Development Directorate.

de Valle, M.N. & Norman, P. (1992) Causal attributions, health locus of control beliefs and lifestyle changes among pre-operative coronary patients. *Psychology & Health,* **7**, 201–211.

Dovidio, J.F. (1984) Helping behaviour and altruism: an empirical and conceptual overview. In L. Berkowitz (Ed.), *Advances in experimental social psychology* (Vol. 27, pp. 362–414). New York: Academic Press.

Downey, G., Cohen Silver, R. & Wortman, C.B. (1990) Reconsidering the attribution-adjustment relation following a major negative event: coping with the loss of a child. *Journal of Personality & Social Psychology,* **59**, 925–940.

DuCette, J. & Keane, A. (1984) "Why me?" An attributional analysis of a major illness. *Research in Nursing and Health,* **7**, 257–264.

Duster, T. (1990) *Backdoor to eugenics.* New York: Routledge.

Elig, T.W. & Frieze, I.H. (1979) Measuring causal attributions for success and failure. *Journal of Personality and Social Psychology,* **37**, 621–634.

Fogle, T. (1995) Information metaphors and the human genome project. *Perspectives in Biology and Medicine,* **38**, 535–547.

Gallup. (1995) Genetic testing: Poll conducted on 1114 members of UK general population: 25–30 October.

Green, D.W. & McManus, I.C. (1995) Cognitive structural models: The perception of risk and prevention in coronary heart disease. *British Journal of Psychology,* **86**, 321–336.

Heaven, P.C.L. (1994) The perceived causal structure of poverty: A network analysis approach. *British Journal of Social Psychology,* **33**, 259–271.

Herzlich, C. (1973) *Health and illness: a social psychological analysis.* London: Academic Press.

Kargbo, D.B, Hobbs, E.D. & Erickson, G.L. (1980) Children's beliefs about inherited characteristics. *Journal of Biological Education,* **14**, 137–146.

Kessler, S. (1988) Invited essay on the psychological aspects of genetic counselling-v-Presentation: a family coping strategy in Huntington's disease. *American Journal of Medical Genetics,* **31**, 617–621.

Knopke, D. & Kuklinski, J.H. (1982) *Network Analysis* (Sage University paper series on Quantitative Applications in the Social Sciences, series No. 07–001) Beverly Hills/London: Sage.

Koslowsky, M., Croog, S.H. & LaVoie, L. (1978) Perceptions of the etiology of illness: causal attributions in a heart patient population. *Perceptual and Motor Skills,* **47**, 465–485.

Landrine H. & Klonoff, E.A. (1992) Culture and health-related schemas: a review and proposal for interdisciplinary integration. *Health Psychology,* **11**, 267–276.

Landrine, H. & Klonoff, E.A. (1994) Cultural diversity in causal attributions for illness. *Journal of Behavioural Medicine,* **17**, 181–193.

Lau, R.R. (1988) Beliefs about control and health behavior. In D.S. Gochman (Ed.), *Health behavior: Emerging research perspectives.* New York: Plenum.

Lau, R.R. & Hartman, K.A. (1983) Common-sense representations of common illnesses. *Health Psychology,* **2**, 167–185.

Lazarus, R.S. & Folkmanm S, (1984) *Stress, appraisal and coping.* New York: Springer.

Leventhal, H. & Diefenbach, M. (1991) The active side of illness cognition. In J.A. Skelton & R.T. Croyle (Eds.), *Mental representations in health and illness.* New York: Springer Verlag.

Leventhal, H. & Nerenz, D.R. (1985) The assessment of illness cognition. In P. Karoly (Ed.), *Measurement strategies in health psychology* (pp. 517–554). New York: Wiley & Sons.

Lewontin, R.C. (1991) *Biology as ideology: the doctrine of DNA.* New York: Harper Perennial.

Lowery, B.J., Jacobson, B.S. & Murphy, B.B. (1983) An exploratory investigation of causal thinking of arthritics. *Nursing Research*, **32**, 157–162.

Lunt, P.K. (1988) The perceived causal structure of examination failure. *British Journal of Social Psychology*, **27**, 171–179.

Lunt, P.K. (1991) The perceived causal structure of loneliness. *Journal of Personality and Social Psychology*, **61**, 26–34.

Marteau, T.M. & Drake, H. (1995) Attributions for disability: the influence of genetic screening. *Social Science and Medicine*, **40**, 1127–1132.

Marteau, T.M. & Riordan, D.C. (1992) Staff attitudes to patients: The influence of causal attributions for illness. *British Journal of Clinical Psychology*, **31**, 107–110.

Meyer, D., Leventhal, H. & Gutmann, M. (1985) Common-sense models of illness: The example of hypertension. *Health Psychology*, **4**, 115–135.

Michela, J.L. & Wood, J.W. (1986) Causal attribution in health and illness. In P.C. Kendall (Ed.), *Advances in cognitive-behavioural research and therapy* (Vol. 5). New York: Academic Press.

Michie, S., McDonald, V. & Marteau, T.M. (1996) Understanding responses to predictive genetic testing: a grounded theory approach. *Psychology and Health*, **11**, 455–470.

Norman, P. (1992) Causal beliefs for coronary heart disease. *Journal of the Institute of Health Education*, **30**, 17–24.

Peterson, C., Semmel, A., von Baeyer, C., Abramson, L.Y., Metalsky, G.I. & Seligman, M.E.P. (1982) The attributional style questionnaire. *Cognitive Therapy and Research*, **6**, 287–300.

Pill, R. & Stott, N. (1986) Concepts of illness causation and responsibility: Some preliminary data from a sample of working class mothers. In C. Currer & M. Stacey (Eds.), *Concepts of health, illness and disease: A comparative approach*. Leamington Spa: Berg Publishers Ltd.

Richards, M.P.M. (1996) Lay and professional knowledge of genetics and inheritance. *Public understanding of science*, **5**, 217–230.

Richards, M.P.M. & Ponder, M. (1996) Knowledge of inheritance and attitudes to new genetic techniques. Manuscript in preparation.

Rose, S., Lewontin, R.C. & Kamin, L.J. (1984) *Not in our genes: biology, ideology and human nature*. Harmondsworth, Middlesex: Penguin Books Limited.

Schiaffino, K.M & Cea, C.D. (1995) Assessing chronic illness representations: The implicit models of illness questionnaire. *Journal of Behavioural Medicine*, **18**, 531–48.

Schmitt, N. & Stults, D. (1986) Metholodology review: analysis of mutltitrait-multimethod matrices. *Applied psychological measurement*, **10**, 1–22.

Senior, V., Marteau, T.M. & Weinman, J. (1996) Impact of genetic testing on the context and structure of causal models of heart disease and arthritis: An analogue study. Manuscript submitted for publication.

Shakespeare, J. (1992) *Communication in Huntington's disease families.* Paper presented at the Third European meeting on Psychosocial Aspects of Genetics, University of Nottingham, September.

Sharrock, R., Day, A., Qazi, F. & Brewin, C.R. (1990) Explanations by professional care staff, optimism and helping behaviour: an application of attribution theory. *Psychological Medicine*, **20**, 849–855.

Shiloh, S. & Berkenstadt, M. (1992) Lay conceptions of genetic disorders. *Birth Defects*, **28**, 191–200.

Stratton, P., Munton, T., Hanks, H., Heard, D. & Davidson, C. (1988) *Leeds attributional coding system manual.* Leeds Family Therapy and Research Centre: Leeds, England.

Taylor, S.E., Lictman, R.R. & Wood, J.V. (1984) Attributions, beliefs about control and adjustment to breast cancer. *Journal of Personality & Social Psychology*, **46**, 489–502.

Tennen, H., Affleck, G. & Gershman, K. (1986) Self-blame among parents with perinatal complications: The role of self protective motives. *Journal of Personality & Social Psychology*, **50**, 690–696.

Tennen, A. & Affleck, G. (1990) Blaming others for threatening events. *Psychological Bulletin*, **108**, 209–232.

Turk, D.C., Rudy, T.E. & Salovey, P. (1986) Implicit models of illness. *Journal of Behavioural Medicine*, **9**, 453–474.

Turnquist, D.C., Harvey, J.H. & Anderson, B.L. (1988) Attributions and adjustment to life-threatening illness. *British Journal of Clinical Psychology*, **27**, 55–65.

Wallston, K.A., Wallston, B.S. & DeVellis, R. (1978) Development of the multidimensional health locus of control (MHLC) scales. *Health Education Monogram*, **6**, 160–170.

Weil, J. (1991) Mothers' postcounseling beliefs about the causes of their children's genetic disorders. *American Journal of Human Genetic*, **48**, 145–153.

Weiner, B. (1971) *Achievement, motivation and attribution theory*. Morristown: New Jersey: General Learning Press.

Weiner, B. (1979) A theory of motivation for some classroom experiences. *Journal of Educational Psychology*, **71**, 3–25.

Weiner, B. (1986) *An attributional theory of motivation and emotion*. New York:Springer.

Weinman, J., Petrie, K.J., Moss-Morris, R. & Horne, R. (1996) The illness perception questionnaire: A new method for assessing the cognitive representation of illness. *Psychology and Health*, **11**, 431–445.

White, P.A. (1992) The anthropomorphic machine: Causal order in nature and the world view of common sense. *British Journal of Psychology*, **83**, 61–96.

Williams, L.J., Cote, J.A. & Buckley, M.R. (1989) Lack of method variance in self-reported affect and perceptions at work: reality or artifact? *Journal of Applied Psychology*, **74**, 462–468.

Wong, P.T.P. & Weiner, B. (1981) When people ask "why" questions and the heuristics of attributional search. *Journal of Personality & Social Psychology*, **40**, 650–663.

9

Processing Risk Factor Information: Defensive Biases in Health-Related Judgments and Memory

Robert T. Croyle, Yi-Chun Sun & Marybeth Hart

> *It needs to be said again and again — in contradistinction to the normative and veridical emphasis in cognitive psychology — that thinking is not necessarily objective, as I noted earlier, especially when strong social and personal values are at stake.* (Lazarus, 1991, p. 146)

Understanding the nature, function and origin of illness representations is a goal shared by many of the contributors to this volume. Although the studies of health-related perceptions and representations described here vary in terms of their conceptual frameworks, research methods and levels of analysis, they share a common theoretical assumption — that mental representations of health and illness play a critical role in health-related adjustment and behaviour. As the body of empirical work in support of this assumption continues to grow in its size and complexity, it is important to refocus attention on the identification of general features and processes of health-related cognition that are observable across a variety of disease domains. The purpose of this chapter is to identify and describe one such characteristic feature of health-related cognition, which we label defensiveness.

Defensiveness can be construed as a type of bias, a feature of cognition that produces variations in judgments and memory as a function of the positivity, self-relevance and ambiguity of a stimulus. The discussion that follows expands on the following propositions: 1) Defensiveness is a bias that characterises a wide range of human judgment and memory. 2) Defensiveness occurs when individuals encounter information that is inconsistent with their goals and is personally relevant. 3) Because many health threats are ambiguous, personally relevant and inconsistent with self-beliefs and goals (e.g., health), defensiveness is pervasive in the health domain.

THE STUDY OF BIAS: A BRIEF HISTORY

Throughout the 1970s and '80s, psychologists were engaged in a vigorous debate concerning human decision-making and judgment. A number of studies conducted in the 1970s showed that everyday human judgments did not follow normative scientific rules of inference. Although major theorists in cognitive and social psychology earlier had proposed that individuals act like "intuitive scientists" when forming inferences from stimulus information (Jones & Davis, 1965; Kelley, 1967), investigators like Tversky and Kahneman (1974) and Ross (1977) reported mounting evidence that questioned the scientist metaphor. Instead of engaging in objective data collection and theory-testing, individuals overgeneralize from biased samples, focus on evidence that confirmed prior theories and apply "arbitrary and capricious" inferences about causality to human events. The debate that followed focused on two competing explanations for these errors and biases in judgment. Whereas some theorists argued that the biases reflected ego-defensive motivations (e.g., Burger, 1981; Zuckerman, 1979), others supported cognitive non-motivational explanations of judgmental errors (e.g., Miller & Ross, 1975; Nisbett & Ross, 1980).

Health psychology and the public health sciences were silent bystanders to this critical debate about biases in judgment. Although the dominant theoretical model employed by public health investigators during this period, the Health Belief Model (Becker, 1974), focused on rational decision making, the determinants and function of the cognitive components of the model were unspecified and largely unexplored. Investigators in behavioural medicine and public health were interested primarily in the predictive value of judgments, not their psychological underpinnings. As a result, the debates among psychologists concerning the nature of judgmental biases and the role of emotional processes were largely ignored, as were criticisms of the Health Belief Model that challenged its psychological assumptions (e.g., Leventhal & Cameron, 1987). The unimpressive record of many large-scale interventions suggests that public health investigators should reconsider their lack of attention to psychological processes underlying health-related judgments.

Psychologists also stand to benefit from the study of biases in health-related judgment. Recent evidence shows that the health domain may be one of the most fruitful contexts within which to study biases in judgments and memory. Most of the common criticisms of laboratory cognitive psychology (e.g., low external validity; triviality of laboratory stimuli; lack of emotional involvement by study participants) are moot when similar processes are investigated comprehensively within the context of health and illness. Issues surrounding health and illness are a feature of everyday life. Health-related judgments and actions have significant personal consequences. For most individuals, health is important, disease is frightening and illness can place tremendous demands on one's cognitive, emotional and physical resources.

In this chapter, we will review and discuss research that examines how individuals process and respond to information about personal health risks. Whereas most laboratory research concerning health-related risk perception has examined judgments of hypothetical risks or environmental hazards (see Fischoff, Bostrom & Quadrel, 1993, for a review), our focus will be on judgments and recall of actual disease risk factor test results. Risk factor information is now being provided to individuals in a variety of ways, via public screening programs, clinical assessment, mass media and genetic testing. The study of psychological responses to risk information can therefore provide insight into a wide range of encounters that individuals have with illness and health care.

By relying on our own work and the work of others, we will argue that substantial evidence supports the notion that health-related judgments and memory are characterised by systematic biases. In this respect, the work to be discussed can be viewed as an extension of more basic research conducted by cognitive and social psychologists. However, the study of biases in health-related judgments and memory provides empirical and theoretical contributions that are both unique and substantial. Although it is the case that individuals actively seek information that can be used to draw accurate inferences about their health status, their interpretations and recall of this information are less than objective. This is especially true when individuals are faced with "bad news," immediate and personally relevant information (such as that provided by a screening test result) suggesting that they have an increased risk of developing a disease. In our view, the evidence we will discuss can be most parsimoniously explained by attributing many of the biases in the processing of personally relevant health-related information to self-defensive motives.

DEFENSIVE BIASES IN HEALTH-RELATED JUDGMENTS

Not only is it true that most individuals prefer health to illness (i.e., health is both a value and a goal), they also *want to believe* they are healthy until presented with overwhelming evidence that they are not. This conclusion is based largely on research conducted by health psychologists in the past decade. However, the broader theoretical foundations for these goals and preferences have a longer history. Research conducted by a diverse group of psychologists over the past two decades has shown that people tend to see themselves in a positive light (Brown, 1991; Greenwald, 1980). The interpretation of these self-related judgments as evidence of bias is supported by the fact that the large majority of us view our abilities and traits as better than average (Alicke, 1985; Brown, 1986), which, of course, is logically impossible. In the health domain, Weinstein (e.g., 1984; 1987) has documented a similar bias, showing that most people perceive their individual risk of disease as lower than average. Although a traditional psychodynamic perspective might view these biases as maladaptive defense mechanisms, several psychologists have advocated a different perspective. Taylor and Brown (1988) have argued that the tendency to view ourselves positively, exaggerate our ability to control our environment and maintain an unrealistic degree of optimism concerning personal events, is an adaptive feature of mental health. But what happens when individuals are faced with an actual, objective health threat? Do they abandon the heuristics and biases observed in so many psychology experiments? Or, does the presence of a health threat actually exacerbate the tendency to minimise and distort self-relevant information?

It's Not Serious: Biased Appraisal of Threat

Social psychologists have clearly established that interpretations of success and failure feedback are biased (Bradley, 1978; Mullen & Riordan, 1988). Individuals tend to take credit for their successes but attribute failures to temporary situational factors. One strategy that people often use to defend the self against negative inferences is to minimise the importance and the relevancy of the dimension on which they receive negative feedback. For example, Tesser and Paulus (1983) found that after receiving negative feedback on an ability dimension, college students reduced the importance of that dimension in defining themselves in order to protect their positive self-concept.

More recently, research conducted in our laboratory has shown that individuals often use similar strategies to cope with threatening feedback regarding their health status. Before we conducted our experimental studies, research had shown that individuals with known risk factors downplay the seriousness of the risk relative to those without the risk factor. For example, Eiser, Sutton and Wober (1979) reported that smokers who responded to their survey were less likely to agree that smoking was dangerous than were non-smokers. The interpretation of these findings was problematic, because the judgments could either be a determinant of the risk behaviour or a response to it. Although Lazarus (1983) and others observed that psychological minimisation was one coping response to health threat, experimental evidence concerning this proposition was lacking. Our work has now established that in many cases, differences in judgment can be a response to risk awareness.

For example, Croyle (1990) conducted a study to examine college students' reactions to randomly assigned false feedback regarding their blood pressure. He found that subjects who were informed that their blood pressure was high rated high blood pressure as a less serious health threat than did subjects who were told that their blood pressure was normal. Similar results were found in an experimental study of appraisals of cholesterol test results. Croyle, Sun and Louie (1993, study 1) found that college students who were led to believe that their cholesterol level was in the borderline high-risk range rated having a high cholesterol level as a less serious health threat than did students who were told their cholesterol level was in the desirable range. The authors interpreted the findings as evidence of the phenomenon described by Lazarus (1983) as psychological minimisation.

Jemmott and his colleagues (Jemmott, Ditto & Croyle, 1986) developed an experimental paradigm using a fictitious enzyme deficiency as a context within which to study individuals' reactions to risk factor information (see Croyle & Ditto, 1990 for a review). The paradigm allows the investigator to maximise internal validity because both knowledge about and experience relevant to the risk factor can be completely controlled. Participants are led to believe that "Thioamine Acetylase (TAA) enzyme deficiency" is a risk factor for a mild but irritating pancreatic disorder. They are also told that a simple diagnostic test has been developed recently to detect the enzyme deficiency. The paradigm allows a direct causal examination of how health judgments are affected by the personal relevance of a health threat, because participants can be randomised to receive different test results and different kinds of information about the risk factor and its consequences.

Laboratory experiments that have utilized the TAA enzyme paradigm provide consistent evidence that health threat appraisals are significantly influenced by the personal implications of a health threat. If the threat implicates the individual who is appraising it, the seriousness of that threat is minimised (Croyle & Sande, 1988; Ditto & Lopez, 1992; Jemmott et al., 1986). Several experiments have been conducted to test possible explanations for the minimisation effect (see Ditto & Croyle, 1995, for a review). Together, these studies have shown that minimisation is a defensive response to health threat. One finding from this line of work that supports the defensiveness explanation will be mentioned here. Ditto, Jemmott and Darley (1988) told subjects they were being tested for TAA deficiency and varied the information provided to them regarding the treatability of the condition. Half of the participants were informed that there was a simple treatment available that reversed the deficiency. The others were not provided with any information regarding treatability. Based on a rational decision-making model, one might expect that individuals who received treatability information would rate the deficiency as less serious than individuals given no information about treatment. However, Ditto *et al.* (1988) found that subjects in the treatment-available condition did not minimise the seriousness of the risk factor. This result makes sense if one assumes that defensive reappraisal is more likely to occur when the individual believes that controllability or "coping potential" (Lazarus, 1991) is low.

Although experimental studies of health threat appraisal have the advantage of high internal validity, they suffer from several criticisms. First, participants in laboratory studies are typically young college students. Therefore, generalization of the research findings to older, more diverse and less healthy individuals can be questioned. Second, because laboratory studies often rely on temporary deception (requiring debriefing before dismissal), long-term responses to health threats cannot be studied. Therefore, we conducted a large-scale prospective study that would address these limitations.

Our research project used cholesterol screening as a context within which to examine judgments of health threat. Through newspaper and radio advertisements, we invited residents of the Salt Lake City area to participate in a free cholesterol screening. Interested residents telephoned to make an appointment and, upon their arrival to the screening site, received a description of the study, signed a consent form and completed a baseline questionnaire. The participant's cholesterol level was then measured by a trained laboratory assistant. Unlike our earlier laboratory studies that provided participants with randomised false feedback, we provided each participant with his or her actual cholesterol test result. After the test was conducted, each participant was asked to answer several questionnaire items, including one designed to measure threat appraisal. As in the laboratory experiments, each participant was asked to rate the seriousness of a high cholesterol level. A total of 554 men and women participated in the study. They ranged in age from 18 to 83 years old. We restricted the study to individuals who had not had their cholesterol tested within the previous six months.

Results from the cholesterol study revealed that the psychological minimisation of health threat is limited neither to the experimental laboratory nor to healthy college students. Participants whose cholesterol levels were in the borderline-high risk (201–239 mg/dl) or the high risk (240 mg/dl and above) range, rated high cholesterol as a less serious threat to health than did participants whose cholesterol levels were in the desirable range (below 200 mg/dl). Minimisation was stronger among those who had never been tested (Croyle *et al.*, 1993, Study 2); this particular finding suggests that minimisation might be more likely when the threat is unexpected.

Next we investigated the duration of the minimisation response. Duration is an important dimension, because, if minimisation is only a short-term response to a health threat, the clinical significance of such a reaction may be limited. In order to pursue this question, we included a follow-up interview in the cholesterol study. Although participants had given consent to be contacted by telephone at some point following their screening visit, they were not informed about the purpose or exact timing of the interview. Through random assignment, participants were contacted by telephone at one, three, or six months after their cholesterol screening test. The follow-up interview included the same seriousness rating item that was asked during the screening visit.

We found that participants' seriousness ratings at follow-up were significantly correlated with the seriousness rating they provided at the time of screening. However, after controlling for the initial seriousness rating, ratings provided in the follow-up interview still provided evidence of minimisation. That is, participants who had a cholesterol level above the desirable range rated having a high cholesterol level as a less serious health threat than did those who had a cholesterol level within the desirable range. This pattern of results held true among participants in the one-month follow-up group and among participants in three-month follow-up group. The minimisation effect was no longer statistically significant at six months. These findings indicated that, contrary to a widely-held assumption among coping theorists regarding the time-limited nature of defensive appraisal, minimisation in response to a health threat can persist over a substantial period of time.

The Test is Inaccurate: Biased Evaluation of Test Validity

A second coping strategy people use in response to risk notification is to derogate the validity or accuracy of the test result. As mentioned earlier, social psychological research concerning attribution processes has shown that research subjects who fail a task often blame external circumstances, such as the validity or difficulty of the task itself. In addition, subjects tend to view tests that provide positive feedback as more valid. For example, Pyszczynski, Greenberg and Holt (1985) randomly assigned subjects to succeed or fail on a "social sensitivity test". Subjects who believed they succeeded rated a study supporting the test's validity more positively than did subjects who failed the test. Do similar biases in the evaluation of validity occur among individuals who are provided with medical test results?

In the health context, research has shown that people do tend to discredit the medical test result and/or testing instruments after receiving information that has a negative implication for their health. In one study that used the fictitious enzyme paradigm, Croyle and Sande (1988) found that participants who were randomly assigned to test positive for TAA deficiency derogated the validity of the test by rating it as less accurate than did participants who tested negative.

Ditto and Lopez (1992) also conducted several experiments using the TAA enzyme paradigm to examine people's verbal and behavioural reactions to threatening health-related information. Ditto and Lopez (1992, study 2), first described to their participants the saliva test for TAA enzyme deficiency and then left participants alone in the room to conduct the test. The self-administration of the test was videotaped. The results of the study revealed that participants who received unfavourable test results expressed their distrust of the test both verbally and behaviourally. Specifically, questionnaire data showed that participants who tested positive for TAA deficiency rated the saliva test as less accurate than did participants who tested negative. Data extracted from the videotapes showed that participants who tested positive for TAA deficiency spent more time in examining the test strips than did participants who tested negative. Participants who tested positive also engaged in more "retesting" than participants who tested negative. For example, the investigators observed subjects "redipping the original test strip into the original saliva sample", "conducting a second test with a new test strip", and "placing the test strip directly on their tongue" (p. 576).

Even stronger evidence in support of the defensive nature of validity evaluations was provided by another experiment conducted by

Ditto and Lopez (1992, study 3). They found that peoples' perceptions of the accuracy of the test were moderated by their perception of the desirability of having TAA deficiency. In that study, every participant was led to believe that they had TAA deficiency. However, half of the participants were led to believe that TAA deficiency was a desirable health consequence (people who have TAA deficiency are less likely to experience pancreatic disease). The other half of the participants were led to believe that TAA deficiency is an undesirable health consequence (people who have TAA deficiency are more likely to experience pancreatic disease). After this manipulation, half of the participants rated the accuracy of the TAA saliva test before they conducted the test and the other half rated the accuracy of the test after they received their test result. Ditto and Lopez (1992) found differential ratings of the accuracy of the test as a function of the desirability of the deficiency, but only among participants who answered the question after they received their test results. Those who believed that TAA deficiency was unhealthy rated the test as less accurate than participants who believed that TAA deficiency was healthful.

Not only was this pattern of findings evidenced by the TAA studies, but a similar pattern of results was also observed within the more familiar context of cholesterol testing. Croyle *et al.* (1993) found that college students who were informed that their cholesterol levels were in the borderline-high risk range rated the test result as less accurate than those who were informed that their cholesterol levels were in the desirable range.

Use of the derogation strategy is not limited to the risk factor screening context. It can also be observed in the ways individuals interpret and respond to descriptions of health-related research such as those that frequently appear in the media. For example, Kunda (1987) and Liberman and Chaiken (1992) found that after reading medical reports describing a causal link between coffee consumption and fibrocystic disease, coffee drinkers were less likely to believe the evidence than were non-drinkers. However, the fact that relative to non-coffee drinkers, coffee drinkers reported that they exerted more effort in trying to understand the message and listed more weaknesses in the report, suggested that their distrust of the message was a result of defensive information processing (Liberman & Chaiken, 1992).

Everybody Else Has It, Too: Biased Perceptions of Risk Factor Prevalence

Biased perception is also manifested in individuals' tendency to overestimate the extent to which others think and act as they do, a bias referred to by social psychologists as false consensus. For example, Ross, Greene and House (1977) found that college students believed that a majority of their peers would favour the same grading policy that they favoured. Nisbett and Kunda (1985) reported that college students overestimated the percentage of people who would share their beliefs (e.g., the degree to which women were allowed to have an abortion on demand), or behaviours (e.g., the frequency of drinking alcoholic beverages).

False consensus is also a powerful bias within the health domain. Individuals with poor health habits perceive those behaviours as more common than do those with good health habits (Sherman *et al.*, 1983; Suls, Wan & Sanders, 1988). Jemmott, Croyle and Ditto (1988, Study 1) surveyed college students and found that those who had experienced a particular illness or symptom judged it as more common in the population than did students who had never experienced the illness or symptom. When judgments were solicited from a sample with more expertise and experience (physicians), the pattern of findings was replicated (Jemmott *et al.*, 1988, Study 2).

False consensus can also be observed in experimental studies of health threat appraisal. In the TAA paradigm, subjects who were told they had TAA deficiency judged it as more prevalent than did those who tested negative (Croyle & Sande, 1988; Ditto & Lopez, 1992, study 2). Compared to people who were told that their cholesterol levels were in the desirable range, college students who were told that their cholesterol levels were in the borderline-high risk range estimated a higher percentage of their peers as having high cholesterol (Croyle *et al.*, 1993).

Are these biased perceptions of the prevalence of health problems the product of a defensive process? In the social psychological domain, there has been a long-running debate concerning cognitive vs. motivational explanations of the false consensus phenomenon. Although non-motivational factors (e.g., the salience of one's own characteristics) play a role, the evidence to date indicates that the bias has important motivational underpinnings, especially when studied in meaningful or involving contexts. If defensive processes are at work, then one would expect the bias to be stronger when the threat value of the information is greater. This is indeed the case. For example, the false consensus bias is exacerbated when the prevalence judgments concern important or undesirable personal characteristics (Marks & Miller, 1987).

It's Only Temporary: Biased Judgments of Chronicity

One of the features of an individual's mental representations of health threats is the time course or chronicity of the disorder. As Leventhal, Nerenz and Steele (1984) noted, individuals tend to believe that a health problem is either acute, cyclical, or chronic. These beliefs can play an important role in a number of health behaviours, including compliance with medication regimens (Meyer, Leventhal & Gutmann, 1985).

There is some evidence that judgments concerning the time course of a health problem can be characterised by defensiveness. In Croyle's (1990, Experiment 2) study of blood pressure testing, participants received randomly-assigned blood pressure readings. In addition to a measure of seriousness judgments, a measure was included to assess judgments concerning the time course of hypertension. Results revealed that high blood pressure test results produced not only minimisation of seriousness, but also more frequent endorsement of a cyclical model of high blood pressure. Furthermore, seriousness judgments were related to judgments regarding time course. The subjects in the high blood pressure group who minimised the threat were the same subjects who endorsed either the acute or cyclical models of high blood pressure.

Summary

Health-related judgments are affected by the personal relevance of the threat that is evaluated. When the threat directly impacts the individual who is forming a judgment, several aspects of the perceiver's mental representation of the threat are affected. Relative to individuals who learn that they do not have a particular risk factor, those who are informed they are at risk question the validity of the test and perceive the risk factor as less serious, more prevalent and less stable.

DEFENSIVE BIASES IN HEALTH-RELATED MEMORY

The idea that unpleasant events are recalled less well than pleasant events has a long history (Singer & Salovey, 1993). Ever since Freud developed his theory of repression, investigators have attempted to understand apparent differences in the accuracy of recall as a function of the nature and emotional qualities of the event.

Given the long history of research concerning the repression construct, it is surprising that so little attention has been paid to the potential impact of defensiveness on health-related memories. The practical importance of accuracy in health-related memories is clear and public health researchers have expressed growing concern regarding the accuracy of recall-based self-reports (Catania *et al.*, 1993; Dwyer, Krall & Coleman, 1987). The effectiveness of medical care relies to a great extent on a patient's ability to recall what a physician has said. Patients cannot comply with recommendations that they cannot recall (Ley, 1986). Consequently, much of the research in behavioural medicine concerning memory has focused on patients' memories of procedural information or treatment recommendations (Croyle & Loftus, 1992; Croyle *et al.*, 1993). However, much less attention has been focused on the recall of risk-related information, such as screening test results.

As in the case of health-related judgments, the study of health-related memories can be informed by work in other domains. Research in experimental social psychology suggests that, like judgments, memory can also be influenced by defensive biases. In 1980, an important paper by Greenwald (1980) synthesized the first wave of this research, arguing that our "totalitarian" egos distort information to create and maintain a positive view of the self. Nevertheless, the published research concerning recall bias is not extensive. Results are somewhat mixed and the laboratory studies tend to focus on relatively small, short-term effects.

We chose to use cholesterol screening as a context within which to study biases in long-term memory. There were several advantages to this. Because we conducted our own screening program, we were able to use a highly standardised protocol. In contrast to an observational research approach in an uncontrolled clinical setting, this allowed us to standardise both our procedures and all of the communication with participants. Although the test results communicated to patients were relatively straight-forward, the context allowed us to examine recall of both quantitative information (total cholesterol number) and qualitative information (cardiovascular disease risk category).

Recall was assessed via telephone interviews. Participants were randomised to either a one, three, or six month post-test interview. Interviewers asked respondents to recall their cholesterol level from memory only. Subjects who first responded to the recall question by saying that they were unsure or did not remember were prodded for their "best guess". In addition to being asked to recall their exact total cholesterol level, they were also asked to recall whether their cholesterol level was in the desirable, borderline-high risk, or high risk category.

Across all follow-up groups, about one third of the respondents accurately recalled their cholesterol level. As expected, there was a significant difference across the three follow-up groups in accuracy. Recall accuracy declined as the recall interval increased (46.4% accuracy at one month, 32.7% at three months and 28.3% at six months).

Although overall accuracy rates have practical significance, the pattern of recall errors has greater theoretical importance. If the error in recall is unbiased, there should be no obvious pattern in the errors — one would expect a simple random distribution. Under these circumstances, the proportion of participants who recall a cholesterol level higher than the actual level should be about the same as the proportion of participants who recall a cholesterol level lower than their actual level. On the other hand, a defensive bias would be manifested if errors are more likely to occur in the favourable direction (e.g., lower cholesterol readings).

Our analyses revealed that the pattern of recall error was not random. Across all three follow-up groups, significantly more of the participants who incorrectly recalled their cholesterol level reported a more desirable number (40.3%) than a less desirable number (21.7%). When analysing the recall error pattern within each follow-up group, the same error pattern was significant within both the one-month and six-month follow-up groups (see Table 1).

Because recalling one's exact cholesterol level has limited clinical significance, we also examined recall of risk category. Treatment guidelines and decisions are based on these categories and the counselling individuals typically receive emphasises their importance. It should be much easier to recall one of three broad categories than a specific three-digit number. Therefore, we were not surprised to find that participants' recall of their risk category was much more accurate than their recall of their exact cholesterol level. Among the participants interviewed, 88.7% recalled their risk category accurately. The analysis of recall errors, however, revealed a pattern of bias similar to the one we found in recall of cholesterol level. Across all three follow-up groups, significantly more of the participants who were incorrect reported a more desirable risk category than a less desirable risk category.

The pattern of recall errors concerning both cholesterol level and risk category suggests that our health-related memories are biased in a particular direction, the direction that allows us to view our health in a positive yet somewhat inaccurate light. If the defensiveness explanation for this effect is valid, then one would expect that the higher an individual's cholesterol level, the greater the motive to distort information recalled from memory. In terms of cholesterol screening, this theoretical perspective would predict that the bias would be stronger among participants whose cholesterol level was in the high risk range as compared to the bias in participants whose cholesterol level was in a more desirable range.

We conducted a logit analysis to examine the relationship between recall bias, cardiovascular disease risk category and follow-up interval. The results revealed that the model that best describes the relationship between the dependent variable (direction of recall error) and the independent variables (level of threat and follow-up interval), was a model containing two main effects. As level of threat increased, participants were more likely to remember their cholesterol level as lower than it actually was. In addition, the longer the interval between screening and recall, the more likely participants were to recall their cholesterol level as lower than it actually was.

In addition to analysing the frequency of different types of recall error, we also examined the magnitude of these errors. We found a linear relationship between the average size of the discrepancy in participants' recall and their disease risk category. Individuals whose cholesterol screening test results placed them in the high risk category showed the strongest tendency to recall cholesterol levels that were lower than those actually received.

Finally, we found suggestive evidence that as memory strength weakens, individuals tend to "fill in" their memories with biased

Table 1   Recall bias: Percent of screening participants within risk category who misremembered their cholesterol test result

Risk Category	Higher than Actual	Lower than Actual
	1-month follow-up	
desirable	17.7	32.5
borderline-high	17.0	34.0
high	2.6	55.3
	3-month follow-up	
desirable	30.6	36.1
borderline-high	29.5	31.8
high	20.5	48.7
	6-month follow-up	
desirable	22.6	43.5
borderline-high	26.2	35.7
high	23.9	54.3

information. Participants who were initially reluctant to report a recalled cholesterol score were encouraged by the interviewer to provide their best guess based on their memory. This "prodded" group of respondents showed an even stronger defensive bias (average discrepancy) in recall than did the non-prodded group.

Summary

The data from the cholesterol screening study provide the strongest evidence to date that long-term, health-related memory is subject to defensive bias. These data are also important outside of the health domain in that they provide some of the best evidence of defensive bias in any study of long-term memory. Although many processes influence long-term memory (and defensive bias is only one of them), it may be that the role of defensiveness in health-related self-reports has been underestimated. Because much of the research concerning the validity of health-related self-reports examines behaviours that are either difficult to verify (e.g., use of condoms) or are trivial in terms of their personal significance (e.g., dietary intake), the research reported here is unique in terms of the use of a highly standardised protocol and its focus on information that is significant to the study participants. The data go beyond the findings from memory researchers in that the recall intervals were longer than those typically seen in memory studies and the material tested for recall concerns one type of personally relevant event that was experienced by every study participant.

DISCUSSION

In this chapter, we reviewed research evidence showing that individuals manifest significant biases in the way they evaluate and respond to personally relevant information about disease risk. When the information has negative implications for the self, it is interpreted and remembered differently than when it has positive implications. Individuals who are informed that they have an elevated risk of disease minimise the seriousness of the health threat posed by the risk factor, estimate the prevalence of the risk factor as relatively high, derogate the validity of the risk factor test and are less likely to endorse a chronic model of the risk factor's time course. Evidence supporting this conclusion comes from both cross-sectional and prospective studies. In addition, data from both controlled experiments and observational studies show that defensive bias characterises both short-term and long-term responses to risk notification.

Perhaps the most striking findings from the cholesterol screening study were the data concerning long-term memory. Individuals who misremembered their cholesterol test results at follow-up displayed a systematic pattern of error. Errors in recall were significantly more likely to occur in the "good news" direction, with subjects recalling healthier cholesterol test results than were actually received (see also Irvine & Logan, 1994). In addition, the errors became larger and more biased as objective threat increased and as the time since the cholesterol test increased. Finally, respondents who were reluctant to answer the recall question and had to be prodded for a response showed a stronger defensive bias than did subjects who responded immediately. This finding, along with the effect of recall interval, suggests that as memory decayed, subjects "filled in" the missing pieces with their preferred belief.

In our view, the biases in health-related judgments and memory discussed here are but a special instance of a general tendency for individuals to minimise, derogate, or forget information that threatens the self-concept. The consistent role of defensiveness in our own research findings can be compared with less consistent evidence in two related bodies of research, one conducted outside of the health domain, the other conducted within the health domain.

Outside of the health domain, social psychologists have shown that defensiveness is only one of several processes that accounts for such phenomena as false consensus, attribution biases and self-enhancing biases in recall. In many circumstances, these biases can be accounted for by general information processing mechanisms (e.g., salience effects) without reference to motivational processes (Nisbett & Ross, 1980). Our work demonstrates that when judgment and memory are examined within the context of actual health threats, the role of motivational processes is more important.

A similar comparison can be made with related research conducted within the health domain. Studies concerning risk perception, judgment and memory that rely on subjects who are not evaluating immediate, personally relevant health threats probably underestimate the role of defensiveness in real-life situations. We reason that defensiveness is most likely to be observed in situations that produce emotion.

The findings reported here concerning memory are important because they help address a common limitation of studies concerning judgment. Because there is no objective standard with which to compare most appraisals of seriousness (Eiser, 1994), the minimisation effects observed in the research we discussed are described as biases rather than errors. The recall data from the cholesterol screening study, however, show that factors associated with differences in judgment (e.g., level of health threat) are also associated with differences in the accuracy of recall.

Nevertheless, Eiser (1994) also has questioned whether such effects should be considered biases, given that most investigators (including ourselves) tend to focus on the patterns of subjects' responses rather than on underlying cognitive structures or processes. The term "bias" does imply something about the way in which information is processed and additional work is needed to determine how personal involvement affects specific cognitive processes. For example, personal involvement might influence both the encoding of new threat-related stimuli and the accessing of knowledge regarding a family history of disease. Experiments conducted by social psychologists suggest that higher levels of involvement induce a more extensive evaluation of the message content (Petty & Cacioppo, 1986), or a "motivated scepticism" regarding evidence that is inconsistent with preferred self-beliefs (Ditto & Lopez, 1992).

The clinical significance of the biases reviewed here requires further investigation. Although physicians are unlikely to make clinical decisions based only on self-reported cholesterol levels, one can cite a wide range of medical care situations in which clinical decision-making (e.g., ordering a medical test) relies heavily on patient self-report. If patients report an inaccurate history, physicians might consider hypotheses that they might otherwise ignore. In addition, these biases might have a significant impact on the data collected by public health investigators. A great deal of epidemiological research relies on self-reports that are not verified by the investigators. The findings discussed here challenge the common assumption that recall-based errors in self-report are randomly distributed.

The relationship between defensive biases and health-related behaviour also remains unclear. Our own work suggests that the relationship between these is neither simple nor direct. Laboratory experiments that have utilized the fictitious enzyme paradigm have shown that psychological minimisation does not preclude the formation of intentions to change behaviour (Croyle & Jemmott, 1991). In fact, the two responses can be shown to be moderated by different variables (Croyle & Hunt, 1991). This makes sense if one views minimisation as a fear control strategy that operates in parallel with deliberate efforts to reduce the threat itself (Leventhal *et al.*, 1984). The picture becomes more complex, however, when one recognizes that active, problem-focused coping is not immune to defensive bias, either. For example, information-seeking is subject to bias in that individuals tend to select or perceive information in ways that confirm their preferred belief (Ditto *et al.*, 1988; Frey, 1981; Pyszczynski & Greenberg, 1987).

Clearly, the key to understanding the function of defensiveness in coping with health threats lies in the dynamic relationships among beliefs, emotions and behaviour. A consensus is emerging that the relationship between judgment and emotion is bidirectional and that coping with health threat involves the regulation of emotion as well as the reduction of threat (Leventhal *et al.*, 1984; Miller, Shoda & Hurley, 1996). In everyday life, it might very well be that defensiveness, applied in moderation, is an effective means of controlling distress while appropriate actions are developed and enacted. Interventions that reduce high levels of distress might reduce and individual's reliance on defensiveness, facilitating objective information processing and action planning, but this remains to be demonstrated within the context of risk factor testing. In the meantime, investigators should focus on examining experimentally the emotional processes that moderate the relationship between health-related judgments and behaviour.

REFERENCES

Alicke, M.D. (1985) Global self-evaluation as determined by the desirability and controllability of trait adjectives. *Journal of Personality and Social Psychology*, **49**, 1621–1630.

Becker, M.H. (1974) The health belief model and sick role behavior. *Health Education Monographs*, **2**, 409–419.

Bradley, G.W. (1978) Self-serving biases in the attribution process: A re-examination of the fact or fiction question. *Journal of Personality and Social Psychology*, **36**, 56–71.

Brown, J.D. (1986) Evaluations of self and others: Self-enhancement biases in social judgments. *Social Cognition*, **4**, 353–376.

Brown, J.D. (1991) Accuracy and bias in self-knowledge: Can knowing the truth be hazardous to your health? In C.R. Snyder & D.F. Forsyth (Eds.), *Handbook of social and clinical psychology: The health perspective.* New York: Pergamon Press.

Burger, J.M. (1981) Motivational biases in the attribution of responsibility for an accident: A meta-analysis of the defensive-attribution hypothesis. *Psychological Bulletin*, **90**, 496–512.

Catania, J.A., Turner, H., Pierce, R.C., Golden, E., Stocking, C., Binson, D. & Mast, K. (1993) Response bias in surveys of AIDS-related sexual behavior. In D.G. Ostrow & R.C. Kessler (Eds.), *Methodological issues in AIDS behavioral research* (pp. 133–162). New York: Plenum Press.

Croyle, R.T. (1990) Biased appraisal of high blood pressure. *Preventive Medicine*, **19**, 40–44.

Croyle, R.T. & Ditto, P.H. (1990) Illness cognition and behavior: An experimental approach. *Journal of Behavioral Medicine*, **13**, 31–52.

Croyle, R.T. & Hunt, J.R. (1991) Coping with health threat: Social influence processes in reactions to medical test results. *Journal of Personality and Social Psychology*, **60**, 382–389.

Croyle, R.T. & Loftus, E.F. (1992) Improving episodic memory performance of survey respondents. In J.M. Tanur (Ed.), *Questions about questions: Inquiries into the cognitive bases of surveys* (pp. 95–101). New York: Russell Sage.

Croyle, R.T., Loftus, E.F., Klinger, M.R. & Smith, K.D. (1993) Reducing errors in health-related memory: Progress and prospects. In Schement, J.R. & Ruben, B.D. (Eds.), *Between communication and information: Information and behavior* (Vol. 4). Piscataway, NJ: Transaction.

Croyle, R.T. & Jemmott, J.B. III. (1991) Psychological reactions to risk factor testing. In Skelton, J.S. & Croyle, R.T. (Eds.), *Mental representation in health and illness* (pp. 85–107). New York: Springer-Verlag.

Croyle, R.T. & Sande, G.N. (1988) Denial and confirmatory search: Paradoxical consequences of medical diagnosis. *Journal of Applied Social Psychology*, **18**, 473–490.

Croyle, R.T., Sun, Y.C. & Louie, D.H. (1993) Psychological minimization of cholesterol test results: Moderators of Appraisal in college students and community residents. *Health Psychology*, **12**, 503–507.

Ditto, P.H. & Croyle, R.T. (1995) Understanding the impact of risk factor test results: Insights from a basic research paradigm. In Croyle, R.T. (Ed.), *Psychosocial effects of screening for disease prevention and detection* (pp. 144–181). New York: Oxford University Press.

Ditto, P.H., Jemmott, J.B. III & Darley, J.M. (1988) Appraising the threat of illness: A mental representational approach. *Health Psychology*, **7**, 183–200.

Ditto, P.H. & Lopez, D.F. (1992) Motivated skepticism: The use of differential decision criteria for preferred and nonpreferred conclusions. *Journal of Personality and Social Psychology*, **63**, 568–584.

Dwyer, J.T., Krall, E.A. & Coleman, K.A. (1987) The problem of memory in nutritional epidemiology research. *Journal of the American Diabetic Association*, **87**, 1509–1512.

Eiser, J.R. (1994) Risk judgments reflect belief strength, not bias. *Psychology and Health*, **9**, 197–199.

Eiser, J.R., Sutton, S.R. & Wober, M. (1979) Smoking, seat-belts and beliefs about health. *Addictive Behaviors*, **4**, 331–338.

Fischoff, B., Bostrom, A. & Quadrel, M.J. (1993) Risk perception and communication. *Annual Review of Public Health*, **14**, 183–203.

Frey, D. (1981) The effects of negative feedback about oneself and cost of information on preferences for information about the source of this feedback. *Journal of Experimental Social Psychology*, **17**, 42–50.

Greenwald, A.G. (1980) The totalitarian ego: Fabrication and revision of personal history. *American Psychologist*, **35**, 603–618.

Irvine, M.J. & Logan, A.G. (1994) Is knowing your cholesterol number harmful? *Journal of Clinical Epidemiology*, **47**, 131–145.

Jemmott, J.B. III, Ditto, P.E. & Croyle, R.T. (1986) Judging health status: Effects of perceived prevalence and personal relevance. *Journal of Personality and Social Psychology*, **50**, 899–905.

Jemmott, J.B. III, Croyle, R.T. & Ditto, P.E. (1988) Commonsense epidemiology: Self-based judgments from laypersons and physicians. *Health Psychology*, **7**, 55–73.

Jones, E.E. & Davis, K.E. (1965) From acts to dispositions: The attribution process in person perception. In L. Berkowitz (Ed.), *Advances in experimental social psychology* (Vol. 2, pp. 220–266). New York: Academic Press.

Kelley, H.H. (1967) Attribution theory in social psychology. In Levine, D. (Ed.), *Nebraska symposium on motivation* (Vol. 15, pp. 192–240). Lincoln: University of Nebraska Press.

Kunda, Z. (1987) Motivated inference: Self-serving generation and evaluation of causal theories. *Journal of Personality and Social Psychology*, **53**, 636–647.

Lazarus, R.S. (1983) The costs and benefits of denial. In S. Breznitz (Ed.), *The denial of stress* (pp. 1–30). New York: International Universities Press.

Lazarus, R.S. (1991) *Emotion and adaptation.* New York: Oxford University Press.

Leventhal, H. & Cameron, L. (1987) Behavioral theories and the problem of compliance. *Patient Education and Counseling*, **10**, 117–138.

Leventhal, H., Nerenz, D.R. & Steele, D.J. (1984) Illness representations and coping with health threats. In A. Baum, S.E. Taylor & J.E. Singer (Eds.), *Handbook of psychology and health* (Vol. 4, pp. 219–252). Hillsdale, NJ: Erlbaum.

Ley, P. (1986) Cognitive variables and noncompliance. *Journal of Compliance in Health Care*, **1**, 171–188.

Liberman, A. & Chaiken, S. (1992) Defensive processing of personally relevant health messages. *Personality and Social Psychology Bulletin*, **18**, 669–679.

Marks, G. & Miller, N. (1987) Ten years of research on the false-consensus effect: An empirical and theoretical review. *Psychological Bulletin*, **102**, 72–90.

Meyer, D., Leventhal, H. & Gutmann, M. (1985) Common-sense models of illness: The example of hypertension. *Health Psychology*, **4**, 115–135.

Miller, D.T. & Ross, M. (1975) Self-serving biases in the attribution of causality: Fact or fiction? *Psychological Bulletin*, **82**, 213–225.

Miller, S.M., Shoda, Y. & Hurley, K. (1996) Applying cognitive-social theory to health-protective behavior: Breast self-examination in cancer screening. *Psychological Bulletin*, **199**, 70–94.

Mullen, B. & Riordan, C.A. (1988) Self-serving attributions for performance in naturalistic settings: A meta-analytic review. *Journal of Applied Social Psychology*, **18**, 3–22.

Nisbett, R.E. & Kunda, Z. (1985) Perception of social distributions. *Journal of Personality and Social Psychology*, **48**, 297–311.

Nisbett, R.E. & Ross, L. (1980) *Human inference: Strategies and shortcomings of social judgment*. Englewood Cliffs, N.J.: Prentice-Hall.

Petty, R.E. & Cacioppo, J.T. (1986) *Communication and persuasion: Central and peripheral routes to attitude change*. New York: Springer-Verlag.

Pyszczynski, T. & Greenberg, J. (1987) Toward an integration of cognitive and motivational perspectives on social inference: A biased hypothesis-testing model. In L. Berkowitz (Ed.), *Advances in Experimental Social Psychology* (Vol. 20, pp. 297–340). San Diego, CA: Academic Press.

Pyszczynski, T., Greenberg, J. & Holt, K. (1985) Maintaining consistency between self-serving beliefs and available data: A bias in information evaluation. *Personality and Social Psychology Bulletin*, **11**, 179–190.

Ross, L.D. (1977) The intuitive psychologist and his shortcomings: Distortions in the attribution process. In L. Berkowitz (Ed.), *Advances in experimental social psychology* (Vol. 10). New York: Academic Press.

Ross, L., Greene, D. & House, P. (1977) The "false consensus effect": An egocentric bias in social perception and attribution processes. *Journal of Experimental Social Psychology*, **13**, 279–301.

Sherman, S.J., Presson, C.C., Chassin, L., Corty, E. & Olshavsky, R. (1983) The false consensus effect in estimates of smoking prevalence: Underlying mechanisms. *Personality and Social Psychology Bulletin*, **9**, 197–207.

Singer, J.A. & Salovey, P. (1993) *The remembered self.* New York: Free Press.

Suls, J., Wan, C.K. & Sanders, G.S. (1988) False consensus and false uniqueness in estimating the prevalence of health-protective behaviors. *Journal of Applied Social Psychology,* **18**, 66–79.

Taylor, S.E. & Brown, J.D. (1988) Illusion and well-being: A social psychological perspective on mental health. *Psychological Bulletin,* **103**, 193–210.

Tesser, A. & Paulus, D. (1983) The definition of the self: Private and public self-evaluation maintenance strategies. *Journal of Personality and Social Psychology,* **44**, 672–682.

Tversky, A. & Kahneman, D. (1974) Judgment under uncertainty: Heuristics and biases. *Science,* **185**, 1123–1131.

Weinstein, N.D. (1984) Why it won't happen to me: Perceptions of risk factors and susceptibility. *Health Psychology,* **3**, 431–457.

Weinstein, N.D. (1987) Unrealistic optimism about susceptibility to health problems: Conclusions from a community-wide sample. *Journal of Behavioral Medicine,* **10**, 481–500.

Zuckerman, M. (1979) Attribution of success and failure revisited, or: The motivational bias is alive and well in attribution theory. *Journal of Personality,* **47**, 245–287.

10
Screening for Cancer: Illness Perceptions and Illness Worry

Linda D. Cameron

Cancer. The very word strikes fear in the hearts and minds of most individuals. Over one million cases are diagnosed each year in the United States alone, where it is second only to heart disease as the leading cause of mortality. And with recent medical advances in the treatment and control of heart disease, infectious illnesses, diabetes and other major causes of mortality, individuals increasingly face the prospect of dying from cancer. Cancer fears are further fuelled by dramatic media accounts and personal memories of protracted, painful suffering by individuals who have died of cancer, as well as from beliefs that its onset and progress are almost uncontrollable. It is little wonder, then, that cancer is often construed as a death sentence and dreaded more than any other disease with the possible exception of AIDS.

Yet these dire perceptions of cancer are unrealistically pessimistic in many respects. Continued advances in cancer treatment and control have led to successful remission for a large proportion of individuals with cancer; in fact, over 40% of cancer patients in the United States have a survival rate of five years or more, with most enjoying normal life expectancies (American Cancer Society, 1993). Moreover, the chances for survival are vastly improved by early detection. For example, 93% of women with breast cancer enter into remission if the cancer is detected early and has not spread to lymph nodes or beyond, while the detection of prostate cancer in its early stages leads to successful control for 88% of patients (American Cancer Society, 1993). Early detection has thus become of paramount importance in the successful treatment and control of cancer and medical organisations around the world have established guidelines for regular cancer screening services for adult men and women. These guidelines generally include regular schedules for mammography, clinician breast examinations and breast self-examinations (BSEs) for breast cancer detection; fecal occult blood test and sigmoidoscopies for the detection of colorectal cancer; Pap tests for cervical cancer; testicular self-examinations for testicular cancer (TSEs); self and clinician screenings for skin cancer; and lung X-rays for regular smokers and others at high risk for lung cancer.

Although cancer screening guidelines have been in place for years, adherence rates remain critically low. Almost 70% of women fail to adhere to national guidelines for mammogram screening (Marchant & Sutton, 1990), while nonadherence with sigmoi-doscopy screening guidelines generally range from 85% to 100% (Davis, Meyer & Love, 1987; McPhee, Richard & Solkowitz, 1986). Utilisation rates for other screening practices are equally discouraging. Concern over poor adherence has spurred over three decades of research aimed at identifying the factors determining decisions to obtain cancer screenings, with a primary focus on educational and sociodemographic characteristics related to screening use. This research has brought to light the critical importance of education about cancer screening services, income and insurance coverage as necessary conditions enabling access to screening services; however, even men and women with the necessary knowledge and ready access to such services demonstrate poor adherence rates. And, as has been found in many health contexts, neither educational programmes that simply provide information about the importance of cancer screening tests nor efforts to increase access to screenings sufficiently increase adherence rates.

It is clear that cancer screening decisions are largely determined by subjective perceptions of cancer and its control, including beliefs about its consequences and treatability, perceptions of the screening tests and beliefs about one's personal risk of cancer. Screening decisions are also shaped by the currents of anxiety and distress surrounding cancer and its detection. Cancer screenings can be frightening experiences and emotions are well known for their powerful ability to alter the course of rational thought. Increasing adherence to cancer screening thus requires an understanding of both the illness perceptions and the emotional experiences underlying the decision-making process.

This chapter will review the research to date, exploring the role of illness perceptions in cancer screening decisions. A striking aspect of this field is that the majority of empirical studies have not been grounded within an organising theory of health behaviour. Indeed, in their excellent review of theoretical models of adherence to breast cancer screening, Curry and Emmons (1994) noted that over 75% of nearly 150 articles reporting empirical research within the previous decade did not use a theoretical framework to guide either the research methods or the interpretation of the findings. Consequently, studies of cancer beliefs and their relationships with screening decisions are often conducted in a haphazard and nonintegrative manner. Of the studies guided by illness perception theories, the vast majority have focused on reasoned perceptions of cancer risk and the relative costs and benefits of screening behaviours, with some attention to the role of social influence in determining screening decisions. Although these studies have been invaluable in identifying and furthering our understanding of the reasoned cognitions involved in cancer screening decisions, they have not addressed the potentially powerful impact of emotions on these decisions.

Following this review is a description of a self-regulatory approach to the problem of cancer screening and its ability to integrate research findings regarding the cognitive and emotional processes underlying cancer screening behaviour. Next, two recent studies demonstrating the utility of the self-regulatory model for advancing our understanding cancer screening decisions are discussed. The chapter concludes with a consideration of potential implications for intervention programmes and directions for future research.

REASONED PERCEPTIONS OF CANCER SCREENING

Perceptions of Vulnerability, Costs, Benefits and Self-Efficacy

As in many other areas of health behaviour research, investigators assessing the cognitive processes underlying cancer screening behaviour have most frequently relied on the health belief model (Becker,

1974) to guide their explorations. The health belief model construes health behaviour as the product of a rational, cost-benefit analysis of the favourability of taking action under conditions of uncertainty. Consequently, our understanding of the cognitions influencing screening decisions is largely based on reasoned perceptions of cancer risk and the relative costs and benefits of screening behaviours (while beliefs about disease severity represent a critical component of the health belief model, they are rarely assessed in studies of cancer screening behaviour due to the lack of variability in perceptions of cancer as an extremely serious disease). Nevertheless, research guided by the health belief model and other rational decision theories has provided valuable insights into the influence of these perceptions on cancer screening intentions and behaviour.

An important aspect of this research is its emphasis on perceptions of vulnerability to cancer, as it highlights the probabilistic nature of the health threat and the wide variability in perceptions of personal cancer risk. Vulnerability perceptions have gained considerable attention and empirical support as critical determinants of health protective behaviour in general since the introduction of the health belief model (cf., Janz & Becker, 1984; Rogers, 1983; Weinstein, 1988). Vulnerability beliefs have been found to be positively associated with just about every cancer screening behaviour, including decisions to obtain mammograms (Aiken *et al.*, 1994a; Champion, 1991; Lerman *et al.*, 1990; Stein *et al.*, 1992), BSEs (Champion, 1991), clinician breast examinations (Lerman *et al.*, 1990), fecal occult blood testing (McCrae & Hill, 1984), Pap tests (Paskett *et al.*, 1990) and screening for skin cancer (Friedman *et al.*, 1993), although some studies have failed to find significant relationships between vulnerability perceptions and cancer screening (cf., Curry & Emmons, 1994 for examples in breast cancer screening research).

Considerable attention has also been given to perceptions of the benefits afforded by cancer screening and perceptions of the costs or barriers to screening. These beliefs have been found to predict a number of screening behaviours, including mammography (Aiken *et al.*, 1994a; Burack & Laing, 1989; Kurtz *et al.*, 1993; Lerman *et al.*, 1990), BSE's (Champion, 1991; Kurtz, *et al.*, 1993), clinician breast examination (Kurtz *et al.*, 1993), skin cancer screening (Friedman *et al.*, 1993) and fecal occult blood testing (McCrae & Hill, 1984). Once again, however, several studies have failed to reveal direct

relationships between reports of cancer screening benefits or barriers and cancer screening use (Murray & McMillan, 1993; Rimer
et al., 1991; Stein *et al.,* 1992).

A final cognitive attribute identified by later versions of the health
belief model as well as by other rational decision theories is self-
efficacy (Rogers, 1983; Rosenstock, Strecher & Becker, 1988).
Perceptions of one's ability to carry out the recommended action
appear to play a particularly important role in self-screening behaviours such as BSEs (Champion, 1991; Friedman *et al.,* 1994), skin
self-examination (Friedman *et al.,* 1993) and TSEs (Brubaker &
Wickersham, 1990).

In general, this research has contributed to our understanding of
illness perceptions related to cancer screening by accentuating the
abstractness and uncertainty of outcomes that are germane to these
types of prevention behaviours. Much of our knowledge about
illness perceptions derives from research regarding responses to
illness conditions once they have begun, as in the case of research
exploring symptom perceptions, seeking health care for problems
and adherence to treatment protocols (cf., Skelton & Croyle, 1991).
In these situations, the individual has entered into a stage of the
disease process in which symptoms and disease consequences
underscore the reality of the health threat and serve as immediate
and powerful triggers to action.

In the case of cancer screening and other prevention behaviours,
however, there are no symptoms or other concrete cues of disease
risk to stimulate protective behaviour and inaction may be further
exacerbated by beliefs that cancer is an improbable event. Although
cancer risk is high from an epidemiological perspective, an individual's risk of getting some form of cancer is an unlikely 1 in 3 and the
odds of getting a specific type of cancer are lower even when considering the most prevalent forms such as breast cancer (1 in 9) and
prostate cancer (1 in 11). These odds are clearly cause for concern,
but for the average individual they are still in favour of not getting
cancer. The probabilistic nature of cancer, in combination with the
absence of symptoms to reinforce its potential, may lead to inatten-
tion to the need for cancer screening and forgetting to take action
even when individuals have reasonable motivations to use screening
services and techniques. These aspects of cancer risk may also facilitate the use of self-serving biases aimed at reducing threat and may

lead to denial, avoidance, delaying use of screening services and the minimisation of personal risk (Croyle, 1992). Unfortunately, the health belief model and other rational decision theories fail to address the potential role of these affect-driven biases in health threat perceptions.

The limitations of research guided by the health belief model and related decision theories have been discussed repeatedly over the last three decades (cf., Curry & Emmons, 1994; Leventhal, 1970; Siebold & Roper, 1979; Wallston & Wallston, 1984) and many criticisms are relevant to current research in the cancer screening domain. The factors (particularly costs and benefits) continue to be poorly defined and so broad as to include a wide variety of cognitions. Moreover, the model does not give attention to the social and affective processes influencing decisions, except to ascribe them to the general categories of costs, benefits, or severity. Finally, the health belief model and other rational decision theories are static in nature and ignore the dynamic processes guiding health behaviours over time (Cameron & Leventhal, 1995; Skelton & Croyle, 1991).

Recently, the transtheoretical model of behaviour change (Prochaska & DiClemente, 1992) has been applied to the study of mammogram use in an effort to provide a more dynamic view of the reasoned perceptions influencing screening behaviours. This model focuses upon changes in illness perceptions over a series of action stages: precontemplation, contemplation, preparation, initiation and maintenance. It is proposed that movement through the stages is determined by the balance of beliefs regarding the pros and cons of taking action (these factors are operationally equivalent to the cost and benefit categories of the health belief model). Several studies have confirmed that the balance of mammography pros and cons endorsed by women is reliably associated with advancement through the behavioural stages (Prochaska *et al.*, 1994; Rakowski, Dube, Marcus *et al.*, 1992; Rakowski, Fulton & Feldman, 1993). However, it is not clear that the positive and negative beliefs about mammography move the individual from one stage to another; instead, these beliefs may simply reflect post hoc rationalisations for one's current use of mammography. Moreover, the pro and con categories do not discriminate between cognitive, social, or emotional factors; consequently, this model may be ignoring important dynamics of the cognitive, social and affective processes underlying cancer detection decisions.

Perceptions of Social Influence

Another body of research exploring the cognitive determinants of cancer screening behaviours has been generated by the use of social psychological theories of attitudes and behaviour, including the theory of reasoned action (Ajzen & Fishbein, 1980), the theory of planned behaviour (Ajzen, 1985) and the Triandis model of choice (Triandis, 1980). Two critical factors distinguish these general attitude-behaviour theories from the health belief model and related theories explicitly designed to explain health behaviours. First, they do not specify a critical role of vulnerability perceptions in the decision process as they were designed to account for general behaviour and not just actions associated with personal risk under conditions of uncertainty. Second, these theories emphasize the importance of social influences on these behaviours. For example, the theory of reasoned action and the theory of planned behaviour identify perceptions of social influence and general attitudes about the behaviour as the two primary determinants of intentions and action; the latter model also identifies perceptions of self-efficacy as guides of intentions and behaviour. Similarly, the Triandis model identifies social influence, perceived consequences of the behaviour and facilitating conditions (which are congruent with the absence of "barriers", noted by the rational decision models) as the critical perceptions guiding behavioural decisions. The Triandis model is unique in that it also identifies the non-reasoned influences of habit and affect on behaviour.

Research fostered by these models has confirmed the importance of social influence on cancer screening decisions. Perceptions of social norms have been found to predict decisions to utilise BSE (McCaul *et al.*, 1993), mammography (Baumann *et al.*, 1993; Montano & Taplin, 1991), TSE (Brubaker & Wickersham, 1990) and Pap tests (Seibold & Roper, 1979). In fact, social influence appears to be a stronger determinant of Pap intentions than reasoned cognitions about these tests (Seibold & Roper, 1979). Interestingly, the social influence of one's physician may be the most powerful facilitator of cancer screening decisions. For example, several studies report that the strongest predictor of mammogram use was physician recommendation (Aiken *et al.*, 1994a; Love *et al.*, 1993; Rimer *et al.*, 1991).

In general, these models have been reasonably successful in predicting screening intentions and behaviours. However, the lack of attention to vulnerability perceptions suggests that these models may be ignoring a potentially critical determinant of health protective behaviours. Moreover, with the exception of selected studies based on the Triandis model, this research fails to consider the potential role of emotions in cancer screening decisions.

A SELF-REGULATORY PERSPECTIVE OF ILLNESS REPRESENTATIONS AND CANCER SCREENING

As the foregoing literature review demonstrates, our understanding of the illness perceptions influencing cancer detection behaviour has benefited considerably from research guided by rational decision models and general attitude-behaviour theories. Yet decisions to engage in cancer detection behaviour clearly involve more than reasoned perceptions regarding vulnerability, costs, benefits, self-efficacy and social influence. The field is ready to move beyond the limited assessment of these reasoned perceptions and to consider more carefully the process by which they are formed and modified, as well as how they interact with emotional dynamics to influence behaviour over time. A self-regulation perspective of cancer-screening decisions offers the opportunity to explore the cognitive and emotional attributes of cancer-related perceptions in this manner.

The self-regulation theory of illness cognition (Leventhal, 1970) proposes that illness representations consist of both reasoned, conceptual cognitions and concrete, emotional memories and experiences and that both conceptual and emotional aspects of these representations guide protective behaviour. This model is consistent with research regarding the general dynamics underlying cognition, in which there is increasing confirmation that the encoding and processing of information involves two parallel, partially independent systems: one that is controlled, abstract, conceptual and "reasoned"; and another that is immediate, concrete, emotional and experiential (see Epstein, 1994 for a review). Both processing systems are seen as integral determinants of behaviour.

The self-regulation model proposes that health-related decisions evolve through a recursive set of stages, beginning with the formation of a health threat representation. Representational attributes include both conceptual perceptions and concrete-emotional information regarding the disease consequences, time-line, associated symptoms, cause, treatment and control. This representation guides the formation and enactment of coping behaviours aimed at resolving the objective health problems, as well as behaviours aimed at reducing emotional distress induced by the health threat. If these objective and emotional coping plans conflict, then behaviour will be determined by the relative salience of each motivation as well as by the immediate environmental constraints. Outcomes of coping efforts are then appraised and used to update the representations or to revise efforts to control the health threat and emotional distress. Illness representations evolve over repeated iterations of the self-regulatory stages and coping efforts increase as the representation and associated distress responses become more elaborated, salient and intrusive (Cameron, Leventhal & Leventhal, 1993).

Social influence processes are actively involved in all stages of self-regulation, as health threat information is shared and discussed with members of one's social network (Croyle, 1992; Leventhal, Nerenz & Steele, 1984). The potential threat and salience of a health problem are directly related with motivations to talk with others about it and solicit relevant information and advice (Zola, 1973; Cameron *et al.*, 1993). Social interactions stimulate the development of cognitive representations and coping plans as information from others is evaluated and integrated. Talking with others may also amplify awareness that the health problem threatens the well-being of many in the social network and is, therefore, a social event that poses consequences for others. Coping intentions and behaviours are likely to be strongly influenced by feelings of obligation to others as well as by faith in their advice.

Vulnerability Perceptions as Catalysts to the Development of Illness Representations

As noted earlier, prevention behaviours aimed at reducing disease risk are rarely associated with salient cues such as symptoms or other signs of disease threat. In the absence of concrete cues, perceptions of disease vulnerability may serve as the triggers for the development of illness representations guiding prevention behaviours. In the case of cancer risk, vulnerability perceptions often develop following exposure to information about possible causes of cancer, risk factors for cancer, or information that similar others have developed cancer. Once a cognitive match between cancer risk information and one's personal status is made, this sense of vulnerability stimulates the further development of the health threat representation by enhancing the accessibility of the illness representation and fostering inclinations to scan for and attend to cancer-relevant information from educational materials, family and friends and health care professionals (Cameron & Leventhal, 1995). In this manner, vulnerability perceptions accelerate the development of beliefs regarding consequences, treatment and control.

Individuals who feel vulnerable to a particular type of cancer thus will have more elaborated health threat representations, which in turn will stimulate the formation and enactment of coping behaviours. At the same time, these vulnerability beliefs lead to the activation and development of fear and worry, which may promote rumination, intrusive ideation and avoidance of cancer detection behaviours despite strong "reasoned" intentions to engage in these behaviours. Cancer screening may be particularly susceptible to avoidance reactions due to fears that such behaviour will result in a cancer diagnosis. From a self-regulatory perspective, then, vulnerability perceptions are important catalysts of health threat representations, prompting the development of elaborated and patterned cognitive and emotional attributes. The importance of vulnerability perceptions in health protective behaviours is well documented; the self-regulatory model furthers our understanding of vulnerability perceptions by delineating their place in the self-regulatory processing of conceptual and concrete-emotional information.

Emotional Distress and Cancer Screening Decisions

A growing body of research supports the self-regulatory hypotheses regarding the emotional currents underlying cancer risk perceptions and screening decisions. First, it is increasingly evident that vulnerability perceptions are not merely "cool", reasoned beliefs as construed by rational decision theories; rather, they induce emotional distress that can reduce psychological well-being and create barriers to regular screening behaviour. In a recent study of women who had first-degree relatives with ovarian cancer, perceptions of cancer vulnerability positively predicted intrusive thoughts and feelings about cancer which, in turn, were associated with increased psychological distress (Schwartz *et al.*, 1995). Similarly, a study of women with a family history of breast cancer revealed that over

50% of the sample experienced intrusive ideation about their cancer risk, with approximately 33% of the women reporting that their worries about cancer had a detrimental effect on their general well-being and daily activities (Lerman *et al.*, 1993).

Although vulnerability perceptions and cancer-related anxiety are often positively associated with cancer screening intentions (e.g., Lerman *et al.*, 1991; Stein *et al.*, 1992), several studies have found that they appear to inhibit use of these screening activities, including the use of mammograms (Kash *et al.*, 1992; Lerman *et al.*, 1993; Lerman *et al.*, 1990), BSEs (Alagna *et al.*, 1987; Kash *et al.*, 1992), Pap tests (Murray & McMillan, 1993) and lung X-rays (Leventhal & Watts, 1966). This pattern of findings suggests that reasoned perceptions of cancer risk promote intentions to engage in screening behaviours in the future, but that these reasoned intentions may be overpowered by mounting anxiety and avoidance motivations as the time of screening approaches.

The potential for cancer worries to interfere with screening use underscores the peculiarity of these protective actions. Unlike health promotion behaviours such as exercise and sunscreen use, screening procedures do not directly reduce disease risk. Instead, as noted earlier, they present the individual with the rather threatening prospect of detecting the presence of cancer. As such, disease detection behaviours are more likely than health promotion behaviours to be influenced by distress and avoidance motivations (Leventhal, 1970; Millar & Millar, 1993).

Millar and Millar (1995) recently explored cognitive and affective responses to disease detection and health promotion behaviours and their findings suggest that emotional processes are particularly active during considerations of detection behaviours. They asked participants to vividly imagine engaging in either a detection behaviour, such as a skin cancer screening, or a promotion behaviour, such as wearing sunscreen. Afterwards, the participants listed the responses that came to mind while thinking about the behaviour and then completed a mood measure. Evaluations of the response lists revealed that, compared to promotion behaviours, detection behaviours prompted more affective responses and fewer cognitive responses. There were also clear differences between detection and promotion behaviours regarding the impact of the cognitive and affective responses on general mood. For detection behaviours, negative affect responses strongly influenced general mood while cognitive responses did not. For health promotive behaviours, general mood was influenced by cognitive responses but not by affective responses. Overall, these results suggest that emotional arousal and processing may have a relatively strong influence on detection behaviours, whereas conceptual processing may predominate in decisions about health protective behaviours. Consequently, cancer screening and other detection behaviours may be especially prone to the influence of distress-induced defence mechanisms such as avoidance. Efforts to increase these protective behaviours may need to attend more to overcoming emotional distress than to instilling reasoned perceptions about the utility of these behaviours.

EVIDENCE FOR THE SELF-REGULATORY ROLES OF CANCER-RELATED PERCEPTIONS AND WORRY IN CANCER SCREENING DECISIONS

Research evidence concerning the role of emotional distress in cancer screening decisions is highly consistent with the self-regulatory model. To date, however, very few studies have explicitly used the self-regulatory model as the theoretical guide for their investigations of cancer screening behaviour. My colleagues and I recently completed two studies explicitly assessing self-regulation hypotheses regarding the conceptual and concrete-emotional processes underlying the development of cognitive representations and their influence on screening decisions. The first study explores the role of vulnerability beliefs as catalysts for the development of cognitive representations of breast cancer risk and its control and the associations between representational attributes and decisions to obtain screening mammograms. The findings support the self-regulatory hypothesis that vulnerability perceptions stimulate the development of screening-related perceptions and emotional responses, which in turn predict mammogram decisions.

The second study uses the context of a clinical trial of tamoxifen chemoprevention therapy for women with breast cancer in remission to explore the impact of symptomatic side effects on the use of BSE. The findings suggest that symptom experiences associated with tamoxifen use may stimulate worry about cancer and increase BSE rates, particularly among women who previously were nonadherent with recommended BSE guidelines. Taken together, these studies suggest that a self-regulatory approach can broaden our understanding of illness perceptions, cancer-related distress and screening behaviours.

Vulnerability Beliefs and the Decisions to Obtain Screening Mammograms

The first study uses data from a longitudinal project assessing the delivery of cancer screening and prevention services to over 5,000 men and women between the ages of 50 and 65 years who are members of primary care practices throughout the upper Midwestern portion of the United States. While the primary objective of this project is to evaluate the effectiveness of two intervention pro-grammes aimed at increasing the delivery of these services, research team members are using the baseline assessment data to assess the roles of cognitive beliefs and affect in predicting cancer screening habits and intentions (Baumann *et al.*, 1993; Love *et al.*, 1993).

We evaluated data concerning mammogram screening intentions and behaviour to test the hypothesis that vulnerability beliefs promote the development of elaborated representations of cancer and its control, which includes both reasoned perceptions (conse-quences, social influence and barriers) and emotional reactions to mammography (Cameron *et al.*, 1996). We predicted that high vul-nerability beliefs would be associated with stronger cognitive beliefs and affective responses, which in turn would predict mam-mogram habits and intentions. In other words, we predicted that the data would reveal a pattern indicating that vulnerability beliefs stimulate the development of representational attributes that promote mammogram habits and intentions.

Participants who had been identified as regular patients at the primary practices were contacted by mail and asked to take part in a longitudinal study of disease prevention. The 58% of the sample who consented were then mailed a questionnaire pamphlet (the response rate for the questionnaire was 90%). The final sample included 3914 women who were primarily Caucasian (98%) and married (79%), with an average education level of a high school degree and an average income of between $20,001 and $30,000; 22% reported a family history of breast cancer. This group of women had reasonable access to mammogram screening services, with 78% reporting full or partial insurance for mammograms, 91%

reporting at least one mammogram in their lives and all having regular contact with their primary care providers. However, only 36% had received yearly mammograms in the prior three year period as recommended for this age-group by the National Cancer Institute and the American Cancer Society.

The questionnaire included measures of representational and emotional attributes, with each measure including two or three items selected on the basis of their high reliability following a pilot test of a larger pool of items; responses to these items were made on 4-point scales. Vulnerability beliefs were assessed with a conceptual item ("How likely are you to get breast cancer?") and a concrete-emotional item ("How worried are you about breast cancer?") so as to tap both aspects of this construct (the two items were highly correlated, $r = .78$). Reasoned perceptions regarding mammogram screening included positive consequences (e.g., "Getting a mammogram regularly is important to me because breast cancer is more curable if found early"), barriers (e.g., "It takes too much time to go to the doctor unless I'm really sick") and social influence (e.g., "My family and friends think I should get a mammogram regularly"). A measure of mammogram-related distress included items such as, "Getting a routine mammogram is scary." Mammogram screening habits were determined by reports of the number of mammograms obtained in the previous three years and intentions were assessed with the item, "How likely are you to get a routine mammogram in the next two years?"

Initial correlational analyses provided some indications of the extent to which demographic characteristics may contribute to vulnerability beliefs and mammogram intentions. Family history of breast cancer was significantly correlated with vulnerability beliefs ($r = .40$), suggesting that this established risk factor is recognised as such by these women and promotes the development of vulnerability beliefs. Mammogram intentions were positively associated with both income ($r = .26$) and education ($r = .19$); neither of these demographic variables was associated with vulnerability beliefs. Consistent with previous research, vulnerability beliefs were positively correlated with both mammogram habits ($r = .14$) and intentions ($r = .14$), although these direct correlations were small.

We used path analytic techniques outlined by Cohen and Cohen (1983) to test the predicted direct and indirect relationships among vulnerability beliefs, mammogram perceptions, distress, habits and

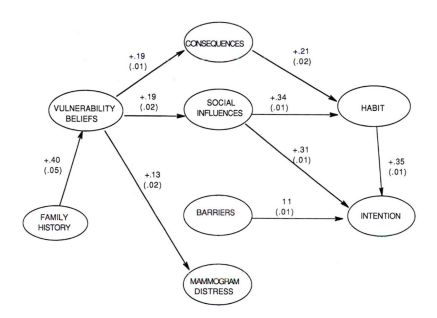

FIGURE 1 Path analysis of vulnerability beliefs, mammogram-related perceptions and distress and mammogram habits and intentions. Path coefficients are standardised regression coefficients; standard errors are shown in parentheses.

intentions. The resulting model, which includes only the significant paths (p's < .0001), is presented in Figure 1. Consistent with self regulatory hypotheses, vulnerability beliefs were directly related to conceptual beliefs about social influence and perceived consequences, although their expected association with perceived barriers was not significant. Vulnerability beliefs were also directly associated with mammogram distress, suggesting that these beliefs also foster the development of concrete-emotional reactions to this screening behaviour. Vulnerability beliefs did not directly predict either mammogram habits or intentions; instead, they were indirectly related to habits and intentions through their associations with social influence and consequences. Mammogram intentions were directly predicted by habit, social influence and barriers, which together accounted for 38% of the variance.

Mammogram distress was not associated with reduced mammogram intentions and it remains to be seen whether mammogram distress leads to delay or avoidance in actually obtaining a mammogram at the two year follow up assessment. Individuals may find it easier to be "rational" about intentions to carry out this type of aversive, yet protective behaviour in the future, while distress-induced avoidance may play a stronger role when it comes time to schedule and attend the mammogram screening. The path model also clarifies the relative influence of family history of breast cancer (objective risk) and vulnerability beliefs (perceived risk) on cognitive representations and mammogram decisions. Family history of breast cancer appears to foster beliefs of vulnerability, but it is only indirectly related to other representational attributes, habits and intentions through its influence on vulnerability beliefs.

This study represents an initial attempt to take a more dynamic, self-regulatory approach to understanding the reasoned perceptions and emotional factors underlying cancer screening decisions. The results are consistent with hypotheses concerning the role of vulnerability perceptions as catalysts for the development of elaborated representations of cancer and its control, which in turn influence screening decisions. These findings parallel those from a previous study, in which the development of an elaborated disease representation (as indicated by strong illness perceptions and emotional responses) was highly associated with decisions to seek medical care for new, undiagnosed symptoms (Cameron *et al.*, 1993). Moreover, they suggest a resolution to the current inconsistencies in the literature regarding the relationship between vulnerability perceptions and screening decisions, whereby some studies find a positive relationship while others do not. The present analyses suggest that the relationship between vulnerability beliefs and mammogram decisions may be mediated by specific representational attributes. Studies that simultaneously regress intentions on vulnerability and a set of other mammogram-related perceptions may find that vulnerability beliefs do not independently predict mammogram decisions and they may erroneously conclude that vulnerability beliefs are an insignificant factor in mammogram behaviour.

As with other surveys assessing illness perceptions and behavioural intentions, our confidence in the directionality of the observed relationships is limited by the simultaneous measurement of the variables. Indeed, given the dynamic nature of health threat representations, coping and appraisals, we expect a degree of recursiveness in the observed relationships. Nonetheless, the path model represents our expectations regarding the dominant influences and helps to clarify the general pattern of relationships among the health threat perceptions, emotional responses and screening behaviour. The consistency of the findings with the self-regulatory hypotheses is promising and encourages inferential explorations of cancer screening decisions using self-regulation theory.

Illness Representations and Symptom Experiences as Triggers for Breast Self-Examination

The previous study explored the role of illness perceptions in screening decisions for women with no previous history of breast cancer. This next study focused on a different population, one that is growing in numbers as cancer treatment becomes increasingly effective and the use of chemoprevention therapy gains popularity. The study participants were women with breast cancer in remission who entered into a clinical trial of tamoxifen, a chemoprevention drug aimed at reducing the recurrence of breast cancer. Chemoprevention therapies for breast cancer, prostate cancer and lung cancer are developing rapidly for use by individuals with cancer in remission as well as in experimental programmes aimed at reducing cancer rates among individuals deemed to be at high risk. Chemoprevention therapy participants possess several characteristics that may influence the self-regulation processes underlying cancer screening behaviour. First, individuals with cancer in remission have active and elaborated illness representations that incorporate extensive conceptual and concrete-emotional knowledge of cancer. These representations may be highly accessible and strongly linked with emotional responses and a repertoire of coping behaviour. A second important characteristic of these participants is that their high risk status intensifies the need for adherence to recommended screening regimens. Third, these participants may be experiencing significant side effects from the chemoprevention drugs and these symptoms may serve as persistent reminders of their cancer risk.

A placebo-controlled toxicity trial of tamoxifen chemotherapy conducted by Richard Love and his associates (cf., Love *et al.*, 1991) provided a unique opportunity to explore self-regulatory processes linking concrete signs of disease risk (tamoxifen side effects) with cancer detection behaviour (BSE). We used data from this study to test the self-regulatory hypothesis that symptom experiences associated with cancer risk trigger the activation of the illness representation, thereby activating cancer worry as well as motivations to engage in health protective behaviours, including cancer screening (Cameron, Leventhal & Love, 1996). Interestingly, the symptoms do not at all signify the presence of breast cancer; instead, they reflect the use of a drug aimed at reducing disease risk. However, we expected that they would increase the frequency of cancer worries and the use of BSE because they serve as concrete reminders of breast cancer risk.

Women with breast cancer in remission ($N = 140$) were randomly assigned to take tamoxifen or a placebo twice a day for the duration of the two-year study. These women were 46 to 64 years old and postmenopausal, with breast cancer in remission for up to 10 years. Measures of physical symptoms, worry about cancer, BSEs and other psychological and behavioural responses were given at three, six and twelve months during the first year of the trial. The symptom report included generic sensations, such as headaches and fatigue, as well as hormonally-related symptoms believed to be induced by tamoxifen: hot flashes, face flushes and vaginal irritation. Participants rated the severity of these symptoms using 10-point scales. A measure of cancer worry consisted of three items assessing the extent to which these worries occurred, caused emotional upset and intruded upon activities during the previous month. Participants also reported the number of BSEs performed in the previous three months.

The retention rate of this toxicity trial was excellent, with only 11% (6 placebo users and 10 tamoxifen users) dropping out of the study during the first year. The following analyses used all available data from participants at each time point. Trait anxiety, assessed during the baseline interview, was used as a covariate in the analyses of worry scores in order to reduce error variance. The distribution of BSE scores were highly skewed, due to a small number of women reporting BSE rates of more than twice per week. These extreme values were truncated and log transformations were conducted on the BSE data before analyses in order to correct for the skewness.

Our first goal was to determine whether tamoxifen causes symptomatic side effects and, in particular, whether it induces reliable increases in the hormonally-related symptoms. As predicted, the tamoxifen users reported significant increases in hormonal symptoms over the entire year (p's $< .01$; see Figure 2). Tamoxifen use was not associated with increases in any other symptoms

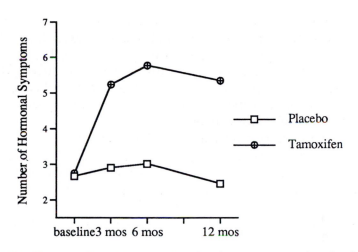

FIGURE 2 Mean number of hormonally-related symptoms, predicted to be exacerbated by tamoxifen, reported by tamoxifen and placebo users during the first year of a chemoprevention trial.

(for a comprehensive evaluation of these findings regarding the symptomatic side effects of tamoxifen see Love, Cameron, Connell & Leventhal, 1991).

The tamoxifen users also reported more frequent and intrusive cancer worries as well as more BSEs in relation to the placebo users. Figure 3 shows that tamoxifen users reported higher cancer worry than did the placebo users during the first six months of the trial (p's < .02), although the group difference was not significant by the end of the year. The tamoxifen users also showed a tendency to engage in more BSEs during the first three months of the trial (p < .10) and they reported significantly more BSEs at the 6 month and 12 month assessments (p's < .05; see Figure 4). These findings are consistent with our prediction that tamoxifen use would induce relatively greater BSE rates because the side effects would trigger the activation of breast cancer representations and related behaviours. However, it is surprising that the group differences are partly due to distinct decreases in BSE reports by the placebo users. One explanation is that participants may have overestimated their BSE rates at baseline due to retrospective biases in

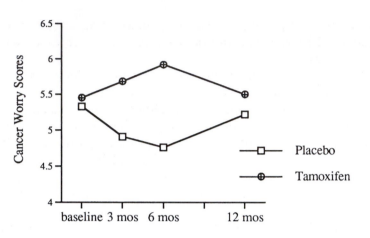

FIGURE 3   Mean cancer worry scores for tamoxifen and placebo users during the first year of a chemoprevention trial.

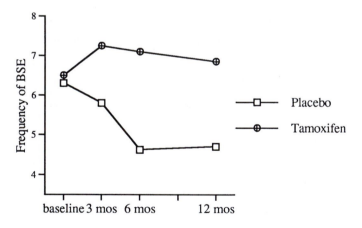

FIGURE 4   Mean number of breast self-examinations conducted within the previous three months by tamoxifen and placebo users during the first year of a chemoprevention trial.

recall. As the trial progressed and they paid closer attention to their BSE habits, their reported frequencies may have regressed to more accurate levels.

A closer examination of the baseline BSE frequencies revealed that, while many women performed BSEs at least once a month, a sizeable proportion of both groups (28% of placebo users and 34% of tamoxifen users) were not adhering to this recommended rate at the time they entered the trial. An important question is whether trial participation leads to BSE rates that fall below recommended levels for placebo users who are already adhering with the guidelines and whether tamoxifen motivates changes in BSE rates for women who are not complying with recommendations. We therefore assessed BSE rates over the year for adherent and nonadherent women in the tamoxifen and placebo conditions.

Figure 5 illustrates the pattern of findings. BSE rates for the adherent placebo users significantly declined over the first year the trial ($p < .05$); the decline in BSE rates for the adherent tamoxifen users was not statistically significant. Nevertheless, both groups

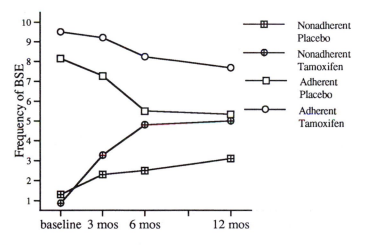

FIGURE 5 Mean breast self-examinations over the previous three months reported by tamoxifen and placebo users who were either adherent or nonadherent to BSE screening guidelines at the onset of the chemoprevention trial.

stayed well above recommended levels over the course of the year; on average, only 6% of participants in both groups reported BSE rates of less than once per month during the year.

More striking is the change in BSE rates for the women who were nonadherent at baseline. Nonadherent tamoxifen users demonstrated a greater increase in BSE rates in relation to the nonadherent placebo users ($p < .05$). Moreover, their average adherence rates met or exceeded recommended levels at each timepoint following baseline, with 74% of the nonadherent tamoxifen users practicing BSE at least once per month by the end of the year, compared to 58% of the nonadherent placebo users. Tamoxifen use appears to have induced important increases in BSE adherence for these women at high risk for breast cancer recurrence.

Because random assignment equalised the groups in terms of social, psychological and physical characteristics, the factor most likely to be responsible for the group differences in cancer worry and BSE use is the increase in symptoms experienced by the tamoxifen users. These findings suggest that tamoxifen-induced side effects serve as reminders of cancer risk for these women and that by activating these illness representations they trigger associated worries about cancer and prompt coping strategies such as BSE. Chemoprevention drug use may lead to changes in cancer screening behaviours and it may increase the frequency and intrusiveness of cancer-related worries due to symptom-induced accessibility of cancer representations.

IMPLICATIONS FOR INTERVENTIONS AIMED AT INCREASING CANCER SCREENING BEHAVIOUR

Our current understanding of reasoned perceptions underlying cancer detection decisions has been applied to the development of intervention programmes aimed at promoting beliefs such as disease vulnerability and the benefits of cancer detection behaviours (e.g., Aiken *et al.*, 1994b; Bastani, Marcus & Maxwell, 1994; Brubaker & Fowler, 1990). These efforts have met with some success, but there is still a considerable gap between actual and ideal adherence rates. These interventions clearly are not addressing some critical components determining the use of screening services. Research reviewed in this chapter indicates a need for intervention programmes to address the potential interference created by emotional distress in cancer screening decisions. The reliable associations between vulnerability beliefs and cancer-related distress suggests that distress-induced avoidance may be especially likely to impede screening use for individuals who believe they are highly vulnerable to cancer. Wellness-oriented messages may help to "cool" strong emotional responses for these individuals, enabling them to focus on the cancer screening in a more reasoned, objective manner and to attend to more positive aspects of the cancer screening experience (such as peace of mind provided by the reassurance that one is free of cancer). Research in other health domains indicates that wellness messages promote protective behaviour among individuals with beliefs of high disease vulnerability, although they may not effectively promote action for those harbouring low vulnerability beliefs (Cameron & Leventhal, 1995; Gintner *et al.*, 1987).

Cancer-related distress may also pose a threat to screening behaviour in the all-too-common situation in which a healthy individual receives a false-positive result from a cancer screening. A significant number of mammograms, Pap tests and other screenings produce inconclusive or false-positive results and individuals who receive them experience significant distress even after subsequent testing rules out cancer (Lerman *et al.*, 1991; Reelick, De Haes & Schuurman, 1984). These individuals may lose their trust in the efficacy of cancer screening tests and fail to return for subsequent screenings. Even if their confidence is not shaken, extreme worry may promote avoidance that delays or even blocks cancer detection behaviour. Climbing utilisation rates will inevitably lead to greater numbers of false-positive screenings, making it increasingly critical that we develop ways to resolve distress induced by these results.

The strong, motivating potential of physician recommendations and other social norms suggests that harnessing these influences may be a powerful means for increasing cancer screening behaviour. Increased attention to primary care services by physicians may significantly increase rates of adherence to cancer screening guidelines. Programmes urging individuals to encourage spouses, parents and significant others to obtain recommended screenings may also prove to be a cost-effective means for increasing screening use. Such interventions would capitalize on the possibility that individuals with family and friends who depend on them are motivated more by their perceived duty to their loved ones than by personal wishes to avoid the emotional threats posed by screening tests. Programmes that combine a social influence approach with efforts to control emotional distress during the screening process promise even greater success in promoting adherence to a recommended schedule of cancer screenings.

The findings that tamoxifen use increases the practice of BSEs support the self-regulatory thesis that symptoms are powerful prompts to protective behaviour (Leventhal, 1970) and have interesting implications for efforts to promote cancer screening. Individuals using chemoprevention therapies may benefit from advice to interpret these side effects as signs that the drugs are working effectively and to use these symptoms as prompts to engage in screening behaviours as a means of obtaining reassuring evidence that the cancer is still in remission. For the vast majority of individuals who are not using chemoprevention drugs, it may be possible to link other sensations with cancer screening behaviour. For example, premenopausal women typically experience hormonally-related changes in breast tissue throughout the menstrual cycle that could be used as cues for BSE. Individuals may be trained to establish an association of skin screening with a particular mole so that it serves as a visual prompt for frequent skin examinations. There appears to be an innate probing response to physical symptoms and the idea of creating associations between naturally-occurring somatic cues and protective action has been prescribed for years by self-regulation theorists (Leventhal, 1970). Efforts to develop and assess techniques aimed at establishing a somatic cue as a prompt for cancer screening behaviour seem to be an ideal venue for testing the efficacy of this concept.

FUTURE DIRECTIONS FOR ILLNESS PERCEPTIONS AND CANCER SCREENING RESEARCH

It is increasingly clear that we need to synthesize the accumulating evidence regarding the perceptions and emotional experiences guiding cancer screening behaviour within a theoretical framework that is consistent with our understanding of general cognition and emotion. The two studies on self-regulatory processes underlying mammogram use and BSE represent preliminary efforts to apply self-regulation theory to the study of cancer screening and they provide encouraging evidence of its potential as an integrative framework. More research guided by a self-regulatory approach to cancer screening promises to advance this field beyond the boundaries of theories emphasising the role of reasoned perceptions.

Given that vulnerability perceptions appear to be important catalysts to the development of cognitive representations about cancer and its control, it is important to determine the origins of these perceptions. What psychological and social factors prompt the development of vulnerability beliefs? Our data and that of others indicate that a family history of cancer promotes perceptions of cancer risk (Evans *et al.*, 1993; Lerman *et al.*, 1995). Family history of cancer may foster vulnerability beliefs by providing conceptual information that the individual may be genetically predisposed to cancer, as well as concrete experiences of family members struggling with the disease. As Lerman and her associates note, vivid memories of cancer experiences may enhance the salience and availability of cancer representations in memory (Lerman *et al.*, 1995). These vivid memories may cause inflated perceptions of personal risk because of the "availability heuristic", a cognitive bias whereby events that are highly salient and easily retrieved from memory are perceived as more likely to occur (Tversky & Kahneman, 1973).

Personality styles represent another potential source of risk perceptions. A recent study found that vulnerability beliefs were strongly associated with dispositional anxiety, hypochondriasis and low self-esteem (Cameron & Leventhal, 1995). However, these personality characteristics were not directly responsible for differences in illness perceptions and behaviours found to be associated with vulnerability beliefs. Instead, these traits appeared to stimulate the development of vulnerability beliefs, which in turn fostered the development of specific cognitions as well as emotional and behavioural responses. Some personality dynamic underlying these interrelated traits may be responsible for the tendency to develop beliefs of disease vulnerability.

Suzanne Miller and her associates have made promising advances toward understanding the role of personality dispositions in the development of vulnerability beliefs. They have identified a self-regulatory style of information processing, called monitoring, that involves a tendency to scan for and process threatening information (Miller, 1987). Monitors appear to be hypervigilant in their attention to health threat cues provided by symptoms and informational messages, and they consequently respond to these cues with significant distress, intrusive ideation and heightened motivations to seek out means for controlling the health threats. Recent evidence suggests that this monitoring style is associated with heightened perceptions of cancer risk and intrusive thoughts about cancer which, in turn, promote worry and distress (Schwartz *et al.*, 1995). Further research on the monitoring style of information processing will undoubtedly help to weave together the threads of anxiety, hypochondriasis, self-esteem, monitoring, sensitization and other personality characteristics running through the literature on responses to health threats and thereby further our understanding of the role of personality styles in the self-regulation of health and well-being.

Finally, research on cancer-related perceptions and screening behaviour remains "diversity challenged", in that the vast majority of studies have focused primarily on the perceptions and behaviours of Caucasian, well-educated samples of moderate to high socioeconomic status. With increasing evidence of differences across sociocultural groups in the performance of cancer screening behaviours (e.g., Hyman *et al.*, 1994), participation in chemoprevention therapies (e.g., Ganz, 1995) and cancer morbidity and mortality rates (e.g., Mebane, Gibbs & Horm, 1990), it is imperative that we diversify our research populations in order to identify the illness perceptions and emotions that contribute to these differences. Recent studies using more diverse samples have found that cancer-related perceptions and their impact on screening decisions do, in fact, vary across ethnic groups (cf., Duke *et al.*, 1994; Michieluite *et al.*, 1994; Price, Colvin & Smith, 1993). Illness representations evolve within the belief systems, social networks and histories of the surrounding cultures and exploring sociocultural differences in illness representations should lead to a greater understanding of their impact on cancer screening decisions and, in turn, cancer morbidity and mortality rates.

REFERENCES

Aiken, L.S., West, S.G., Woodward, C.K. & Reno, R.R. (1994a) Health beliefs and compliance with mammography screening recommendations in asymptomatic women. *Health Psychology*, **13**, 122–129.

Aiken, L.S., West, S.G., Woodward, C.K., Reno, R.R. & Reynolds, K.D. (1994b) Increasing screening mammography in asymptomatic women: Evaluation of a second-generation, theory-based program. *Health Psychology,* **13,** 526–538.

Alagna, S.W., Morokoff, P.J., Bevett, J.M. & Reddy, D.M. (1987) Performance of breast self-examination by women at high risk for breast cancer. *Women and Health,* **12,** 29–46.

Ajzen, I. (1985) From intentions to actions: A theory of planned behavior. In J. Kuhl & J. Beckman (Eds.), *Action control: From cognition to behavior* (pp. 11–39). New York: Springer-Verlag.

Ajzen, I. & Fishbein, M. (1980) *Understanding attitudes and predicting social behavior.* Englewood Cliffs, NJ: Prentice-Hall.

American Cancer Society. (1993) *Cancer facts and figures — 1993.* Atlanta, GA: American Cancer Society.

Bastani, R., Marcus, A.C. & Maxwell, A.E. (1994) Prospective evaluation of an intervention to increase mammography screening in Los Angeles: *Preventive Medicine,* **23,** 83–90.

Baumann, L.J., Brown, R.L., Fontana, S.A. & Cameron, L.D. (1993) Testing a model of mammography intention. *Journal of Applied Social Psychology,* **23,** 1733–1756.

Becker, M. H. (Ed.) (1974) The health belief model and personal health behavior. *Health Education Monographs,* **2,** 324–473.

Brubaker, R.G. & Fowler, C. (1990) Encouraging college males to perform testicular self-examination: Evaluation of a persuasive message based on the revised theory of reasoned action. *Journal of Applied Social Psychology,* **20,** 1411–1422.

Brubaker, R.G. & Wickersham, D. (1990) Encouraging the practice of testicular self-examination: A field application of the theory of reasoned action. *Health Psychology,* **9,** 154–163.

Burack, R.C. & Laing, J. (1989) The acceptance and completion of mammography by older black women. *American Journal of Public Health,* **79,** 721–726.

Cameron, L.D., Helberg, C.P., Brown, R.L. & Baumann, L.J. (1996) Vulnerability beliefs and decisions to obtain screening mammography. Manuscript in preparation.

Cameron, L.D. & Leventhal, H. (1995) Vulnerability beliefs and the processing of health threat information: A self-regulatory perspective. *Journal of Applied Social Psychology,* 1859–1883.

Cameron, L.D., Leventhal, E. & Leventhal, H. (1993) Symptom representations and affect as determinants of care seeking in a community-dwelling, adult sample population. *Health Psycho-logy*, **12**, 171–179.

Cameron, L.D., Leventhal, H. & Love, R.R. (1996) Chemoprevention side effects as triggers for cancer worry and protective behavior. Manuscript in preparation.

Champion, V.L. (1991) The relationship of selected variables to breast cancer detection behaviors in women 35 and older. *Oncology Nursing Forum*, **18**, 733–739.

Cohen, J. & Cohen, P. (1983) *Applied multiple regression/correlation analysis for the behavioral sciences*. Hillsdale, NJ: Lawrence Erlbaum.

Croyle, R.T. (1992) Appraisal of health threats: Cognition, motivation and social comparison. *Cognitive Therapy and Research*, **16**, 165–182.

Curry, S.J. & Emmons, K.M. (1994) Theoretical models for predicting and improving compliance with breast cancer. *Annals of Behavioral Medicine*, **16**, 302–316.

Davis, J.E., Meyer, D.L. & Love, R.R. (1987) Cancer prevention and screening activities in primary care practice. *Preventive Medicine*, **16**, 277.

Duke, S.S., Gordon-Sosby, K., Reynolds, K.D. & Gram, I.T. (1994) A study of breast cancer detection practices and beliefs in Black women attending public health clinics. *Health Education Research*, **9**, 331–342.

Epstein, S. (1994) Integration of the cognitive and the psychodynamic unconscious. *American Psychologist*, **49**, 709–724.

Evans, D.G., Burnell, L.D., Hopwood, P. & Howell, A. (1993) Perception of risk in women with a family history of breast cancer. *British Journal of Cancer*, **67**, 612–634.

Friedman, L.C., Bruce, S., Webb, J.A. & Weinberg, A.D. (1993) Skin self-examination in a population at increased risk for skin cancer. *American Journal of Preventive Medicine*, **9**, 359–364.

Friedman, L.C., Nelson, D.V., Webb, J.A. & Hoffman, L.P. (1994) Dispositional optimism, self-efficacy and health beliefs as predictors of breast self-examination. *American Journal of Preventive Medicine*, **10**, 130–135.

Ganz, P.A., Day, R., Ware, J.E., Redmond, C. & Fisher, B. (1995) Base-line quality-of-life assessment in the National Surgical Adjuvant Breast and Bowel Project Breast Cancer Prevention Trial. *Journal of the National Cancer Institute*, **87**, 1372–1382.

Gintner, G., Rectanus, E., Achord, K. & Parker, B. (1987) Parental history of hypertension and screening attendance: Effects of wellness appeal versus threat appeal. *Health Psychology*, **6**, 432–444.

Hyman, R.B., Baker, S., Ephraim, R. & Moadel, A. (1994) Health Belief Model variables as predictors of screening mammography utilization. *Journal of Behavioral Medicine*, **17**, 391–406.

Janz, N.K. & Becker, M.H. (1984) The health belief model: A decade later. *Health Education Quarterly*, **11**, 1–47.

Kash, K., Holland, J., Halper, M. & Miller, D. (1992) Psychological distress and surveillance behaviors of women with a family history of breast cancer. *Journal of the National Cancer Institute*, **84**, 24–30.

Kurtz, M.E., Given, B., Given, C.W. & Kurtz, J.C. (1993) Relationships of barriers and facilitators to breast self-examination, mammography and clinical breast examination in a worksite population. *Cancer Nursing*, **16**, 251–259.

Lerman, C., Daly, M., Sands, C., Balshem, A., Lustbader, E., Heggan, T., Goldstein, L., James, J. & Engstrom, P. (1993) Mammography adherence and psychological distress among women at risk for breast cancer. *Journal of the National Cancer Institute*, **85**, 1074–1080.

Lerman, C., Lustbader, E., Rimer, B., Daly, M., Miller, S., Sands, C. & Balshem, A. (1995) Effects of individualized breast cancer risk counseling: A randomized trial. *Journal of the National Cancer Institute*, **87**, 286–292.

Lerman, C., Rimer, B., Trock, B., Balshem, A.A. & Engstrom, P. (1990) Factors associated with repeat adherence to breast cancer screening. *Preventive Medicine*, **19**, 279–290.

Lerman, C., Trock, B., Rimer, B., Jepson, C., Brody, D. & Boyce, A. (1991) Psychological side effects of breast cancer screening. *Health Psychology*, **10**, 259–267.

Leventhal, H. (1970) Findings and theory in the study of fear communication. In L. Berkowitz (Ed.), *Advances in experimental social psychology* (Vol. 5, pp. 140–208). New York: Academic.

Leventhal, H., Nerenz, D.R. & Steele, D.J. (1984) Illness representations and coping with health threats. In A. Baum, S.E. Taylor & J.E. Singer (Eds.), *Handbook of psychology and health* (Vol. 4 pp. 219–252). Hillsdale, NJ: Erlbaum.

Leventhal, H. & Watts, J. (1966) Sources of resistance to fear-arousing communications on smoking and lung cancer. *Journal of Personality*, **34**, 155–175.

Love, R.R., Brown, R.L., Davis, J.E., Baumann, L.J., Fontana, S.A. & Sanner, L.A. (1993) Frequency and determinants of screening for breast cancer in primary care group practices. *Archives of Internal Medicine*, **153**, 2113–2117.

Love, R.R., Cameron, L.D., Connell, B.L. & Leventhal, H. (1991) Symptoms associated with tamoxifen treatment in post-menopausal women. *Archives of Internal Medicine*, **151**, 1842–1847.

Love, R., Wiebe, D., Newcomb, P., Cameron, L., Leventhal, H., Jordan, C., Feyzi, J. & DeMets, D. (1991) Cardiovascular risk factor effects of tamoxifen in postmenopausal women. *Annals of Internal Medicine*, **115**, 860–864.

Marchant, D.J. & Sutton, S.M. (1990) Use of mammography — United States, 1990. *Morbidity and Mortality Weekly Report*, **30**, 621–630.

McCaul, K.D., Sandgren, A.K., O'Neill, H.K. & Hinsz, V.B. (1993) The value of the theory of planned behavior, perceived control and self-efficacy expectations for predicting health-protective behaviors. *Basic and Applied Social Psychology*, **14**, 231–252.

McCrae, F. & Hill, D. (1984) Predicting colon cancer screening behaviour from health beliefs. *Preventive Medicine*, **13**, 115–126.

McPhee, S.J., Richard, R.J. & Solkowitz, S.N. (1986) Performance of cancer screening in a university general internal medicine practice: Comparison with the 1980 American Cancer Society guidelines. *Journal of General Internal Medicine*, **1**, 275.

Mebane, C., Gibbs, T. & Horm, J. (1990) Current status of prostate cancer in North American black males. *Journal of the National Medical Association*, **82**, 782–788.

Michielutte, R., Sharp, P.C., Dignan, M.B. & Blinson, K. (1994) Cultural issues in the development of cancer control programs for American Indian populations. *Journal of Health Care for the Poor and Underserved*, **5**, 280–295.

Millar, M.G. & Millar, K. (1993) Affective and cognitive responses to disease detection and health promotion behaviors. *Journal of Behavioral Medicine*, **16**, 1–23.

Millar, M.G. & Millar, K. (1995) Negative affective consequences of thinking about disease detection behaviors. *Health Psychology*, **14**, 141–146.

Miller, S.M. (1987) Monitoring and blunting: Validation of a questionnaire to assess styles of information seeking under threat. *Journal of Personality and Social Psychology*, **52**, 345–353.

Montano, D.E. & Taplin, S.H. (1991) A test of an expanded theory of reasoned action to predict mammography participation. *Social Science and Medicine*, **32**, 733–741.

Murray, M. & McMillan, C. (1993) Health beliefs, locus of control, emotional control and women's cancer screening behavior. *British Journal of Clinical Psychology*, **32**, 87–100.

Paskett, E.D., Carter, W.B., Chu, J. & White, E. (1990) Compliance behavior in women with abnormal Pap smears. *Medical Care*, **28**, 643–656.

Price, J.H., Colvin, T.L. & Smith, D. (1993) Prostate cancer: Perceptions of African-American males. *Journal of the National Medical Association*, **85**, 941–947.

Prochaska, J.O. & DiClemente, C.C. (1992) Stages of change in the modification of problem behaviors. In M. Herson, R.M. Eisler & P.M. Miller (Eds.), *Progress in behavior modification* (pp. 184–218). Newbury Park, CA: Sage.

Prochaska, J.O., Velicer, W.F., Rossi, J.S., Goldstein, M.G., Marcus, B.H., Rakowski, W., Fiore, C., Harlow, L., Redding, C.A., Rosenbloom, D. & Rossi, S.R. (1994) Stages of change and decisional balance for 12 problem behaviors. *Health Psychology*, **13**, 39–46.

Rakowski, W., Dube, C.E., Marcus, B.H., Prochaska, J.O., Velicer, W.F. & Abrams, D.B. (1992) Assessing elements of women's decisions about mammography. *Health Psychology*, **11**, 111–118.

Rakowski, W., Fulton, J.P. & Feldman, J.P. (1993) Women's decision-making about mammography: A replication of the relationship between stages of adoption and decisional balance. *Health Psychology*, **12**, 209–214.

Reelick, N.F., De Haes, W.F.M. & Schuurman, J.H. (1984) Psychological side-effects of the mass screening on cervical cancer. *Social Science and Medicine*, **18**, 1089–1093.

Rimer, B.K., Trock, B., Lerman, C., King, E. & Engstrom, P. (1991) Why do some women get regular mammograms? *American Journal of Preventive Medicine*, **7**, 69–74.

Rogers, R. (1983) Cognitive and psychological processes in fear appeals and attitude change: A revised theory of protection motivation. In J. Caccioppo & R. Petty (Eds.), *Social psychophysiology* (pp. 153–176). New York: Guilford Press.

Rosenstock, I.M., Stretcher, V.J. & Becker, M.H. (1988) Social learning theory and the Health Belief Model. *Health Education Quarterly*, **15**, 175–183.

Schwartz, M., Lerman, C., Miller, S., Daly, M. & Masny, A. (1995) Coping disposition, perceived risk and psychological distress among women at increased risk for ovarian cancer. *Health Psychology*, **14**, 232–235.

Seibold, D.R. & Roper, R.E. (1979) Psychological determinants of health care intentions: Test of the Triandis and Fishbein models. In D. Nimmo (Ed.), *Communications yearbook 3* (pp. 625–643). New Brunswick, NJ: Transaction Books.

Skelton, J.A. & Croyle, R.T. (Eds.) (1991) *Mental representations in health and illness.* New York: Springer-Verlag.

Stein, J.A., Fox, S.A., Murata, P.J. & Morisky, D.E. (1992) Mammography usage and the Health Belief Model. *Health Education Quarterly*, **19**, 447–462.

Triandis, H.C. (1980) Values, attitudes and interpersonal behavior. In H.E. Howe, Jr. (Ed.), *Nebraska Symposium on Motivation* (pp. 195–259). Lincoln: University of Nebraska Press.

Tversky, A. & Kahneman, D. (1973) Availability: A heuristic for judging frequency and probability. *Cognitive Psychology*, **5**, 207–232.

Wallston, B.S. & Wallston, K.A. (1984) Social psychological models of health behavior: An examination and integration. In A. Baum, S.E. Taylor & J.E. Singer (Eds.), *Handbook of psychology and health* (Vol. 4 pp. 219–252).

Weinstein, N. (1988) The precaution adoption process. *Health Psychology*, **7**, 355–386.

Zola, I. (1973) Pathways to the doctor — From person to patient. *Social Science and Medicine*, **7**, 677–689.

Section 3
Illness Perceptions in Illness and Treatment

11
Illness Representations and the Self-Management of Diabetes

Sarah E. Hampson*

One reason why diabetes has become a target of research in health psychology is because understanding patients' perspectives on their disease should lead to ways to foster better self-management (Cox & Gonder-Frederick, 1992). Although health-care providers play a vital role, the responsibility for diabetes management ultimately rests with the patient. People with diabetes, not surprisingly, often find the regimen burdensome and frustrating (Raymond, 1992). Research on the patient's perspective has studied patients' beliefs and feelings about their disease from a variety of different theoretical perspectives such as the health belief model (e.g., Bond, Aiken & Somerville, 1992), social learning theory (e.g., Glasgow, 1995) and ethnography (e.g., Peyrot, McMurry & Hedges, 1987). Although not explicitly used by many investigators of diabetes self-management, Leventhal's self-regulation model (e.g., Leventhal, Nerenz & Steele, 1984) provides a useful framework for presenting studies focusing on patients' beliefs and emotions about diabetes and the links between these cognitions and self-management behaviours. Before examining the research on patients' representations, this chapter begins by

*Preparation of this chapter was supported in part by grant DK35528 from the National Institute of Diabetes, Digestive and Kidney Diseases, USA. I would like to thank Clare Bradley, Russell E. Glasgow and Timothy C. Skinner for their helpful comments on an earlier draft.

providing some background information on the nature of diabetes and its management.

DIABETES

Diabetes mellitus is a relatively common chronic disease for which there is as yet no known cure. Medical advances in this century, most notably the discovery of insulin, have made it possible to control the disease. Nevertheless, diabetes is the seventh leading cause of death in the USA and is a major risk factor for heart disease (Klein, Moss & Klein, 1992). As a diagnostic category, diabetes includes a number of diseases that all share the common symptom of elevated levels of blood glucose (Cox *et al.*, 1986). The two main forms of diabetes are insulin-dependent diabetes mellitus (IDDM) and non-insulin dependent diabetes mellitus (NIDDM). About 3% of the adult population of the U.K. (i.e. 1.4 million) have diagnosed diabetes, 10–25% of which is IDDM (BDA, 1995). Figures for the USA are broadly comparable (Harris, 1985).

In IDDM, which is also referred to as Type I diabetes, the beta cells of the pancreas are destroyed resulting in an inadequate or nonexistent supply of insulin, which is essential for regulating energy metabolism (Tsalikian, 1990). Insulin controls the storage and release of glucose as well as the uptake of glucose by peripheral tissues such as muscle. Without insulin, or with insufficient insulin, the body is unable to utilise the glucose that is ingested or released by the liver. As a result, blood glucose levels rise producing hyperglycaemia. This in turn can result in excessive urination, thirst and weight loss, which are the most common presenting symptoms of IDDM. If left untreated, the absence of glucose metabolism leads to a breakdown of body fat which produces a build-up of ketones. High blood glucose and high ketone levels can cause diabetic ketoacidosis, which may eventually lead to coma and death. IDDM is widely believed to be caused by some form of autoimmune process in which the beta cells of the pancreas are destroyed. This autoimmune process is probably the result of both genetic and environmental factors. The onset of IDDM usually occurs in childhood or adolescence, although it can develop at any age.

Management of IDDM consists of replacing the lost endogenous insulin production with exogenous insulin, combined with the management of diet, exercise and the testing of blood glucose levels. The automatic, continuous homeostatic process for those with normal insulin production must be replaced by the conscious regulation of insulin, food intake and energy expenditure. The goal of management is to keep blood glucose levels within the normal range (i.e., 80–150 mg/dl, or 4–7 mM/L). Insulin is injected one to four times a day, or is released continuously by an insulin pump. Meals of known caloric value must be eaten at regular intervals and physical activity will require additional calories. Blood glucose testing should be done at least once a day and involves pricking a finger to obtain a drop of blood that is placed on a specially treated test strip, which is then read by an electronic meter. There is a constant danger of reducing blood glucose levels to below the normal range resulting in hypoglycaemia. This condition can be serious, producing seizures and coma if left untreated. In sum, the person with IDDM must manipulate the components of self-management in order to steer a course between the Scylla of hyperglycaemia and the Charybdis of hypoglycaemia.

By far the most common form of diabetes is NIDDM. Onset of NIDDM is typically after age 40 and the prevalence increases with age. In NIDDM, there are two problems related to insulin: impaired beta cell functioning resulting in insufficient insulin and insulin resistance in the peripheral tissue (muscle) and splanchnic (liver and gut) impairing glucose uptake (DeFronzo, Bonadonna & Ferrannini, 1992). Obesity aggravates insulin resistance and over 80% of people with NIDDM in the United States are estimated to be over 120% recommended body weight (Zimmerman, 1990). There is a major hereditary component to NIDDM.

The management of NIDDM can, for some people, be accomplished through diet and exercise alone. Weight loss and physical activity appear to decrease insulin resistance thus allowing endogenous insulin to reduce hyperglycaemia. People with NIDDM are encouraged to eat a diet that is low in fat, particularly saturated fat, and high in fibre (American Diabetes Association, 1994). However, for many patients medication is also necessary. Sulfonylureas are taken orally to reduce hyperglycaemia. More recently, metformin is being used as an alternative to sulfonylureas (UK Prospective Diabetes Study Group, 1995). When blood glucose persists at above normal levels, insulin is needed. The components of self-management for people with NIDDM are therefore the same as for those with IDDM.

People with NIDDM need to modify their diet, engage in physical activity and take their medication (either insulin or pills, or both). Moreover, by regular testing of their blood glucose levels they can monitor the effectiveness of their self-management activities and make informed adjustments.

For both IDDM and NIDDM, the goal of keeping blood glucose levels within the acceptable range is designed to ward off both short-term and long-term complications (Cox *et al.*, 1986). Diabetes can lead to damage to various parts of the body as a result of impairments to the blood vessels and nervous system. Diabetic retinopathy can result in blindness if left untreated and diabetic nephropathy can result in renal failure. In addition to these microvascular complications, diabetes also leads to macrovascular impairment associated with heart disease. Diabetic neuropathy (complications of the nervous system) damages both the peripheral and autonomic nervous systems. Peripheral damage to the nerves in the feet causes pain and eventually loss of sensation. This numbness means that the feet are susceptible to damage, which can lead to ulceration and infection. In the worst cases, amputation of the extremities is required.

It has long been suspected that poor glycaemic control is associated with the development of diabetic complications. The results of the recent Diabetes Control and Complications Trial (DCCT) in the USA (Diabetes Control and Complications Research Group, 1993) and a similar study in Sweden (Reichard, Nilsson & Rosenqvist, 1993) now confirm that for patients with IDDM, intensive management that keeps blood glucose levels closer to the normal range prevents long-term microvascular complications. Moreover, the relationship between control and complications was such that even modest reductions in blood glucose levels were associated with reductions in complications, suggesting that even if near-perfect control is too ambitious a goal for patients it is still important to improve blood glucose control as much as possible. Although the DCCT was limited to IDDM, it is widely held that the findings will generalise to NIDDM and there is a study underway in the United Kingdom to test this assumption (UK Prospective Diabetes Study, 1991). These findings present a challenge to people with diabetes and to practitioners providing their diabetes care. They indicate that the difficult task of diabetes self-management is even more important than was previously believed because future health status depends critically upon good control now. Participants in the DCCT agreed to multiple daily insulin injections and blood glucose testing, as well as weekly and sometimes daily contact with providers. Researchers and practitioners are exploring ways of translating this intensive treatment into a more practical and widely disseminable approach (McCulloch *et al.*, 1994).

Having briefly described the main types of diabetes and their self-management, I will now turn to an examination of studies of diabetes cognitions and their relations to self-management. Research on people's beliefs and feelings about their diabetes has been conducted under various guises, many of which can be recast in terms of the Leventhal illness representations framework. In the next section, I will present studies of diabetes cognitions and their relations to self-management, organised in terms of the five components of illness representations (Identity, Cause, Time-line, Consequences, Control/ Cure) identified by Leventhal and others (e.g., Lau & Hartman, 1983; Leventhal & Diefenbach, 1991; Leventhal *et al.*, 1984). In the final section, I will present comprehensive studies of diabetes illness representations that have explicitly adopted the Leventhal framework.

STUDIES OF DIABETES-RELATED HEALTH COGNITIONS

The studies reviewed in this section have examined constructs that bear a strong conceptual resemblance to illness-representation components. Because they have not explicitly adopted the Leventhal model, typically only a subset of the constructs examined in each study can be mapped onto only a subset of the five components of illness representations. This review is not intended to be comprehensive. A selection from the many relevant studies was made in order to illustrate how other theories of health cognitions have generated findings that can be interpreted under the Leventhal framework.

Symptoms or Identity

Leventhal's self-regulation model can be applied both to the initial identification of a disease and to the subsequent monitoring of changes as the disease progresses, is managed, or is cured. Leventhal *et al.* (1984) illustrate how illness representations guide the interpretation of symptoms and health-care seeking in the initial identification of a disease. They tell the story of an overworked executive on a weekend break who develops symptoms of what he initially thinks is indigestion but later (correctly) suspects is a heart attack. For IDDM, a person may well go through a similar period of experiencing alarming symptoms before seeking medical help (e.g., weight loss, excessive thirst and urination, or even coma). People with NIDDM may have less dramatic symptom experiences and their condition can be a surprise discovery in a routine check-up. Indeed, precise estimates of the prevalence of NIDDM are impossible because of such undetected cases, which have been estimated to be at least as many as the known cases (Harris *et al.*, 1987).

The self-regulation model continues to play an important part after the initial diagnosis of diabetes. The representation of symptoms may be a determining factor in self-management decisions. Both hyperglycaemia and hypoglycaemia produce unpleasant sensations that can be vividly described by patients (Peyrot *et al.*, 1987). However, there tends to be little consistency across patients in the symptoms they associate with high and low blood glucose levels. The self-management of diabetes would be much easier if abnormal blood glucose levels elicited distinctive and reliable symptoms. Patients would then know from monitoring their symptoms (instead of monitoring by testing their blood glucose) when they needed to take measures to increase or decrease their blood glucose.

There is some evidence to suggest that people with diabetes are able to detect abnormal blood glucose levels. Within-subject methodologies have shown that IDDM patients exhibit fairly stable yet idiosyncratic clusters of self-reported symptoms that reliably discriminate between hyper and hypoglycaemia (Gonder-Frederick & Cox, 1990, 1991; Moses & Bradley, 1985; Pennebaker, 1982). However, patients may need training to recognise the association between the way they feel and their blood glucose levels (Gonder-Frederick & Cox, 1990). There have been fewer studies of symptom awareness with NIDDM patients. Diamond, Massey and Covey (1989) found that NIDDM patients were better at detecting hyperglycaemia than hypoglycaemia, presumably because they have much more experience of the former than the latter. Although estimated blood glucose levels based on symptom awareness were correlated with actual levels, the estimates were too inaccurate for self-regulation purposes.

Whether or not patients are accurate in their beliefs about the relation between their symptoms and their blood glucose levels, most patients believe they can recognise symptoms of abnormal blood glucose and are likely to perform some form of self-management activity as a consequence of these symptom experiences. For example, Bond *et al.* (1992), using the health belief model, found that self-management behaviours among adolescents with IDDM were predicted by beliefs about the meaning of symptoms (which formed the "cues to action" component of the health belief model).

Many people with diabetes are nervous about lowering their blood glucose because they fear having a hypoglycaemic episode, which can result in embarrassment, accidents, or even coma and hospitalisation (Cox *et al.*, 1987). Consequently, their beliefs and emotions concerning symptoms can result in patients deliberately keeping their blood glucose levels higher than normal to reduce the possibility of a hypoglycaemic episode (Cox *et al.*, 1986; Surwit, Feingloss & Scovern, 1983). Moreover, patients who have had hyperglycaemia for a long time may actually feel worse when their blood glucose approaches normal levels, which serves to reinforce their tendency to keep their blood glucose levels high.

While the accuracy of symptom awareness associated with changes in blood glucose levels remains controversial, the benefits of checking for symptoms resulting from diabetic neuropathy of the feet are undisputed (Litzelman *et al.*, 1993). People with diabetes are encouraged to inspect their feet every day for sores or wounds that they may not be able to feel because of diabetic neuropathy. Careful monitoring for these symptoms can prevent the onset of complications that could eventually lead to amputation and it has been estimated that 50% of these amputations could be avoided if the symptoms were recognised earlier. However, when patients have lost or reduced sensation in their feet, they do not have pain symptoms to prompt them to check their feet or to ask others to do so. In this case, other aspects of symptom representation, which are probably less strong prompts than physical cues (e.g., knowledge of the potential seriousness of minor foot injuries), must be relied upon to direct behaviour. Patients may benefit from a system of reminders to themselves to check their feet and health care providers have been shown to significantly increase their rate of foot inspections if their patients have already removed their shoes and socks before the consultation (Litzelman *et al.*, 1993).

These studies described above have all addressed an aspect of the symptoms of diabetes and the effects of people's beliefs and feelings about their symptoms on their diabetes-related behaviour. The findings suggest that perceptions of diabetes symptoms play an important part both at the initial identification of the disease and in its ongoing management. In particular, symptoms of abnormal blood glucose levels may lead patients to take actions (e.g., eat a snack) to alleviate the symptoms in the short term. However, because of the imprecise relation between symptom experience and actual blood glucose levels, these actions may be inappropriate. Moreover, to avoid or postpone the long-term complications of diabetes, patients should be actively preventing episodes of high or low blood glucose levels rather than responding to abnormal levels when they occur.

Cause

Beliefs about the cause of illness have commonly been studied within an attribution theory framework (Lewis & Daltroy, 1990). Attribution theory classifies beliefs about cause into internal versus external attributions that vary on stability and globality. An internal attribution of causality locates the cause within the person and may involve self blame. An external attribution locates the cause outside the person (e.g. other people, environmental factors).

In Western society, having a causal theory about one's illness has been found to be related to better adjustment and coping (e.g. Turnquist, Harvey & Andersen, 1988). Sissons Joshi (1995) used an attribution theory approach in a comparative study of lay beliefs about diabetes in England versus India. Using a structured interview, she asked people to describe what they believe caused their disease. All participants were taking insulin and half of the sample in each culture had a family history of diabetes. The most common causes cited were heredity, diet, stress and shock. Only about a third of the patients in both England and India who reported a family history of diabetes actually gave heredity as a cause of their diabetes. Apparently, a genetic account was perceived as inadequate and other factors were needed to explain why they had developed the disease while other relatives remained healthy. Diet was given as a cause by twice as many Indian as English patients and a much higher percentage of the Indian (38%) than the English (6%) sample blamed themselves for their diabetes because of their overeating or eating of too much sugary food. Although the majority of participants in both countries were able to generate possible causes for their illness, slightly more Indian (45%) than English (34%) participants were unable or unwilling to engage in this kind of causal reasoning. For these Indian participants, causality did not appear to be an important aspect of their illness representation. Sissons Joshi asked participants about their adjustment to their diabetes and found that for English participants there was a tendency for the poorly adjusted to be those who could not nominate a cause for their diabetes. In contrast, for Indian participants there was no indication that adjustment was associated with having a causal theory. These findings underline the importance of studying the cultural context of illness representations.

As part of a comprehensive interview assessing representations of diabetes using a modification of the Leventhal framework, we asked diabetes patients about their beliefs about the cause of their diabetes (Hampson, Glasgow & Toobert, 1990; Hampson, Glasgow & Foster, 1995). The results of these studies are presented in more detail later in the chapter. However, unpublished findings on causal beliefs from our most recent study are relevant here and are described below. This study was conducted in the USA with white participants with NIDDM (N = 81, mean age = 70 years). They were given a structured interview on their representations of diabetes.

Several questions were asked about their beliefs about the cause of their diabetes. Over two thirds of participants (68%) spontaneously mentioned heredity, which was the most frequently cited cause. In addition, just over half the participants gave stress (53%), weight (58%) and diet (55%) as causes of their diabetes, either in their open-ended response to the cause question or when prompted. These were the four most likely causes for participants to mention and are similar to those found by Sissons Joshi, except that we did not find that people attributed their diabetes to shock. It may be that such attributions were coded by us as stress. Although 62% of the participants said that they had contributed to some extent to the development of their diabetes, the sample was fairly evenly split on whether they actually blamed themselves for having diabetes (43% said they blamed themselves, 57% said they blamed no one). In our sample, the participants appeared to be fairly knowledgeable about the possible causes of their diabetes and to show considerable variability on whether or not their causal attributions involved self-blame. However, as we shall see later in the chapter, beliefs about self-blame were not strongly related to their diabetes self-management.

Perhaps it is not surprising that beliefs about the original cause for one's diabetes (which may have been first diagnosed decades ago) are unrelated to the more immediate day-to-day aspects of living with the disease such as following the treatment regimen. Possibly of more interest would be people's theories about what causes their blood glucose levels to be high or low. For example, if they do not believe that exercise causes their blood glucose levels to be reduced, perhaps they would be less likely to engage in the physical activity aspects of their regimen. However, in this example, the beliefs about cause are really beliefs about the effectiveness of treatment or self-management activities (i.e., outcome expectancies). Beliefs about the initial cause of a disease may be more related to behaviours concerned with the identification of the disease than with the subsequent management of it. Similarly, beliefs about initial cause may also be more relevant for acute than for chronic conditions.

Time-Line or Course and Consequences

Beliefs about disease course are potentially important predictors of self-management of chronic illness. For example, Meyer, Leventhal and Gutmann (1985) showed that believing that hypertension is an acute condition was associated with dropping out of treatment. Beliefs associated with the course of diabetes do not appear to have been studied under one or more of the alternative cognitive models to the illness representation framework, presumably because none of the alternative approaches include a construct similar to this component of the Leventhal model. In our studies (Hampson *et al.*, 1990; Hampson *et al.*, 1995), we gave up asking people about their beliefs about the course of their diabetes when we discovered that the large majority (89%) believed that their diabetes was a chronic illness with no known cure. Other possible aspects of beliefs about the course of the disease, such as the likelihood of developing diabetes complications, were found to cluster with items intended to measure the consequences of diabetes. The consequences component is also difficult to map onto constructs from other theoretical frameworks. In our studies, we have assessed beliefs about consequences by asking people to rate the adverse impact of their diabetes on various aspects of their lives. These items, along with items assessing the perceived seriousness of their diabetes and the degree of worry and anxiety about their diabetes now and in the future, were all highly intercorrelated. We labelled this cluster of beliefs Seriousness, as is discussed later in this chapter.

The lack of variance on beliefs about Course among white, middle-class Americans reflects these patients' medically accurate understanding of their disease. More variation in beliefs about course and consequences have been obtained in samples with greater ethnic and educational diversity. For example, Quatromoni *et al.* (1994) used focus groups to study Caribbean Latinos' beliefs about their diabetes. Two consistent themes related to Time-line and Consequences were identified. These participants demonstrated little understanding of the long-term consequences of their diabetes. They also had a fatalistic attitude toward the course of their diabetes. Fatalism has been found to be an important component of Mexican American's beliefs about their diabetes (Schwab, Meyer & Merrell, 1994) and Sissons Joshi (1995) found a fatalistic attitude among members of an Indian sample. A fatalistic attitude could be viewed as part of beliefs about Control or Cure, if events believed to be determined by fate are seen as unalterable, demonstrating that it is sometimes difficult to map beliefs and feelings found in other studies onto the five components of the Leventhal model. Indeed, attitudes such as fatalism may be part of several components of diabetes representations.

Treatment or Control

Diabetes is a chronic illness, therefore the treatment component of the illness representation consists of beliefs and feelings associated with diabetes management and control rather than its cure. Beliefs about diabetes treatment are probably the most highly researched aspect of diabetes illness representations. Studies from several different theoretical perspectives can be construed as investigations of the treatment component of illness representation.

Social cognitive theory (Bandura, 1977, 1986) introduced the concept of efficacy and outcome expectations and their effects on behaviour to health psychology. Efficacy expectations are beliefs that one can perform specifed behaviours, and outcome expectations refer to beliefs about the consequences of performing these behaviours (Bandura, 1977). In diabetes self-management, self-efficacy refers to beliefs about one's ability to follow regimen recommendations such as dietary and exercise advice or to take medication and test blood glucose appropriately. Outcome expectations are beliefs about the effects these behaviours will have on one's diabetes control, or quality of life, or how one feels. Both kinds of expectations may be viewed as part of the treatment component of diabetes representations. Kingery and Glasgow (1989) examined self-efficacy and outcome expectations and found them both to be predictive of exercise self-management but not of other aspects of self care. Self-efficacy was more predictive than outcome expectations. Subsequently, other studies have found that self-efficacy beliefs are predictive of various aspects of diabetes self-management, particularly diet and exercise (Hurley & Shea, 1992; Kavanagh, Gooley & Wilson, 1993).

Outcome expectations have been investigated in studies testing the health belief model (Becker & Maiman, 1975; Rosenstock, 1974). According to the early version of this model, health behaviour is determined by beliefs about vulnerability, disease severity, the costs versus benefits of the health behaviour and the cues to perform the health behaviour. Within the health belief model, "benefits" incorporate outcome expectations (i.e., beliefs about the effectiveness of the activity for managing diabetes). In a study of adolescents with IDDM, Bond *et al.* (1992) found that the perceived benefits to costs ratio was predictive of adherence. Brownlee-Duffeck *et al.* (1987) assessed the components of the health beliefs model in a sample of younger and older patients with IDDM and related these measures to regimen adherence and metabolic control. Perceived benefits of adhering were associated with higher levels of adherence and better metabolic control, but only among the older patients.

Other constructs in the health belief model that have been found to be associated with diabetes management do not appear to correspond directly to components of illness representations. In a cross-sectional study of a sample of people with insulin-treated diabetes (either IDDM or NIDDM), Cerkoney and Hart (1980) found that beliefs about the seriousness of diabetes and responding to cues to action, were associated with adherence. Bradley and her colleagues have developed scales to assess constructs from the health belief model for people with IDDM and NIDDM (for a review, see Lewis & Bradley, 1994). These scales assess perceived benefits and barriers to treatment and perceived severity of and vulnerability to diabetes. However, research on the predictive utility of these scales has been limited to predicting glycaemic control without studying their long-term relationships with self-management behaviours. Anderson, Fitzgerald and Oh (1993) found that NIDDM patients with higher adherence acknowledged the seriousness of diabetes and recognised the relation between glucose control and complications. In a study of older NIDDM patients, Polly (1992) found that perceived severity was associated with metabolic control and perceived barriers were associated with adherence. In sum, constructs from the health belief model (in particular perceived seriousness or severity of diabetes and perceived benefits of treatment) have been predictive of both self-management behaviours (i.e. adherence) and metabolic control, for both IDDM and NIDDM patients.

Another theoretical perspective that overlaps with the illness representation framework is that of perceived control (Peterson & Stunkard, 1989). The Treatment component may include beliefs about the controllability of an illness and greater perceived control is generally associated with better adjustment and health outcomes. Accordingly, people who do not believe that they can control their diabetes should be less likely to attempt to do so, which suggests that control beliefs should be predictive of the performance of self-management behaviours. Bradley and her colleagues have developed measures of various types of perceived control (e.g., personal control, medical control) that can be used with people with either form of diabetes (for a review, see Bradley, 1994). These measures have predicted glycaemic control prospectively (Bradley *et al.*, 1987) and well-being and treatment satisfaction concurrently (Bradley *et al.*, 1990). For example, for NIDDM patients, stronger perceived control over their diabetes was found to be associated with better glycaemic control, lower body weight and better psychological adjustment. However, in this cross-sectional study, perceived control may have been the result of these positive outcomes rather than their cause.

COMPREHENSIVE STUDIES OF DIABETES REPRESENTATIONS

Our investigations appear to be the only published studies that have assessed the five components of illness representation explicitly using the Leventhal framework and then have related patients' illness representations to the various aspects of their self-management of diabetes. Both of these studies followed Glasgow and Anderson's (1995) recommendations for improving methodology in diabetes research by being prospective and controlling for demographics and medical history variables, which enables stronger conclusions to be drawn about the role of illness representations as determinants rather than as correlates of self-management.

In our first study, we examined 46 women's representations of their NIDDM (Hampson *et al.*, 1990). Their mean age was 57 years and they had all been diagnosed with diabetes for at least one year. We referred to their representations as "personal models" of their illness, using terminology from medical anthropology (e.g., Kleinman 1980). Personal models were assessed using a comprehensive Personal Models of Diabetes Interview (PMDI) following the recommendations provided by Leventhal and Nerenz (1985). A variety of open-ended and fixed response questions was developed covering a wide range of beliefs, including the five components of illness representation. The questions also addressed the emotional aspects of illness representations by asking participants to describe their feelings about their diabetes and its treatment. Care was taken to develop rapport with the patients and most of the interviews lasted about an hour.

Data on illness representations can be used to describe the majority or typical beliefs of the sample. In this way, the lay or folk model of a disease may be identified. A second use of such data is to use them to derive underlying constructs that identify beliefs on which individuals differ. These individual difference measures may then be related to other variables such as self-management. A descriptive analysis of the sample indicated that these women's personal models of diabetes were in broad agreement with the medical science view of the disease. A large majority (89%) perceived their diabetes as a chronic illness and most believed that it could be controlled to some extent by following the diabetes regimen. As other researchers have found, 80% of our subjects believed that they could tell when their diabetes was in poor control without testing their blood glucose.

Guided by the five components of the illness representations framework and by an examination of the intercorrelations among the interview responses, composite variables were formed by combining responses to several interview questions to assess Symptoms, Cause,

Time-line, Consequences and Treatment Effectiveness. The composites for Time-line and Consequences were highly correlated and so were combined to form a Seriousness construct. Symptoms (four items, alpha = .54) included the number of symptoms of hypoglycaemia reported and beliefs about other health problems perceived as being related to diabetes. Cause (three items, alpha = .61) assessed the extent to which the patient blamed herself for the onset of her diabetes (e.g. "Being overweight helped cause my diabetes"). Seriousness (seven items, alpha = .76) included self-ratings of the patients' perceived seriousness of and emotional reactions to their diabetes, as well as their assessments of the consequences of their diabetes for various aspects of their lives. Treatment Effectiveness (seven items, alpha = .64) was composed of the perceived importance of the various regimen components for controlling diabetes and patients' feelings about following the regimen. The intercoder reliability correlations for these four constructs was .90 for Symptoms, .74 for Cause, .98 for Seriousness and .99 for Treatment Effectiveness.

Individuals' scores on each of these constructs were related to their diabetes self-management assessed by the Summary of Self Care Activities (Toobert & Glasgow, 1994) on a separate occasion but within two weeks of the personal models assessment. This self-report measure has been validated against more objective measures using different methods (e.g., four-day food records). Using hierarchical multiple regression, age and whether or not the patient was taking insulin were entered at the first step and the four personal model constructs were entered at the second step. Personal models contributed significantly (R^2 = .19) to the prediction of dietary self-management (adherence to recommended amount of calories) and marginally to adherence to recommended exercise (R^2 = .13), but not to the more medical components of the regimen (blood-glucose self-monitoring and medication taking). For both diet and exercise, Treatment Effectiveness was the most important predictor of level of self-management. However, personal models constructs were not predictive of glycosylated haemoglobin levels, which provide a biologic measure of blood glucose control over the preceding two to three months. It is not unusual for psychosocial variables to be predictive of self-management behaviours but to fail to predict blood glucose control (Glasgow, 1991; Johnson, 1992). A likely reason for this inconsistency is that glycosylated haemoglobin levels are determined by several biomedical and other factors in addition to psychosocial ones (e.g., insulin compliance, stress and other aspects of the disease process).

The above findings demonstrate that the five components of illness representations found by Leventhal and others for various diseases can also be extended to NIDDM. However, our interview measure did not produce a meaningful distinction between Course (or Time-line) and Consequences, which formed a single internally consistent construct that we called Seriousness. Possibly the chronic nature of diabetes and the long-term threat of serious complications, results in these two components merging together in the representation. In a similar study of osteo arthritis (another common chronic condition of older persons), we also found that Course and Consequences merged together (Hampson, Glasgow & Zeiss, 1994).

Given the small and exclusively female sample used in our first study, we felt it wise to replicate the study on a larger sample including both men and women. In this second study, involving 78 people with NIDDM, we also looked at the short-term stability of personal models and we related them to self-management behaviours assessed both concurrently with the personal models assessment and prospectively four months later (Hampson *et al.*, 1995). The PMDI was improved by removing items that, in the previous study, produced little or no variance and making other minor wording and order changes. This current version of the PMDI can now be completed within 45 minutes by most participants. Possibly as a result of these improvements, the internal consistencies (coefficient alphas) of the personal model constructs were better than those found in the first study. However, as before, Symptoms was the least reliably measured construct and was dropped from further analysis. The alpha reliabilities for the remaining three constructs were .70 for Cause (three items), .79 for Seriousness (eight items) and .75 for Treatment Effectiveness (4 items). The test-retest correlations over one month were .82, .79 and .80, respectively, indicating reasonable stability in the illness representation over this time period.

Patients' personal models were related to their self-reports of dietary intake and levels of physical activity, using the same measure as in the first study. Using hierarchical multiple regression, demographic and medical history variables were entered at step 1, followed by the three personal model constructs at step 2. These analyses examined the concurrent predictions between personal models and self-management and the four-month prospective relations. The pattern of results was broadly similar across both analyses. Replicating our first study, personal models constructs significantly improved the prediction of diet both concurrently ($R^2 = .31$) and prospectively ($R^2 = .18$). Moreover, they significantly improved the prediction of physical activity levels concurrently ($R^2 = .26$), but not at four months ($R^2 = .20$). Examination of the contributions of each of the constructs to the prediction of self-management indicated that, as found before, Treatment Effectiveness was the most important predictor. Interestingly, in the prospective analysis, Cause and Treatment Effectiveness significantly predicted glycosylated haemoglobin levels ($R^2 = .30$).

Together, these two studies have demonstrated that the illness representations framework can be extended to NIDDM, both as a way of describing individual differences in diabetes beliefs and feelings and as a means of contributing to the understanding of diabetes self-management. The next step is to target illness representations in interventions to enhance diabetes self-management. There is some evidence of the feasibility of such an intervention. Wooldridge *et al.* (1992) intervened on adult diabetes patients and achieved increases in perceived severity of diabetes, self-efficacy and perceived benefits of treatment. However, these increases were not related to the improvements in glycaemic control observed for some participants, nor did health beliefs predict levels of self-reported adherence.

We have developed a brief questionnaire version of the PMDI to provide a more practical assessment tool. This measure has been used to assess personal models in the tailoring of a personalised intervention targeting low-fat diet for older diabetes patients (Glasgow *et al.*, 1995). Assessment of personal models formed part of a more comprehensive assessment of nutrition and psychosocial factors affecting diet and the personalised intervention involved negotiating specific behavioural goals. The intervention was demonstrated to be effective relative to the control condition in producing behavioural and biologic changes related to diet that were sustained over three months follow-up (Glasgow, Toobert & Hampson, 1996). Among the intervention group, those who believed more strongly in Treatment Effectiveness showed greater improvement in their self-reported food habits at follow-up, after controlling for initial scores on food habits (partial $r = -.23$, $p < .05$), but Treatment Effectiveness was not associated with the other measures of dietary outcomes.

This intervention was not designed to change illness representations. The interventionist and physician were informed about the patient's strength of belief in Treatment Effectiveness and Seriousness of their diabetes, but they were not given any explicit directions on how to use this information. Future interventions could target beliefs in an attempt to change them, or could deliver different types of intervention depending on the patient's illness representation. However, illness representations are only one of a host of psychosocial and biomedical factors that can be expected to contribute to self-management and glycaemic control (Glasgow, 1995). Therefore, interventions that target illness representations alone are not likely to be successful.

CONCLUSIONS

Together, the studies guided by different theoretical perspectives on health cognitions and the work that explicitly adopted the Leventhal approach, provide a demonstration that people hold a variety of beliefs about their diabetes, some of which are associated with the extent to which they adhere to recommended treatment regimens and self-management behaviours. Beliefs about Treatment (i.e. "costs" and "benefits" according to the health belief model), followed by beliefs about Seriousness, appear to be most strongly associated with self-management. On the basis of face validity, it was possible to find similarities among the various health cognitions and the components of illness representations. There are many similarities across the various social cognition models of health beliefs and, from the studies reviewed here and elsewhere in this book, it appears that the Leventhal framework may provide the basis for an overarching taxonomy of health cognitions. Such a taxonomy would be useful because it would assist in identifying similar constructs across different theories and perhaps it would prevent the unnecessary proliferation of measures.

However, despite its promise as a taxonomy of health cognitions, the illness representation approach has a number of limitations. To date, almost all the measures of illness representations have been interviews or questionnaires, which assume that people can verbalise their beliefs and feelings about their disease. However, Leventhal has always argued that illness representations will include important nonverbal elements (Leventhal, Meyer & Nerenz, 1980). We need to develop more creative approaches to assessing representations that can measure those aspects of which the person is not necessarily aware. For example, we have developed a card-sorting technique to assess the dimensional complexity of people's illness representations (Hampson & Glasgow, 1996) and used this method to compare "experts" (those with diabetes) versus "novices" (those without diabetes). Nonverbal measures may also prove useful for assessing the emotional aspects of illness representations. The Leventhal framework differs from the other theories of health cognitions in its emphasis on emotional aspects, yet these have tended to be inadequately assessed.

Other models of health cognitions (e.g., the health belief model) have been criticised for being only a collection of variables and not a truly integrated theory. The Leventhal framework is in danger of being open to the same criticism if we are content simply to identify the presence of the five components in people's representations of various diseases without examining their inter-relationships and their role within the self-regulation model. Research also needs to go beyond the description of illness representations to test whether and how these representations are predictive of significant, long-term health-related behaviour and how these relationships are affected by disease characteristics. The studies of diabetes representations have demonstrated that some modification to the five components is probably necessary and the same may be true for other diseases as well. Moreover, the relation between the components of the illness representation and illness-related behaviour appears to differ across diseases. For example, although beliefs about Treatment are most strongly related to diabetes self-management, beliefs about Seriousness (or Intensity) are most strongly related to the self-management of osteo arthritis (see Pimm's chapter in this book). We need to develop the self-regulation model to incorporate these disease-based differences in its operation.

REFERENCES

American Diabetes Association (1994) Nutrition recommendations and principles for people with diabetes mellitus. *Diabetes Care*, **17**, 519–522.

Anderson, R.M., Fitzgerald, J.T. & Oh, M.S. (1993) The relationship between diabetes-related attitudes and patients' self-reported adherence. *The Diabetes Educator*, **19**, 287–292.

Bandura, A. (1977) Self-efficacy: Toward a unifying theory of behavioral change. *Psychological Review*, **84**, 191–215.

Bandura, A. (1986) *Social foundations of thought and action: A social cognitive theory*. Englewood Cliffs: Prentice Hall.

Becker, M.H. & Maiman, L.A. (1975) Sociobehavioral determinants of compliance with health and medical care recommendations. *Medical Care*, **13**, 10–23.

Bond, G.G., Aiken, L.S. & Somerville, S.C. (1992) The Health Belief Model and adolescents with insulin-dependent diabetes mellitus. *Health Psychology*, **11**, 190–198.

Bradley, C. (1994) Measures of perceived control of diabetes. In C. Bradley (Ed.), *Handbook of psychology and diabetes* (pp. 291–331). Switzerland: Harwood Academic.

Bradley, C., Lewis, K.S., Jennings, A.M. & Ward, J.D. (1990) Scales to measure perceived control developed specifically for people with tablet-treated diabetes. *Diabetic Medicine*, **7**, 685–694.

Bradley, C., Gamsu, D.S., Moses, J.L., Knight, G., Boulton, A.M., Drury, J. & Ward, J.D. (1987) The use of diabetes specific perceived control and health belief measures to predict treatment choice and efficacy in a feasibility study of continuous subcutaneous insulin infusion pumps. *Psychology and Health*, **1**, 133–146.

British Diabetic Association (1995) *Fact Sheet*. London: BDA.

Brownlee-Duffeck, M., Peterson, L., Simonds, J.F., Goldstein, D., Kilo, C. & Hoette, S. (1987) The role of health beliefs in the regimen adherence and metabolic control of adolescents and adults with diabetes mellitus. *Journal of Consulting and Clinical Psychology*, **55**, 139–144.

Cerkoney, K.A. & Hart, L.K. (1980) The relationship between the health belief model and compliance of persons with diabetes mellitus. *Diabetes Care*, **3**, 594–598.

Cox, D.J. & Gonder-Frederick, L. (1992) Major developments in behavioral diabetes research. *Journal of Consulting and Clinical Psychology*, **60**, 628–638.

Cox, D.J., Gonder-Frederick, L., Pohl, S. & Pennebaker, J.W. (1986) Diabetes. In K.A. Holroyd & T.L. Creer (Eds.), *Self-management of chronic diseases* (pp. 305–346). Orlando, Florida: Academic Press.

Cox, D.J., Irvine, A., Gonder-Frederick, L., Nowacek, G. & Butterfield, J. (1987) Quantifying fear of hypoglycemia: a preliminary report. *Diabetes Care*, **10**, 617–621.

DeFronzo, R.A., Bonadonna, R.C. & Ferrannini, E. (1992) Pathogenesis of NIDDM. *Diabetes Care*, **15**, 319–368.

Diabetes Control and Complications Trial Research Group. (1993) The effect of intensive treatment of diabetes on the development and progression of long-term complications in insulin-dependent diabetes mellitus. *New England Journal of Medicine*, **329**, 977–986.

Diamond, E.L., Massey, K.L. & Covey, D. (1989) Symptom awareness and blood glucose estimation in diabetic adults. *Health Psychology*, **8**, 15–26.

Glasgow, R.E. (1991) Compliance to diabetes regimens: conceptualization, complexity and determininants. In J.A. Cramer & B. Spilker (Eds.), *Patient compliance in medical practice and clinical trials* (pp. 209–224). New York: Raven.

Glasgow, R.E. (1995) A practical working model of diabetes management and education. *Diabetes Care*, **18**, 117–126.

Glasgow, R.E. & Anderson, B.J. (1995) Future directions for research on pediatric chronic disease management. *Journal of Pediatric Psychology*, **20**, 389–402.

Glasgow, R.E., Toobert, D.J. & Hampson, S.E. (1996) Effects of a brief, office-based intervention to facilitate diabetes dietary self-management. *Diabetes Care*, **19**, 835–842.

Glasgow, R.E., Toobert, D.J., Hampson, S.E. & Noell, J.W. (1995) A brief office-based intervention to facilitate diabetes self-management. *Health Education Research: Theory and Practice*, **10**, 467–478.

Gonder-Frederick, L.A. & Cox, D.J. (1990) Symptom perception and blood glucose feedback in the self-treatment of IDDM. In C.S. Holmes (Ed.), *Neuropsychological and behavioral aspects of diabetes* (pp. 154–174). New York: Springer-Verlag.

Gonder-Frederick, L. & Cox, D.J. (1991) Symptom perception, symptom beliefs and blood glucose discrimination in the self-treatment of insulin-dependent diabetes. In J.A. Skelton & R.T. Croyle (Eds.), *Mental Representations in health and illness* (pp. 220–246). New York: Springer-Verlag.

Hampson, S.E. & Glasgow, R.E. (1996) Dimensional complexity of representations of diabetes and arthritis. *Basic and Applied Social Psychology*, **18**, 45–59.

Hampson, S.E., Glasgow, R.E. & Foster, L.S. (1995) Personal models of diabetes among older adults: Relation to self-management and other variables. *The Diabetes Educator*, **21**, 300–307.

Hampson, S.E., Glasgow, R.E. & Toobert, D.J. (1990) Personal models of diabetes and their relation to self-care activities. *Health Psychology,* **9**, 632–646.

Hampson, S.E., Glasgow, R.E. & Zeiss, A. (1994) Personal models of osteoarthritis and their relation to self-management and quality of life. *Journal of Behavioral Medicine*, **17**, 143–158.

Harris, M.I. (1985) Prevalence of noninsulin-dependent diabetes and impaired glucose tolerance. *Diabetes in America: Diabetes Data Complied 1984* (DHHS, NIH Publication No. 85–1468). Washington, DC: US Government Printing Office.

Harris, M.I., Hadden, W.C., Knowler, W.C. & Bennett, P.H. (1987) Prevalence of diabetes and impaired glucose tolerance and plasma glucose levels in U.S. populations aged 20–74 Yr. *Diabetes*, **36**, 523–534.

Hurley, C.C. & Shea, C.A. (1992) Self-efficacy: A strategy for enhancing diabetes self-care. *The Diabetes Educator*, **18**, 146–150.

Johnson, S.B. (1992) Methodological issues in diabetes research: Measuring adherence. *Diabetes Care*, **15**, 1658–1667.

Kavanagh, D.J., Gooley, S. & Wilson, P.H. (1993) Prediction of adherence and control of diabetes. *Journal of Behavioral Medicine*, **16**, 509–522.

Kingery, P.M. & Glasgow, R.E. (1989) Self-efficacy and outcome expectations in the self-regulation of non-insulin dependent diabetes mellitus. *Health Education*, **20**, 13–19.

Klein, B.E., Moss, S.E. & Klein, R. (1992) Use of cardiovascular disease medications and mortality in people with older onset diabetes. *American Journal of Public Health*, **82**, 1142–1144.

Kleinman, A. (1980) *Patients and healers in the context of culture.* Berkeley: University of California Press.

Lau, R.R. & Hartman, K.A. (1983) Common sense representations of common illnesses. *Health Psychology*, **2**, 167–185.

Leventhal, H. & Diefenbach, M. (1991) The active side of illness cognition. In J.A. Skelton & R.T. Croyle (Eds.), *Mental representations in health and illness* (pp. 220–246). New York: Springer-Verlag.

Leventhal, H. & Nerenz, D. (1985) Assessment of illness cognition. In P. Karoly (Ed.), *Measurement strategies in health* (pp. 517–554). New York: Wiley.

Leventhal, H.D., Meyer, D. & Nerenz, D. (1980) The commonsense representation of illness danger. In S. Rachman (Ed.), *Contributions to medical psychology* (Vol 2) (pp. 7–31). Oxford: Pergamon Press.

Leventhal, H., Nerenz, D. & Steele, D.J. (1984) Illness representations and coping with health threats. In A. Baum, S.E. Taylor & J.E. Singer (Eds.), *Handbook of psychology and health* (pp. 219–252). Hillsdale, N.J.: Lawrence Erlbaum Associates.

Lewis, K.S. & Bradley, C. (1994) Measures of diabetes-specific health beliefs. In C. Bradley (Ed.), *Handbook of psychology and diabetes* (pp. 247–289). Switzerland: Harwood Academic.

Lewis, F.M. & Daltroy, L.H. (1990) How causal explanations influence health behavior: Attribution theory. In K.Glanz, F.M. Lewis & B.K.Rimer (Eds.), *Health behavior and health education* (pp. 92–114). San Francisco: Jossey-Bass.

Lewis, K.S., Jennings, A.M., Ward, J.D. & Bradley, C. (1990) Health Belief scales developed specifically for people with tablet-treated Type 2 diabetes. *Diabetic Medicine*, **7**, 148–155.

Litzelman, D.K., Slemenda, C.W., Langefeld, C.D., Hays, L.M., Welch, M.A., Bild, D.E., Ford, E.S. & Vinicor, F. (1993) Reduction of lower extremity clinical abnormalities in patients with non-insulin dependent diabetes mellitus. *Annals of Internal Medicine*, **119**, 36–41.

McCulloch, D.K., Glasgow, R.E., Hampson, S.E. & Wagner, E. (1994) A systematic approach to diabetes management in the post-DCCT era. *Diabetes Care*, **17**, 765–769.

Meyer, D., Leventhal, H. & Gutmann, M. (1985) Common-sense models of illness: The example of hypertension. *Health Psychology*, **4**, 115–135.

Pennebaker, J.W. (1982) *The psychology of physical symptoms*. New York: Springer Verlag.

Peterson, C. & Stunkard, A.J. (1989) Personal control and health. *Social Science and Medicine*, **28**, 819–828.

Moses, J.L. & Bradley, C. (1985) Accuracy of subjective blood glucose estimation by patients with insulin-dependent diabetes. *Biofeedback and Self-Regulation*, **10**, 301–314.

Polly, R.K. (1992) Diabetes health beliefs, self-care behaviors and glycemic control among older adults with non-insulin dependent diabetes mellitus. *The Diabetes Educator*, **18**, 321–327.

Peyrot, M., McMurry, J.F. & Hedges, R. (1987) Living with diabetes: the role of personal and professional knowledge in symptom and regimen management. *Research in the Sociology of Health Care*, **6**, 107–146.

Quatromoni, P.A., Mibauer, M., Posner, B.M., Carballeira, N.P., Brunt, M. & Chipkin, S.R. (1994) Use of focus groups to explore nutrition practices and health beliefs of urban Caribbean Latinos with diabetes. *Diabetes Care*, **17**, 869–873.

Raymond, M. (1992) *The human side of diabetes: Beyond doctors, diets and drugs.* Chicago: The Noble Press.

Reichard, P., Nilsson, B-Y. & Rosenqvist, U. (1993) The effect of long-term intensified insulin treatment on the development of microvascular complications of diabetes mellitus. *New England Journal of Medicine*, **329**, 304–309.

Rosenstock, I.M. (1974) Historical origins of the health belief model. *Health Education Monographs*, **2**, 328–335.

Schwab, T., Meyer, J. & Merrell, R. (1994) Measuring attitudes and health beliefs among Mexican Americans with diabetes. *The Diabetes Educator*, **20**, 221–227.

Sissons Joshi, M. (1995) Lay explanations of the causes of diabetes in India and the UK. In I. Markova & R.M. Farr (Eds.), *Representations of health, illness and handicap* (pp. 163–188). UK: Harwood Academic.

Surwit, R.S., Feingloss, M.N. & Scovern, A.W. (1983) Diabetes and behavior: A paradigm for health psychology. *American Psychologist*, **83**, 255–262.

Toobert, D.T. & Glasgow, R.E. (1994) Assessing diabetes self-management: The summary of diabetes self-care activities questionniare. In C. Bradley (Ed.), *Handbook of psychology and diabetes* (pp. 351–375). Switzerland: Harwood Academic.

Tsalikian, E. (1990) Insulin-dependent (Type I) diabetes mellitus: Medical overview. In C.S. Holmes (Ed.), *Neuropsychological and behavioral aspects of diabetes* (pp. 3–11). New York: Springer-Verlag.

Turnquist, D.C., Harvey, J.H. & Andersen, B.L. (1988) Attributions and adjustment to life-threatening illness. *British Journal of Clinical Psychology*, **27**, 55–65.

UK Prospective Diabetes Study Group (UKPDS) 13 (1995) Relative efficacy of randomly allocated diet, sulphonylurea, insulin, or metformin in patients with newly diagnosed non-insulin dependent diabetes for three years. *British Medical Journal*, **310**, 83–88.

UK Prospective Diabetes Study, (UKPDS) VIII (1991) Study design, progress and performance. *Diabetologia*, **34**, 877–890.

Wooldridge, K.L., Wallston, K.A., Graber, A.L., Brown, R.N. & Davidson, P. (1992) The relationship between health beliefs, adherence and metabolic control of diabetes. *The Diabetes Educator*, **18**, 495–500.

Zimmerman, B.R. (1990) Non-insulin dependent (Type II) diabetes: Medical overview. In C.S. Holmes (Ed.), *Neuropsychological and behavioral aspects of diabetes* (pp. 177–183). New York: Springer-Verlag.

12

Self-Regulation and Psycho-educational Interventions for Rheumatic Disease

Theo J. Pimm*

INTRODUCTION

This chapter discusses the application of Leventhal's self-regulatory model to rheumatic disease (Leventhal *et al.*, 1980; Leventhal *et al.*, 1992; Leventhal & Schaefer, 1992). In recent years research in rheumatic disease has suggested that psychological factors may play an important role in mediating between the disease and its outcome. This chapter considers whether the self-regulatory model provides a useful framework for guiding research in this field. The nature of rheumatic diseases and the challenges they present are considered first followed by a discussion about application of the self-regulatory model to rheumatic disease. Next research that has investigated the role that self-regulatory processes may play in adaptation to rheumatic disease is reviewed. Finally psycho-educational interventions that have been developed for rheumatic disease are discussed and whether an understanding of self-regulatory processes could improve the design and outcome of psycho-educational interventions is considered.

*Our research is supported by Arthritis and Rheumatism Council grants PO503 and PO520. I would also like to thank Sharon Hill for her invaluable help in preparing this chapter.

RHEUMATIC DISEASES

Rheumatic disorders include over 120 different diseases affecting the muscular-skeletal structures. Some of the commonest include osteo arthritis (OA), rheumatoid arthritis (RA) and systemic lupus erythematosus (SLE). There are an estimated 37 million people with rheumatic diseases in the US (Lawrence *et al.*, 1989). OA is the most common form of arthritis with 12% of people over the age of 25 being affected (Brandt & Flusser, 1991). The prevalence of OA increases steeply with age and 60% of people over age 65 have at least one joint showing moderate or severe changes on X-ray (Croft, 1990). Other rheumatic diseases are also common. For instance, RA affects over eight million people in the US (Lambert & Lambert, 1987). Approximately 4% of the population have probable RA and 1% definite RA (Hazes & Silman, 1990)

The cause of most rheumatic diseases is unknown, most are chronic, progressive, incurable and the prognosis is uncertain. The emphasis of treatment is on management of symptoms, controlling disease progression and optimizing physical function rather than prevention or cure. Rheumatic diseases are a major cause of disability. They are the leading cause of activity limitation in the US (Kelsey, 1982). The 1988 OPCS survey estimated that three million people in the UK had a disability associated with musculoskeletal disorders (Martin & White, 1988). It is the single greatest cause of disability in the elderly with 53% of adults over age 65 reporting arthritis to be a significant health problem (Controller General, 1979). Over half of the population who are over 85 years had joint problems and most of these reported some disability (Badley & Tennant, 1989). Rheumatic diseases restrict people's ability to perform social and occupational roles e.g. 50% of RA patients suffer significant work disability within 5 years of disease onset (Yelin *et al.*, 1980).

Given the distressing symptoms and disabilities associated with rheumatic diseases it is not surprising that they may lead to difficulties in phychological adjustment (e.g. depression, anxiety and reduced life satisfaction). Prevalence estimates for depression vary considerably. In a review of several large scale surveys of clinic and community samples DeVellis (1993) concludes that levels of depression and depressive symptomatology are higher in people with rheumatic disease than for people without chronic illnesses but are similar to those found in people with other chronic illnesses. However, in an analysis of three cross-sectional studies of RA Zautra *et al.* (1995) report that increased negative affect and reduction in positive affect are significant and independent consequences of RA.

Disease activity and severity are positively related to emotional distress (Zautra *et al.*, 1995). However the relationship between disease status and psychological adjustment is complex. For example depression is related to pain, but controlling for pain there is considerable variation in psychological adjustment. Given similar levels of pain some people do well while others fare poorly (Smith *et al.*, 1991). In addition psychological adjustment to different rheumatic diseases may differ. Hawley and Wolfe (1992) report higher levels of emotional distress in fibromyalgia than in RA, which in turn were higher than in OA. Addressing emotional wellbeing in rheumatic disease is important not only because it plays a key role in people's quality of life but also because depression is associated with poorer physical health outcomes such as days spent in bed.

APPLICATION OF THE SELF-REGULATORY MODEL TO RHEUMATIC DISEASE

There is increasing evidence that non-biological factors play a role in the outcome of rheumatic disease. The relationship between objective measures of disease severity and activity (radiographic measures of joint damage and biochemical markers of auto-immune activity) and pain and emotional distress is poor (Dekker *et al.*, 1992; Summers *et al.*, 1988). Fries and Belamy (1991) suggest that a biopsychosocial model of health may be more helpful for understanding the disability associated with rheumatic disease than the traditional medical model. Psycho-social factors such as educational level, socio-economic status, patient and professional beliefs (perceived control and self-efficacy), emotional state, coping strategies and social support, availability of community resources and access to health care are all thought to contribute to health outcome (Shipley & Newman, 1993).

With no cure for many rheumatic diseases and with medical treatments only being partially effective it is important to explore the self-regulatory processes that mediate between the disease, pain, disability and psychological adjustment. Understanding how some people successfully manage rheumatic disease, minimising pain and disability and optimizing psychological adjustment will help in the development of interventions to assist people who are managing relatively poorly.

A number of features of rheumatic disease may play important roles in shaping the cognitive, emotional and behavioural processes underlying how the person manages symptoms and adapts to disability. The diagnosis may take some time to establish leading to uncertainty and potential emotional distress. They are chronic, progressive, incurable, the cause is frequently unknown and the long term course is uncertain. People with rheumatic disease may experience unpredictable symptom flares of severe pain, fatigue, stiffness and immobility, permanent disability and disfigurement. Further, the illness frequently leads to major consequences for the person's life, affecting work, leisure and social relationships.

The self-regulatory model would suggest that the impact of a rheumatic disease will be mediated by a person's cognitive representation e.g., perceptions of pain, disability and dependence. These will influence their emotional response, coping behaviours and appraisals. In rheumatic disease, coping can include attempts to relieve symptoms or reduce disability, such as taking medication, rest, exercise, or to reduce the emotional impact of the illness such as positive self talk, and seeking emotional support from others. Appraisals include perceptions of one's ability to perform coping behaviours and evaluation of their success in regulating emotional well being, symptoms such as pain and fatigue and functional ability. Modifications of Leventhal's model suggest that self-regulatory processes in turn influence health outcomes such as work status and social relationships (Johnston, 1996).

REVIEW OF RESEARCH ON THE ROLE OF SELF-REGULATORY PROCESSES IN RHEUMATIC DISEASE

This section discusses research that has investigated self regulatory processes in rheumatic diseases. Three major components of the self-regulatory model (illness representations, coping behaviours and appraisals) will be discussed in turn. Relationships between these components and potential antecedents will be explored.

Specifically the review addresses a number of questions. What are people's thoughts about their rheumatic disease? How do people cope with it and how do they appraise their attempts at self-regulation? How do these cognitive and behavioural factors interact? What variables influence these components and how do they affect health outcomes?

Illness Representations

There is an extensive literature exploring the illness representations of people with rheumatic disease. A variety of terms are used to describe conceptually similar psychological constructs including cognitive representations, illness cognitions and lay beliefs. The self-regulatory model proposes that illness cognitions derive from an implicit model of illness based on illness related beliefs, knowledge, experience and information from other people. Illness cognitions lie along five broad cognitive dimensions: *Identity* which includes the label and perceived symptoms of the illness such as pain and fatigue; the perceived *cause* of the illness and exacerbations/remissions; the *time-line* or whether the illness is expected to be acute, episodic or chronic; the *consequences* of the illness for the person's life such as loss of independence; and beliefs about the *curability/controllability* of the illness.

The nature of the specific rheumatic disease, its onset, course, severity and activity may all influence the self regulatory process. According to the self-regulatory model the influence of disease factors on emotional responses, coping behaviours and health outcomes, should be mediated by illness representations. The onset of rheumatic disease presents the person with an array of confusing and serious symptoms which are difficult to understand. Lacking a suitable pre-existing cognitive representation may result in what Bishop (1991) has referred to as "cognitive overdrive". This involves the search for an explanation and considerable distress. One possibility is that a long pre-diagnosis search for a stable cognitive representation could affect later self-regulation. The emotional distress and repeated unsuccessful attempts to cope with the illness may lead to increasing helplessness and reduced self-efficacy. These ideas suggest that the relationship between the onset of illness, the development of a stable cognitive representation, coping behaviour and psychosocial adjustment is worth further study.

Park (1994) has suggested that people with OA may form a cognitive representation of their illness more readily than people with auto-immune rheumatic diseases, such as RA, which present with a more confusing array of symptoms and in which diagnosis may take some considerable time. There is some evidence that people with different types of rheumatic disease may differ in their illness representations. Andersson and Ekdahl (1992) reported that, compared with OA patients, RA patients' self-appraisal of disease was more strongly related to functional abilities and length of time since diagnosis. Moreover people with RA with longer disease duration were more accepting of their illness, suggesting that cognitive representations may be dynamic, changing over time, as postulated by Leventhal *et al.* (1992). Though people with OA and RA reported similar levels of pain they report different pain coping strategies, with OA using more disease minimization and avoidance. These differences in coping strategies suggest that people with OA and RA may also differ in their illness representations.

It seems likely that people experiencing similar challenges associated with a particular rheumatic disease may develop some common illness representations. Hampson *et al.* (1994) reports the shared beliefs of people with OA: 75% viewed OA as fairly/moderately serious, with unpredictable symptoms (81% reported pain varied daily); as chronic (93% expected to have OA permanently); incurable (79% believe a cure is unlikely). In this sample 94% believed it is important to prevent OA getting worse and that it can be managed using medical treatments (95% believe treatment makes them feel better and 88% felt no aspect of their treatment made them feel worse).

These shared beliefs have implications for interactions between health professionals and patients. For example the person with a rheumatic disease may regard pain as the most important indication of the seriousness of their disease while health professionals may view inflammation and joint damage as more important indications of disease severity. Such differences between the perceptions of patients and health professionals may produce misunderstandings disrupt communication. Similarly differences in the treatment expectations of patients and health professionals may lead to dissatisfaction with treatment outcome. Patient expectations should be taken into account when setting goals and evaluating treatment efficacy. These shared beliefs should also inform the design of psycho-educational interventions ensuring that they are sensitive to the needs and beliefs of participants.

With respect to identity, pain is a key concept in people's experience of rheumatic disease (Hampson *et al.*, 1994; Lorig *et al.*, 1984; van Lankveld *et al.*, 1994). However other symptoms are also perceived as significant aspects of people's illness experience. Pimm *et al.* (1995) assessed 90 people with RA using the Illness Perceptions Questionnaire (Weinman *et al.*, 1996) and found that in addition to pain they reported frequent fatigue, sleep difficulties, stiff/ sore joints and loss of strength as salient features of their illness.

Research suggests that the perceived consequences of rheumatic disease, perceived limitations and loss of independence, are very salient features of people's illness representation (Hampson *et al.*, 1994; Lorig *et al.*, 1984; van Lankveld *et al.*, 1994). For example, in two studies of RA van Lankveld *et al.* (1994) found that people perceived the most stressful aspects of their illness to be pain, limitations and dependence. Perceptions of pain, limitations and dependence while being only weakly related to assessments of disease activity and severity were strongly related to measures of quality of life, even after controlling for the objective measures.

Individual differences in people's perceptions of rheumatic disease may help to explain differences in emotional distress, levels of self care behaviours and health outcomes. Hampson *et al.* (1994) suggest that the extent to which people, with rheumatic disease, view their illness as chronic, serious (strong identity and significant consequences) and that treatments are important, influences their adherence to medical treatment and performance of self management behaviours.

They also found that people who perceived OA as more intense, (reporting more symptoms and perceiving OA as more serious) use more self-management strategies on typical and bad days, both concurrently and prospectively. Perceiving OA as more intense was also associated with greater use of health services and poorer quality of life (worse physical function, role function, health perception and pain).

The perceived time course of an illness may influence self-regulation. In a qualitative study of women with chronic illness, mainly arthritis, Belgrave (1990) categorized views about their illness. Some women viewed themselves as ill, seeing coping with disease as a major burden, whereas others considered themselves to be basically healthy and the occasional difficulties they experienced were part of aging. People perceiving themselves as "ill", a chronic time-line perspective, as opposed to being "basically healthy but coping with an episode of illness" (i.e. an acute, episodic time-line), may adopt more elaborate self-regulatory strategies. It might be expected that people with auto-immune rheumatic disorders would be more likely to conceptualize themselves as "ill", given the diffuse, systemic nature of their symptoms. In contrast, people with OA might view themselves as basically healthy individuals with problems, because of the focused, mechanical nature of their illness. Thus the perceived time course of the illness may influence self-management behaviours and in turn, these perceptions may be influenced by experience of a specific rheumatic disease. Further the perceived time course of an illness may influence emotional responses. People who adopt an acute/episodic time-line may become more emotionally distressed over time by repeated symptom flares, whereas someone who adopts a chronic time-line may make a more successful psychological adjustment to the chronic stressors of rheumatic disease. This might explain the differences found between OA and RA in emotional adjustment (Hawley & Wolfe, 1992).

Some studies have investigated causal attributions in rheumatic disease. Affleck *et al.* (1987) found that people reported a variety of causes for their RA (heredity 34.7%, auto-immune factor 24.4%, personal behaviour 22.8%, psychological stress 22.8%) but these were not related to functional ability or psychological adjustment. However those who were unable to identify any cause for their RA were more helpless and had poorer functional ability and psychological adjustment. They also investigated attributions about the cause of symptom flares (psychological stress 45.5%, changes in weather 34%, excessive physical activity 34.1%) and remissions (changes in medication 49.4% and absence of psychological stress 21%). Attributing the cause of current disease activity to psychological stress was associated with poorer functional ability and psychological adjustment. Attributing the cause of flares to excessive physical activity was associated with less helplessness, whereas attributing the cause of remissions to changes in medication was linked with greater helplessness. This may suggest that attributing the cause of current disease activity to areas over which one has some personal control may be more adaptive. It is interesting to note that few people report attributions about the cause of remissions that would support a sense of personal control. In general this study suggests that, in people with established RA, attributions about the cause of current disease activity play a greater role in adaptation to RA than attributions about the cause of the disease.

The perceived controllability of rheumatic disease has also received considerable attention. People with RA are as likely as people with cancer to believe that they have little personal control over their health and hold more external locus of control beliefs than people with other chronic illnesses such as diabetes and hypertension (Felton & Revenson, 1984). Wallston and his colleagues have conducted a large longitudinal study of RA which examined perceived control. In a review of data from this study and other published research on perceived control in rheumatic disease Wallston (1993) concludes that people with rheumatic disease do not tend to view control over their health as strictly internal or external but as residing in both their own actions and what others do to and for them.

Cross sectional studies show that stronger internal health locus of control beliefs are associated with greater life satisfaction and quality of life. However, in longitudinal studies, they do not predict improved life satisfaction or quality of life over time (Wallston, 1993). Research shows that people who have high internal and powerful others and low chance/fate locus of control report less depression over time than people with other patterns of locus of control beliefs (Roscam, 1986). Thus, in influencing psychological wellbeing in rheumatic disease, locus of control is not as important as the perception that health status can be controlled. When the person believes that not only themselves but other people play an important role in the management of their illness this may be particularly conducive to the development of a successful relationship between the health care professional and patient.

In an elegant study Affleck *et al.* (1987b) provided evidence that perceiving personal control over relatively more controllable aspects of rheumatic disease and perceiving that powerful others have control over relatively uncontrollable aspects is more adaptive. Perceiving greater personal control over daily symptoms was associated with better positive mood in people with moderate or severe RA. Perceiving greater personal control over the course of RA was associated with negative mood in people with severe RA. The importance of participation in treatment by people with RA is emphasized by their finding that perceiving greater personal control over treatment is associated with better mood and perceiving greater health professional control over daily symptoms is associated with negative mood in RA.

Affleck *et al.* (1992) studied daily reports of pain, activity limitations and mood over 75 days in people with RA. They found that initial perceived control over pain was positively associated with decreased pain over time. The dynamic nature of self-regulation is emphasized by the finding that pain reports moderated the relationship between initial perceived control beliefs and mood, people who initially assumed they had control over daily pain and then experienced increased pain became more distressed over time.

A different form of perceived control, helplessness, has been shown to be an important determinant of depression in RA (Stein *et al.*, 1988). Smith and Wallston (1992) provide further evidence supporting a self-regulatory model in a longitudinal study of 239 people with RA. They found evidence for a maladaptive pattern of self-regulation involving helplessness cognitions, passive coping with pain and psychosocial impairment. In a later report from the same study, Smith *et al.* (1994) found that greater cognitive distortion (over-generalization, selective abstraction, personalization and catastrophizing) and helplessness were associated with greater depression. Cognitive distortions and helplessness were stable over time and only cognitive distortions predicted change in depression.

Some studies have investigated the relationship between cognitive representations. Hampson *et al.* (1994) found a strong relationship between reporting more symptoms and perceiving OA to be more serious. They suggest this may form an intensity construct. The same finding of a strong relationship between symptom frequency and perceived consequences was found in a longitudinal study of RA using the IPQ (Pimm *et al.*, 1995). Perceived intensity may have implications for treatment adherence and self-management as people who reported more symptoms and viewed OA as more serious were more negative about the treatments used to manage it (Hampson *et al.*, 1994). Other relationships have been reported between illness representations. People who attribute the cause of OA to themselves are more likely to believe that the things they do to manage it are helpful (Hampson *et al.*, 1994).

Schiaffino and Revenson (1992) conducted an important longitudinal study of early RA investigating the relationships between causal attributions, perceived control and self-efficacy and disability and depression. The results suggested that self-efficacy may mediate the positive relationship between perceived control and functional ability. However there was much stronger evidence for moderating relationships between the cognitive variables in relation to adaptation. That is the interaction between perceived control, self-efficacy and causal attributions are critical for understanding current and subsequent depression and disability. Specifically they found different relationships for depression and disability. When people perceived RA to be uncontrollable, internal stable global attributions for the cause of a symptom flare were associated with greater depression. When perceived control was low, the same attributions were associated with less disability and when perceived control was high, internal stable global attributions were made self-efficacy was negatively associated with depression but positively associated with disability. They suggest that these results can be understood using Leventhal's acute/chronic time-line construct. One pattern reflects those with an acute model of RA, who report significant disability, but believe the cause is temporary and due to external factors, perhaps bad luck. As they think that something can be done about it and so there is no reason to be depressed. Although people with this acute pattern may not be depressed, successful management depends on adopting a chronic label so they are unlikely to develop adaptive self-care behaviours. The second pattern reflects a chronic model of RA, in which people see the cause of the flare as related to internal factors that are likely to be permanent and are causing significant disability. However, when the person is confident that they can do something to help the situation they will not be depressed. These studies suggest that elucidating the complex relationships between illness cognitions may provide valuable insights into differences in the patterns of adaptation to rheumatic disease.

Coping

Leventhal's model proposes that people engage in coping behaviours as part of the dynamic process of disease regulation. These self-regulatory behaviours are influenced by the person's representation of the illness and appraisals of coping efforts. Most studies of coping with rheumatic disease have used general cognitive stress and coping models (Lazerus & Folkman, 1984) or models for coping with chronic pain (Brown & Nicassio, 1987). The general cognitive model of coping in which the individual appraises both the situation with which they have to cope and the available coping resources, is compatible with the self-regulatory model of illness (Park, 1994). There has been a great deal of interest in examining the relationship between coping behaviour and pain, disability and emotional adjustment in rheumatic disease. However the cognitive and appraisal processes that provide the context in which coping strategies are selected and evaluated have received less attention (Mann & Zautra, 1992; Newman & Revenson, 1993; Zautra & Mann, 1992).

Coping efforts are aimed at avoiding or reducing the negative consequences of the illness. There are two major categories of coping behaviour. Problem focused coping includes planning and instrumental behaviours to mitigate problems, such as pain and disability, caused by the disease (e.g. pacing). Emotion focused coping includes coping strategies to manage thoughts and feelings associated with the disease (e.g. redefining the situation). In rheumatic disease coping behaviours include self-care behaviours recommended by health professionals, such as splint use or taking medication, but also include self-directed coping strategies such as information seeking, diet and prayer.

Over the course of a rheumatic disease people have to deal with a variety of challenges that may influence coping responses. Early in the disease or during flares of disease activity they need to manage new or increased symptoms such as pain and stiffness and new restrictions on their activities. Later in the disease and during periods when the disease is stable they have to manage the current level of disability and uncertainty about future health.

In the early stages of a rheumatic disease people may need to develop and try out new coping strategies as previous coping strategies may no longer be appropriate or sufficient to manage the novel and chronic stresses associated with the disease. Studies suggest that the coping strategies people adopt early in the course of RA show little change over the first couple of years (Revenson *et al.*, 1989). Further, in people with advanced RA, coping strategies were also found to be relatively stable over a similar time period (Newman *et al.*, 1990). However coping strategies may change over longer time periods, Newman *et al.* (1993) found that people with longer disease duration were more passive in their coping and did not favour the use of any particular coping strategies.

These results have implications for the timing and targeting of interventions aimed at reducing maladaptive coping and enhancing adaptive coping strategies. First, in the early stages of a rheumatic disease, intervention may be helpful as people are developing new coping strategies. Minimal intervention at this time may encourage people to try out alternative adaptive strategies preventing later adjustment difficulties and improving current quality of life. Second, in established rheumatic disease if the person has a relatively stable but unhelpful coping repertoire (e.g. passive coping), intervention may be beneficial as they are unlikely to change significantly with experience.

Most research has focused on how people cope with rheumatic disease in general rather than specific aspects of the illness. Revenson and Felton (1989) report that RA patients most commonly use wish-fulfilling fantasies, threat minimization and cognitive restructuring to cope with their illness. A higher reported use of any strategy was related to heightened positive affect six months later. Other studies have examined patterns of coping with specific aspects of the illness stressor such as pain (Keefe *et al.*, 1989) and disability (Newman *et al.*, 1990). In a study of early RA Schiaffino and Revenson (1991) found that people favour particular coping strategies which they use to manage both pain and disability. People use different coping strategies to manage other illness stressors. In a study that investigated how people cope with specific problems related to RA, Blalock *et al.* (1993) found that people relied less heavily on behavioural coping strategies when dealing with problems involving social relationships than when dealing with problems involving daily activities, leisure activities, or work. They also report that there was little consistency in individuals' use of either cognitive or behavioural strategies across different problem areas. The coping strategies used to deal with problems such as pain differ from those used to cope with emotional stressors. Cohen *et al.* (1986) found that direct actions were frequently used to cope with pain but rarely used to cope with threats to self esteem.

There is some evidence for individual differences in the types of coping strategies used to manage specific aspects of rheumatic disease. Newman *et al.* (1990) examined the overall patterns of coping behaviour in people with established RA. Using cluster analysis they classified people into four groups. *Group 1* used denial, avoidance of others during pain, reorganising routine and seeking support from friends; *group 2*, the largest group, had a passive pattern of coping, not strongly adopting/rejecting any coping strategy; *group 3*: had the most open and active coping pattern, they did not use denial, wish fulfilment, distraction, prayer, or religion but confronting disease, refusing to reorganise routine, engaging in physical activity and expressing feelings; *group 4* used rest, diet, religion and prayer. The groups did not differ on demographic variables, laboratory or clinical measures of disease, suggesting that other factors such as people's representations of their illness or appraisals of coping may account for different patterns of coping. Further work is needed on how illness representations and appraisal affect the selection of coping strategies.

There is considerable evidence that coping strategies are associated with emotional well-being in rheumatic disease. In their review Mann and Zautra (1992) report that using passive coping strategies such as restricting daily activities, sleeping, wishful thinking and self-blame are associated with greater emotional distress. Active coping strategies, information seeking and cognitive restructuring, distracting oneself from pain and maintaining activities despite pain, are associated with less emotional distress although not as consistently. Using a wider range of coping strategies has also been associated with better emotional well-being (Blalock *et al.*, 1993) suggesting that flexibility of coping may be important for adjustment to rheumatic disease.

Coping strategies have also been shown to be associated with pain and disability. Using passive coping strategies to manage pain (focusing on the pain, restricting social activities) are associated with poor functional ability and depressed mood (Brown *et al.*, 1989; Keefe *et al.*, 1989). Use of active coping strategies has been related to less pain and disability. Newman *et al.* (1990) found that people in group 3 who had an open and active coping pattern reported less pain and stiffness, physical disability and better emotional well being. One prospective study of daily pain, coping and mood in RA found that people who used relaxation more frequently as part of their daily coping repertoire had less daily pain and those reporting more coping efforts showed improved pain and mood over time (Affleck *et al.*, 1992).

In their analysis of three cross-sectional studies of RA, Zautra *et al.* (1995) report data consistent with a model in which coping mediates between the perceived severity of RA and positive and negative affect. People who reported more pain and activity limitation use more maladaptive coping strategies and maladaptive coping strategies were associated with less positive affect and greater negative affect. People who report more activity limitation use less adaptive coping strategies which were associated with less positive affect.

In sum, there is some evidence that coping efforts are related to cognitive representations and appraisals and that coping efforts may be important predictors of pain, disability and emotional well being in rheumatic disease. However prospective studies are needed to explore the complex reciprocal relationships between these variables.

Appraisals of Coping Efforts

Research suggests that appraisals of the effectiveness of coping efforts play an important role in the self-regulation of rheumatic disease. Three appraisals have received attention in the literature: catastrophizing, self-efficacy and perceived competence.

With respect to catastrophizing Keefe *et al.* (1987) investigated how people with OA coped with knee pain using the Coping Strategies Questionnaire (CSQ) (Rosenstiel & Keefe, 1983). Two factors from the CSQ, labelled "Coping Attempts" and "Pain Control and Rational Thinking" (PCRT), accounted for 60% of the variance in responding. PCRT measures the extent to which people catastrophize about future outcomes and beliefs about pain controllability. Keefe *et al.* (1987) found that the PCRT was the most significant factor in predicting both physical and psychological disability. Findings from studies of RA have provided more evidence that catastrophizing is an important dysfunctional process in the self-regulation of rheumatic disease. Keefe *et al.* (1989) investigated the relationships between catastrophizing, pain, disability and depression in RA longitudinally. Catastrophizing was stable over time and after controlling for auto-regressive effects at time one, they reported that catastrophizing continued to predict pain, disability and depression. Similarly, Beckham *et al.* (1991) found that the PCRT explained significant variance in physical disability, pain, psychological disability, depression and hassles in RA patients, after controlling for disease status. Although most studies regard the PCRT as measuring a form of coping within Leventhal's framework, it might be seen as reflecting cognitive representations of the illness and appraisals of coping. It is possible that catastrophizing influences outcome through an effect on coping behaviour. Dekker *et al.* (1992) suggest that the effect of catastrophizing on pain and disability may be mediated through avoidance of exercise, resulting in muscle weakness. These results have implications for intervention since training patients not to catastrophize and to restructure beliefs about disease controllability may reduce pain, disability and emotional distress.

Research on self-efficacy has provided some very exciting results in recent years. This research has been facilitated by the development of an arthritis specific self-efficacy measure. The Arthritis Self-Efficacy Scale assesses people's belief in their ability to perform specific self-management behaviours to manage the consequences of arthritis ie. pain, other symptoms of arthritis, such as fatigue and frustration and physical disability (Lorig *et al.*, 1989b).

Self-efficacy is related to health outcomes and self-management behaviours in arthritis. Perceiving greater self-efficacy is associated with lower pain (Lorig *et al.*, 1989b; Taal *et al.*, 1993). Perceiving greater self-efficacy is associated with lower disability both concurrently and subsequently (Lorig *et al.*, 1989; Schiaffino *et al.*, 1991; Taal *et al.*, 1993).

The relationship between self-efficacy and emotional well-being is more complex. Schiaffino *et al.* (1991) found that at low pain self efficacy was unrelated to depression one year later but at high pain self-efficacy was associated with greater future depression. Self-efficacy is related to adaptive coping behaviours since it predicted problem focused coping one year later in RA (Schiaffino *et al.*, 1991). Problem focused coping mediated the relationship between initial self-efficacy and later disability. Self efficacy also predicts adherence to health recommendations in RA (Taal *et al.*, 1993).

A related construct is perceived competence. While self-efficacy judgements are situation/task specific, perceived competence denotes a more general belief in one's ability to interact effectively with the environment. Smith *et al.* (1991) investigated Perceived Competence and adjustment in a longitudinal study of RA. There was evidence from the cross-sectional analyses that perceived competence mediated the relationship between antecedents, such as locus of control beliefs and social support and outcomes such as depressed mood and life satisfaction. People who maintained a belief in their general competence consistently reported being more satisfied with their lives and less depressed than did those who doubted their competence. Evidence from the longitudinal analyses showed consistent but weaker support for the mediational model. Positive changes in perceived competence over the first six months were associated with later improvements in life satisfaction and pain.

PSYCHO-EDUCATIONAL INTERVENTIONS

Treatment for rheumatic diseases has traditionally included pharmacotherapy, physical therapy and surgery. Over the past twenty years there has been considerable interest in the development and evaluation of psycho-educational interventions. There are a number of reasons for this. Medical care is only partially effective in relieving symptoms (Hirano *et al.*, 1994) and preventing disease progression. Thus many people are left with distressing symptoms, disabilities and uncertainty about the future course of their illness. Medical management frequently fails to address psychological well-being, social or occupational function. To optimize the quality of life of people with rheumatic disease there is a major need for interventions that address residual distressing symptoms, physical function, emotional well-being and restricted social roles. Since treatment of rheumatic disease makes major demands on health service resources, psycho-educational interventions could lead to more efficient use of resources by reducing the need for medical consultations, provision of equipment and use of analgesics.

Perhaps the most important rationale for psycho-educational intervention comes from the research described earlier. Active participation in treatment decisions and procedures helps people combat helplessness, develop a sense of self-efficacy and enhance emotional well-being. People seek to understand their illness developing a working model of what the illness is, its effects, why it has happened, how long it will last and whether it can be cured or controlled. These models influence emotional responses to the disease, coping strategies and health outcomes. Therefore interventions aimed at assisting people to develop adaptive models of their disease and encourage active participation may produce significant health outcome benefits.

There are four main aims of psycho-educational interventions in rheumatic disease. First, improving or maintaining optimal health status. The most important areas of health status include: pain and other symptoms such as fatigue, physical function, emotional well-being, social interaction and occupation and disease activity (Tucker & Kirwan, 1991). Second, to assist people to change health related cognitions and behaviours that have been found to be important in mediating between the disease and its outcome. Third, to improve the use of health service resources. Fourth, to improve the acceptability or satisfaction with treatment.

Many different types of psycho-educational intervention for rheumatic disease have been developed and evaluated in controlled research studies. These include the use of structured information giving sessions; training in self-management skills, biofeedback, cognitive behaviour therapy, psychotherapy and social support (DeVellis & Blalock, 1993). Some other novel interventions have also recently been developed but await further evaluation. These include the use of medication organisers to minimize the effect of poor cognitive function on medication adherence (Parke, 1994) and spouse/family therapy to address the impact of rheumatic disease on family members (Revenson, 1993).

There have now been over 100 peer reviewed published studies of psycho-educational interventions for rheumatic disease (Lorig, 1995). Reviews of psycho-educational interventions have shown that they can produce therapeutic benefits reducing pain, disability, depression and tender joint count (Hawley, 1995; Hirano *et al.*, 1994; Lorig *et al.*, 1987; Mullens *et al.*, 1987). Psycho-educational interventions can produce an additional 15–30% improvement in symptoms, an effect size similar to non-steroidal anti-inflammatory drugs (Hirano *et al.*, 1994). There is also consistent evidence that psycho-educational interventions can significantly increase knowledge about arthritis and practice of self-care behaviours such as exercise and relaxation (Hawley, 1995; Hirano *et al.*, 1994; Lorig *et al.*, 1987; Mullens *et al.*, 1987). Self-management interventions have been shown to reduce the frequency of medical consultations producing significant cost savings for OA and RA (Lorig *et al.*, 1993).

There is converging evidence supporting the view that cognitive and behavioural factors may be important proximal variables mediating between psycho-educational intervention and health outcome benefits. The research reviewed above suggests that cognitive representations, coping behaviours and appraisals are associated with pain, disability and emotional well-being concurrently and prospectively. Several studies have also examined the effect of psycho-educational interventions on cognitive and behavioural factors but relatively few studies have directly manipulated cognitions or coping behaviours to investigate whether they mediate the therapeutic benefits of psycho-educational interventions.

The literature suggests that appropriate re-structuring of the person's illness representation is necessary if self-regulation of pain, disability and emotional distress is to be improved. Interventions may fail to show benefits because they produce unhelpful changes in illness representations. In one study Parker *et al.* (1984) presented RA patients with a seven-hour educational programme. Although patients' knowledge about the disease increased, the intervention group reported more pain and disability than the control group. The presentations may have had a negative influence on illness cognitions by highlighting the salience of pain and the possible negative effects of RA. People make their own interpretations of their experiences in psycho-educational interventions and these are not always those anticipated by health professionals. It is important to consider how an intervention will affect people's illness representations and how such a change will lead to improvements in the person's ability to successfully self-regulate the illness.

There is some evidence that psycho-educational interventions produce adaptive changes in cognitions and coping behaviours. Goeppinger and her colleagues found modest decreases in learned helplessness scores, which persisted for 12 months (Goeppinger *et al.*, 1989). Parker *et al.* (1988) primarily studying elderly men with RA, report that participants in a cognitive-behavioural pain management programme catastrophized significantly less and reported increased perception of control over pain compared to attention placebo or no treatment control groups. Although the cognitive-behavioural intervention produced changes in catastrophizing and beliefs about pain controllability, it did not produce therapeutic benefits in pain or depression. In a subsequent longitudinal study Parker *et al.* (1989) report that changes in catastrophizing and beliefs about pain controllability were associated with changes in pain, physical function and arthritis helplessness. These studies suggest that changes in catastrophizing and beliefs about pain control are important but not sufficient to produce improvements in health status.

Radojevic *et al.* (1992) found that behaviour therapy, behaviour therapy with family support and education with family support interventions for RA all produced increases in the use of active coping strategies compared to a no treatment control group. The group receiving behaviour therapy with family support showed the greatest change. However these differences were not evident at 2-month follow up.

Lorig and her colleagues have conducted a series of studies to establish which variables are associated with the benefits of their arthritis self management course (ASMC) (Lorig & Gonzalez, 1992). The ASMC has a positive effect in terms of pain, disability, knowledge and self care behaviours (Lorig *et al.*, 1989a). These benefits were not mediated by behaviour change as increased use of self care behaviours (e.g. exercise and relaxation) were only weakly associated with changes in health status (e.g. pain, disability and depression). However self-efficacy was found to be a particularly important factor in the outcome of self management intervention. Changes in self-efficacy during the ASMC were strongly associated with improvements in health status (Lorig *et al.*, 1989b). Several other studies have described positive changes in self-efficacy following psycho-educational interventions (Davis *et al.*, 1994; Lorig & Holman, 1989; O'Leary *et al.*, 1988; Taal *et al.*, 1993).

Thus, changing self-efficacy or confidence in one's ability to manage the illness, seems to be an important mechanism by which psycho-educational interventions assist people to improve self-regulation of rheumatic disease. To test this hypothesis they redesigned the ASMC to enhance participants' self-efficacy beliefs, introducing strategies such as modelling and behavioural contracts. They reported that this revised course was particularly effective and that significant, positive changes in self-efficacy were noted (Lorig & Gonzalez, 1992).

In sum, there is considerable evidence that key components of the self-regulatory model play a crucial role in the outcome of psycho-educational interventions. However the relative importance of cognitive representations, coping efforts and appraisals in the outcome of psycho-educational intervention is unclear. Further, the precise mechanisms by which psycho-educational interventions enable people to successfully manage the consequences of rheumatic disease are poorly understood. Studies based on psychological theory have led to the development of the most successful psycho-educational interventions (DeVellis & Blalock, 1993; Hirano *et al.*, 1994). However no study has explicitly used the self-regulatory model to guide investigation of how illness cognitions, coping behaviours and appraisals may interact during psycho-educational intervention.

Psycho-educational intervention can be viewed as a method for experimentally manipulating self-regulatory processes. Studying the interaction between self-regulatory variables over the course of a psycho-educational intervention may provide insight into the dynamic processes by which a person can enhance their self-management of chronic rheumatic disease. This in turn could lead to the development of improved psycho-educational interventions. Intervention studies also provide an opportunity to test the self-regulatory model. Such studies enable us to investigate whether the self-regulatory model provides a useful framework for understanding self-management of rheumatic disease.

With colleagues, I have been conducting a study to investigate whether the self-regulatory model provides useful insights into the processes by which self management interventions assist people with RA to improve their health outcomes. In particular we are addressing two research questions: (1) Does a psycho-educational intervention for people with RA, adapted for the UK, have therapeutic benefits, reducing pain, disability and emotional distress?; (2) Are therapeutic benefits mediated by illness representations, coping behaviours and appraisals of coping efforts?

We have developed a self-management intervention based on the US Arthritis Self Management [Help] Course for people with RA in the UK. The intervention is delivered jointly by health professionals and lay people with RA using an intervention manual. Participants are given a copy of the Arthritis Help Book (Lorig & Fries, 1990). The intervention consists of six weekly two-hour meetings and incorporates both educational and cognitive-behavioural methods to assist people in making adaptive changes in cognitions and coping. The intervention has explicit aims and objectives which are discussed with participants during agenda setting sessions. Information about RA and techniques for coping with it are taught. There is a particular emphasis on the management of pain, physical disability and emotional distress. The format of the groups is interactive, participants being encouraged to share the difficulties they experience and to identify helpful/unhelpful cognitions and coping strategies. A number of methods are used to explore and develop more adaptive cognitions, coping behaviours and appraisals including self monitoring, cognitive restructuring, problem solving, goal setting, modelling, graded implementation of new behaviours, reinforcement through group feedback and relapse prevention strategies.

A pilot study showed that the intervention produced significant changes in psycho-educational variables including increased knowledge about RA, knowledge about medication, ability to perform self management skills and a reduction in perceived helplessness (Pimm *et al.*, 1992). A second pilot study investigated whether the intervention had therapeutic benefits and changed illness representations. Results showed significant reductions in pain and the perceived curability/controllability of RA following the intervention (Pimm *et al.*, 1994a; Pimm *et al.*, 1994b).

We are currently conducting a single blind randomized controlled trial of the intervention with 120 people with RA, recruited from a busy rheumatology out-patient clinic. Participants are assessed on five occasions over a year at 0, 8, 16, 26 and 52 weeks. Half of the sample are randomly allocated to receive the intervention after an eight week baseline and half to receive standard medical care. Assessments include measures of disease activity and severity, self report measures of pain, disability and emotional distress. Illness representations are assessed using the Illness Perceptions Questionnaire (Weinman *et al.*, 1996), coping strategies are assessed on a version of the COPE (Carver *et al.*, 1989) adapted for RA. Appraisal of coping efforts are assessed using the Arthritis Self-Efficacy scales. All the intervention groups have now been completed and it is hoped that we will be able to report the results of this study in late 1997.

CONCLUSIONS AND RECOMMENDATIONS FOR FURTHER RESEARCH

Rheumatic diseases are frequently associated with severe pain, disability and depression despite medical management. There is considerable evidence that psychological factors, in particular cognitions, coping behaviours and appraisals, play a crucial role in adaptation to rheumatic disease. This review suggests that Leventhal's self-regulatory model provides a useful framework for future research. Prospective studies are needed to investigate how cognitive and behavioural factors interact over time during the process of adaptation to an unpredictable and progressive rheumatic disease.

Psycho-educational interventions can assist people in managing rheumatic diseases and research suggests that the benefits of these interventions are associated with changes in cognitions, coping behaviours and appraisals. This work suggests that future intervention studies guided by the self-regulatory model may provide valuable insights into the processes by which psycho-educational interventions enhance adaptation to rheumatic disease. Such studies will also provide a useful test of the self-regulatory model. Although this research is likely to identify potential targets for psycho-educational intervention, research is also needed to explore methods for producing adaptive changes in cognitive and behavioural factors.

REFERENCES

Affleck, G., Pfeiffer, C., Tennen, H. & Fifield, J. (1987a) Attributional processes in rheumatoid arthritis patients. *Arthritis & Rheumatism*, **30**, 927–931.

Affleck, G., Tennen, H., Pfeiffer, C. & Fifield, J. (1987b) Appraisals of control and predictability in adapting to a chronic disease. *Journal of Personality and Social Psychology*, **53**, 273–279.

Affleck, G., Tennen, H., Urrows, S. & Higgins, P. (1992) Neuroticism and the pain-mood relation in rheumatoid arthritis: Insight from a prospective daily study. *Journal of Consulting and Clinical Psychology*, **60**, 119–126.

Andersson, S.I. & Ekdahl, C. (1992) Self-appraisal and coping in out-patients with chronic disease. *Scandinavian Journal of Psychology*, **33**, 289–300.

Badley, E.M. & Tennant, A. (1989) The rising tide of joint troubles with increasing age: Findings from a postal survey of the population. *British Journal of Rheumatology*, **28**, 32.

Beckham, J.D., Keefe, F.J., Caldwell, D.S. & Roodman, A.A. (1991) Pain coping strategies in rheumatoid arthritis: Relationship to pain, disability, depression and daily hassles. *Behaviour Therapy*, **22**, 113–124.

Belgrave, L.L. (1990) The relevance of chronic illness in the everyday lives of elderly women. *Journal of Aging and Health*, **2**, 475–500.

Bishop, G.D. (1991) Understanding the understanding of illness. Lay disease representations. In J.A. Skelton & R.T. Croyle (Eds.),

Mental representations in health and illness. Springer-Verlag: New York.

Blalock, S.J., DeVellis, B.M., Holt., K. & Hahn, P.M. (1993) Coping with rheumatoid arthritis: Is one problem the same as another? *Health Education Quarterly*, **20**, 119–132.

Brandt & Flusser, (1991) Osteoarthritis. In: N. Bellam (Ed.), Prognosis in the Rheumatic Diseases (pp. 11–36). London: Kluwer.

Brown, G.K., Nicassio, P.M. & Wallston K. (1989) Pain coping strategies and depression in RA. *Journal of Consulting and Clinical Psychology*, **57**, 652–657.

Carver, C.S., Scheier, M.F. & Weintraub, J.K. (1989) Assessing coping strategies: A theoretically based approach. *Journal of Personality & Social Psychology*, **56**, 267–83.

Cohen, J.L., Sauter, S.V.H., DeVellis, R.F. & DeVellis, B.M. (1986) Evaluation of arthritis self-management courses led by laypersons and by professionals. *Arthritis & Rheumatism*, **29**, 388–393.

Controller General. (1979) *Entering a nursing home — Costly implications for Medicaid and the elderly* (PAD 80–12). Washington, DC General Accounting Office.

Croft, P. (1990) Osteoarthritis: Review of the UK data on the rheumatic diseases-3. *British Journal of Rheumatology*, **29**, 391–395.

Cunningham, L.S. & Kelsey, J.L. (1984) Epidemiology of musculoskeletal impairments and associated disability. *American Journal of Public Health*, **74**, 574–9.

Davis, P., Busch, A.J., Lowe, J.C., Taniguchi, J. & Dikowich, B. (1994) Evaluation of a rheumatoid arthritis patient education program: impact on knowledge and self-efficacy. *Patient Education and Counselling*, **24**, 55–61.

Dekker, J., Boot, B., van der Woude, L.H.V. & Bijlsma, J.W.J. (1992) Pain and disability in osteoarthritis: a review of biobehavioural mechanisms. *Journal of Behavioural Medicine*, **15**, 189–214.

DeVellis, B.M. (1993) Depression in rheumatological diseases. *Bailliere's Clinical Rheumatology*, **7**, 241–258.

DeVellis, R. & Blalock, S. (1993) Psychological and educational interventions to reduce arthritis disability. *Bailliere's Clinical Rheumatology*, **7**, 397–416.

Felton, B.J. & Revenson, T.A. (1984) Coping with chronic illness: A study of illness controllability and the influence of coping strategies on psychological adjustment. *Journal of Consulting and Clinical Psychology*, **52**, 343–353.

Fries, J.F. & Bellamy, N. (1991) Introduction. In N. Bellamy (Ed), *Prognosis in the rheumatic diseases* (pp. 1–10). London: Kluwer.

Goeppinger, J., Arthur, M.W., Baglioni, A.J. Jr., Brunk, S.E. & Brunner, C.M. (1989) A re-examination of the effectiveness of self-care education for persons with arthritis. *Arthritis & Rheumatism*, **32**, 706–716.

Hampson, S.E., Glasgow, R.E. & Zeiss, A. (1994) Personal models of OA and their relation to self-management activities and quality of life. *Journal of Behavioural Medicine*, **17**, 143–158.

Hawley, D. (1995) Psycho-educational interventions in the treatment of arthritis. *Bailliere's Clinical Rheumatology*, **9**, 803–823.

Hawley, D.J., Wolfe, F. & Cathey, M.A. (1992) The Sense of Coherence Questionnaire in patients with rheumatic disorders. *The Journal of Rheumatology*, **19**, 1912–1918.

Hazes, J.M. & Silman, A.J. (1990) Review of UK data on the rheumatic diseases-2. Rheumatoid arthritis. *British Journal of Rheumatology*, **29**, 310–2.

Hirano, P.C., Laurent, D.D. & Lorig, K. (1994) Arthritis education studies, 1987–1991: A review of the literature. *Patient Education and Counselling*, **24**, 9–54.

Johnston, M. (1996) Models of disability. *The Psychologist*, **9**, **5**, 205–210.

Keefe, F.J., Brown, G.K., Wallston, K.A. & Caldwell, D.S. (1989) Coping with rheumatoid arthritis: Catastrophising as a maladaptive strategy. *Pain*, 51–56.

Keefe, F.J., Caldwell, D.S., Queen, K.T., Gil, K.M., Martinez, S., Crisson, J.E., Ogden, W. & Nunley, J. (1987) Pain coping strategies in osteoarthritis patients. *Journal of Consulting and Clinical Psychology*, **55**, 208–212.

Kelsey, J. (1982) Epidemiological aspects of muscoskeletal disorders. *Monographs in epidemiology and biostatistics*, Vol. 3 New York: OUP.

Lambert, V.A. & Lambert, C.E. Jr. (1987) Coping with rheumatoid arthritis. *Nursing Clinics of North America*, **22**, 551–8.

Lawrence, R.C., Hochberg, M.C., Kelsey, J.L., McDuffie, F.C., Medsger, T.A. Jr., Felts, W.R. & Shulman, L.E. (1989) Estimates of the prevalence of selected arthritic and musculoskeletal diseases in the United States. *The Journal of Rheumatology*, **16**, 427–441.

Lazarus, R.S. & Folkman, S. (1984) *Stress, appraisal and coping*. Springer, New York.

Leventhal, H., Diefenbach, M. & Leventhal, E.A. (1992) Illness cognition: Using common sense to understand treatment adherence and affect cognition interactions. *Cognitive Therapy & Research*, **16**, 143–163.

Leventhal, H., Leventhal, A.E. & Schaefer, P.M. (1992b) Vigilant coping and health behaviour. In M.G. Ory, R.P. Abeles & P.D. Lipman (Eds.), *Ageing, health and behaviour* (pp. 109–140). Newbury Park: Sage.

Leventhal, H., Meyer, D. & Nerenz, D. (1992) The commonsense representations of illness danger. In S. Rachman (Ed.), *Contributions to medical psychology*, Vol. 2 (pp. 7–30). New York: Pergamon Press.

Lorig, K. (1995) Patient education: treatment or nice extra? *British Journal of Rheumatology*, **34**, 703–706.

Lorig, K., Chastain, R., Ung, E., Shoor, S. & Holman H.R. (1989a) Development and evaluation of a scale to measure perceived self-efficacy in people with arthritis. *Arthritis & Rheumatism*, **32**, 37–44.

Lorig, K.R., Cox, T., Cuevas, Y., Kraines, R.G. & Britton, M.C. (1984) Converging and diverging beliefs about arthritis: Caucasian patients, Spanish speaking patients and physicians. *The Journal of Rheumatology*, **11**, 76–79.

Lorig, K. & Fries, J.F. (1990) *The arthritis helpbook*. Addison-Wesley: CA.

Lorig, K. & Gonzalez, V. (1992) The integration of theory with practice: a 12 year case study. *Health Education Quarterly*, **19**, 344–368.

Lorig, K. & Holman, H.R. (1989) Long-term outcomes of an arthritis self-management study. Effects of reinforcement efforts. *Social Science & Medicine*, **29**, 221–224.

Lorig, K., Konkol, L. & Gonzalez, V. (1987) Arthritis patient education: A review of the literature. *Patient Education and Counselling*, **10**, 207–252.

Lorig, K., Mazonson, P.D. & Holman, H.R. (1993) Evidence suggesting that health education for self-management in patients with chronic arthritis has sustained health benefits while reducing health care costs. *Arthritis & Rheumatism*, **36**, 439–446.

Lorig, K., Seleznick, M., Lubeck, D., Ung, E., Chastain, R.L. & Holman, H.R. (1989b) The beneficial outcomes of the arthritis self-management course are not adequately explained by behaviour change. *Arthritis & Rheumatism*, **32**, 91–95.

Manne, S.L. & Zautra, A.J. (1992) Coping with arthritis: current status and critique. *Arthritis & Rheumatism*, **35**, 1273–1280.

Martin & White (1988) *The prevalence of disability among adults.* London; HMSO; 1.

Mullen, P.D., Laville, E., Biddle, A.K. & Lorig, K. (1987) Efficacy of psycho-educational interventions on pain, depression, and disability with arthritis adults; A meta-analysis. *Journal of Rheumatology*, **15**, 33–39.

Newman, S., Fitzpatrick, R., Lamb, R. & Shipley, M. (1990) Patterns of coping in RA. *Psychology and Health*, **4**, 187–200.

Newman, S.P. & Revenson, T.A. (1993) Coping with rheumatoid arthritis. *Bailliere's Clinical Rheumatology*, **7**, 259–80.

O'Leary, A., Shoor, S., Lorig, K. & Holman, H.R. (1988) A cognitive behavioural treatment for rheumatoid arthritis. *Health Psychology*, **7**, 527–544.

Park, D.C. (1994) Self-regulation and control of rheumatic disorders. In S. Maes, H. Leventhal & M. Johnston (Eds.), *International review of health psychology* (Vol. 3) New York: John Wiley & Sons Ltd.

Parker, J.C., Singsen, B.H., Hewett, J.E., Walker, S.E., Hazelwood, S.E., Hall, P.J., Holsten, D.J. & Rodon, C.M. (1984) Educating patients with rheumatoid arthritis: a prospective analysis. *Archives of Physical Medicine Rehabilitation*, **65**, 771–774.

Parker, J.C., Frank, R.G., Beck, N.C., Smarr, K.L., Buescher, K.L., Phillips, L.R., Smith, E.I. Anderson, S.K. & Walker, S.E. (1988) Pain management in rheumatoid arthritis patients: a cognitive behavioural approach. *Arthritis & Rheumatism*, **31**, 593–601.

Parker, J.C., Smarr, K.L., Buescher, K.L., Phillips, L.R., Frank, R.G., Beck, N.C. Anderson, S.K. & Walker, S.E. (1989) Pain control and rational thinking. *Arthritis & Rheumatism*, **32**, 984–990.

Pimm, T.J., Amos, M & Byron, M.A. (1992) Evaluation of outpatient education programme for people with rheumatoid arthritis. *British Journal of Rheumatology*, **31**, 77.

Pimm, T.J., Byron, M.A. & Amos, M. (1994a) Coping with rheumatoid arthritis: A pilot study of the therapeutic benefit of a self management intervention. *Scandinavian Journal of Rheumatology*, Suppl. 97.

Pimm, T.J., Byron, M.A., Curson, D. & Weinman, J. (1994b) Personal illness models and the self management of arthritis. *Arthritis & Rheumatism*, **37**, 9(Suppl).

Pimm, T.J., Byron, M.A. & Curson, D. (1995) Illness representations: change during cognitive behavioural therapy for Rheumatoid Arthritis. Paper presented at BPS Special Group Health Psychology (SGHP) Conference Bristol.

Radojevic, V., Nicassio, P. & Weisman, M. (1992) Behavioural intervention with and without family support for rheumatoid arthritis. *Behaviour Therapy*, **23**, 13–20.

Revenson, T.A. & Felton, B.J. (1989) Disability and coping as predictors of psychological adjustment to rheumatoid arthritis. *Journal of Consulting and Clinical Psychology*, **57**, 344–348.

Revenson, T.A. (1993) The role of social support with rheumatic disease. *Bailliere's Clinical Rheumatology*, **7**, 377–396.

Roscam, S. (1986) *Application of a Health Locus of Control typology approach toward predicting depression and medical adherence in rheumatoid arthritis*. Unpublished doctoral dissertation. Nashville T.N., Vanderbilt University.

Rosenstiel, A. & Keefe, F.J. (1983) The use of coping strategies in chronic low back pain patients: Relationship to pain characteristics and current adjustment. *Pain*, **17**, 33–44.

Schiaffino, K.M. & Revenson, T.A. (1992) The role of perceived self-efficacy, perceived control and causal attributions in adaptation to rheumatoid arthritis: distinguishing mediator from moderator effects. *Personality and Social Psychology Bulletin*, **18**, 709–718.

Schiaffino, K.M., Revenson, T.A. & Gibofsky, A. (1991) Assessing the role of self-efficacy beliefs on adaptation to RA. *Arthritis Care and Research*, **4**, 150–157.

Shipley, M. & Newman, S.P. (1993) Psychological aspects of rheumatic diseases. *Bailliere's Clinical Rheumatology*, **7**, 215–9.

Smith, C.A., Dobbins, C.J. & Wallston, K.A. (1991) The mediational role of perceived competence in psychological adjustment to rheumatoid arthritis. *Journal of Applied Social Psychology*, **21**, 1218–1247.

Smith, C.A. & Wallston, K.A. (1992) Adaptation in patients with chronic rheumatoid arthritis: Application of a general model. *Health Psychology*, **11**, 151–162.

Smith, T.W., Christensen, A.J., Peck, J.R. & Ward J.R. (1994) Cognitive distortion, helplessness and depressed mood in rheumatoid arthritis: a four-year longitudinal analysis. *Health Psychology*, **13**, 213–217.

Stein, M.J., Wallston, K.A., Nicassio, P.M. & Casner, N.M. (1988) Factor structure of the Arthritis Helplessness Index. *The Journal of Rheumatology*, **15**, 427–432.

Summers , M.N., Haley, W.E., Reveille, J.D. & Alarcon, G.S. (1988) Radiographic assessments and psychologic variables as predictors of pain and functional impairment in osteoarthritis of the knee or hip. *Arthritis & Rheumatism,* **31**, 204–209.

Taal, E., Rasker, J.J., Seydel, E.R. & Wiegman, O. (1993) Health status, adherence with health recommendations, self-efficacy and social support in patients with rheumatoid arthritis. *Patient Education and Counselling*, **20**, 63–76.

Tucker, M. & Kirwan, J.R. (1991) Does patient education in rheumatoid arthritis have therapeutic potential? *Annals of the Rheumatic Diseases*, **50**, 422–428.

van Lankveld, W., van Pad Bosch, P., van de Putte, L., Naring, G. & van der Staak, C. (1994) Disease-specific stressors in rheumatoid arthritis: coping and well-being. *British Journal of Rheumatology*, **33**, 1067–73.

Wallston, K.A. (1993) Psychological control and its impact in the management of rheumatological disorders. *Bailliere's Clinical Rheumatology*, **7**, 281–95.

Weinman, J. Petrie, K.J. Moss-Morris, R. & Horne, R. (1996) The Illness Perception Questionnaire: A new method for assessing the cognitivie representation of illness. *Psychology & Health*, **11**, 431–445.

Yelin, E., Meenan, R., Nevitt, M. & Epstein, W. (1980) Work disability in rheumatoid arthritis: effects of disease, social and work factors. *Annals of Internal Medicine*, **93**, 551–6.

Zautra, A.J. & Manne, S.L. (1992) Coping with rheumatoid arthritis: a review of a decade of research. *Annals of Behavioural Medicine*, **14**, 31–39.

Zautra, A.J., Burleson, M.H., Smith, C.A., Blalock, S.J., Wallston, K.A., DeVellis, R.F., DeVellis, B.M. & Smith, T.W. (1995) Arthritis and perceptions of quality of life: An examination of positive and negative affect in rheumatoid arthritis patients. *Health Psychology*, **14**, 399–408.

13

Illness Representations and Breast Cancer: Coping with Radiation and Chemotherapy

Deanna L. Buick*

INTRODUCTION

Breast cancer is consistently reported to be the most common malignancy in women of developed countries (Bennett *et al.,* 1990; Vecchia, Decarli & Parazzini, 1987). The aetiology of the disease remains poorly understood and appropriate management is controversial. A number of possible risk factors have been identified including family history of breast cancer, few or late pregnancies, age at first menarche and prolonged menstruation (e.g., Kelsey, 1993; Spicer & Pike, 1994). In addition, a number of studies have suggested psychological-based risk factors including Type C personality (Baltrusch & Santagostino, 1989; Temoshok & Dreher, 1992) and stress (Baltrusch, Stangel & Titze, 1991; Cheang & Cooper, 1985). Whilst advances in early detection and medical intervention procedures may account, in part, for the increase in women diagnosed with early stage breast cancer, research has done relatively little to investigate the parallel psychological ramifications of these advances.

*Preparation of this chapter was supported by a grant from the New Zealand Health Research Council.

The increased prevalence of breast cancer and early medical intervention emphasizes the need for more research which addresses how people cope with the disease and its treatment. The current literature indicates a wide array of psychological response to cancer diagnosis and surgery. These individual differences suggest that patients hold different perceptions of the cancer experience, implicating cognitive factors as a major determinant of psychological response. Taylor (1983) has proposed that successful adjustment to cancer involves the amendment of assumptions and perceptions concerning one's self and world. Anecdotal evidence also supports the role of patients' perceptions in understanding illness behaviour (e.g., Bond & Wellisch, 1990). However, good quantitative research that corroborates this for patients undergoing radiation and chemotherapy, explicitly, is limited. We suggest that patients' illness perceptions form a primary component of the cognitive-interpretive framework within which the cancer experience is defined and understood. This hypothesis implicates illness perceptions in the mediation of psychological and behavioural responses to cancer treatment. The aim of this chapter is, therefore, threefold. First, this chapter will review the research to date which explores the cognitive basis to psychological adjustment associated with breast cancer and its treatment. Second, two studies will be presented which provide empirical-based evidence for the utility of the self-regulatory model of behaviour within the cancer field. Third, the practical implications of illness perceptions for patient care and clinical intervention will be considered in the closing section of this chapter.

POST-SURGICAL TREATMENT FOR BREAST CANCER

Breast cancer is treated using several methods either separately or in combination; surgical resection, chemotherapy, radiation, hormone therapy and immunotherapy[1]. Radiation and chemotherapy have become common treatments for breast cancer. Radiation has come to play an important role in the treatment of early stage breast cancer, allowing for more conservative surgical intervention. The intent of

---

[1]Cameron's chapter on 'Screening for Cancer: Ilness Perceptions and Illness Worry' addresses the role of self-regulatory behaviour in a clinical trial of tamoxifen.

radiation therapy is, therefore, to target the sub-clinical population of cancer cells which may remain following surgical resection, thereby reducing the chances of recurrence. Resection of the tumour without subsequent irradiation results in a 15 to 40% risk of local recurrence (Fisher, Bauer & Margolese, 1985; Lagios *et al.,* 1982). Adjuvant radiation involves radiating the breast for four to five weeks for a total of 4000 to 5000 radiation absorbed dose (RAD), which may be followed by an electron beam boost to the original tumour site. In addition to destroying malignant tissue, radiation also affects normal tissue which can cause a number of side effects, some so severe, that patients terminate treatment (Frytak & Moerter, 1981). Common physical side effects include fatigue, skin irritation and peeling, burns and hair loss in the irradiated area. The extent and severity of the side effects are site-, dose-, tissue volume- and fractionated-dependent. Over 70% of patients receiving radiation to the trunk area report some degree of nausea and vomiting, resulting in a loss of appetite and weight (Welch, 1980). The side-effects usually begin after the first treatment and increase in severity with additional treatments as the tolerance of the normal tissue to withstand the radiation is surpassed.

Cancer chemotherapy involves the administration of chemicals that are toxic to rapidly dividing cells, a primary feature of tumorigenesis. Whereas surgery and radiation are used to treat cancer localised to a small part of the body, chemotherapy is a systemic treatment aimed at destroying cancer cells which have metastasised in other areas of the body, distant from the original tumour site. The majority of chemotherapeutic agents work by disrupting cellular reproduction. As a result of its effect on normal tissues, a course of chemotherapy can produce some of the most adverse side effects of any form of cancer treatment, including: nausea, vomiting, hair loss, skin rashes, loss of appetite, disruption of sexual functioning, immunosuppression, weight gain, cessation of menstruation, neuropsychiatric effects and negative affects such as anxiety and depression (DeVita, 1985; Holland & Lesko, 1990; Knobf, 1986). Side effects vary widely, however, depending on the drug combination, dosage, number of cycles and whether the treatment is given in association with radiation. In addition to treatment side-effects, many patients develop conditioned negative responses to chemotherapy. Twenty to 65% of patients experience these conditioned side-effects (Burish & Carey, 1984).

The treatment of breast cancer appears, therefore, to be more inimical than the symptoms of the disease. This is one of the characteristics which delineates cancer from other chronic illnesses. Research suggests, however, that patients persist with therapy even in the face of adverse side effects. For example, Taylor, Lichtman and Wood (1984a) reported that few women refused chemotherapy and most complied with the regimen. The high rate of compliance coupled with the vast individual differences in psychological adjustment to treatment suggest a role for psychological factors. Disparate or even irrational responses can be interpreted by understanding the patients' perceptions of the disease and the meaning attributed to each aspect of the treatment. These meaning constructs or representations of the disease and its treatment may determine, to a large extent, patients' emotional responses and coping strategies (Petrie, Buick, Weinman & Booth, 1996). There is very little research which has addressed the importance of cognitive factors in mediating patients' adjustment to post-surgical radiation and chemotherapy.

PSYCHOLOGICAL REACTIONS TO TREATMENT

Clinical descriptions of patients' reactions to treatment are available (Peck & Boland, 1977; Rotman *et al.,* 1977; Smith & McNamara, 1977; Welch, 1980; Yonke, 1967). Radiation therapy produces significant anxiety, physiological arousal, discomfort and fatigue for patients (Andersen *et al.,* 1984). Emotional distress comprising anxiety and depression have also been reported among chemotherapy patients (Knobf, 1986; Nerenz *et al.,* 1984). In a longitudinal study of women receiving chemotherapy or radiation following surgery for breast cancer, we found that overall, chemotherapy patients reported greater levels of distress than radiation patients (Buick, 1996). As can be seen from Figure 1, patients undergoing chemotherapy reported an accumulation in distress as they progressed through treatment. Heightened levels of negative affect were maintained up to three months post-treatment. Our recent follow-up of these women at one year suggests a subsequent decrease in distress. Radiation patients showed the opposite pattern of results: the level of distress decreased across treatment. Figure 1 also shows patients' reported positive affect across therapy. Chemotherapy patients reported a decrease in positive affect following treatment.

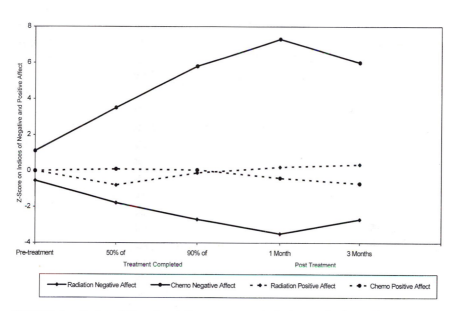

FIGURE 1   Patients' Emotional Response to Radiation and Chemotherapy Over Time

These results are consistent with Sinsheimer and Holland (1987) who reported increased depressive symptoms and decreased hope in chemotherapy patients on completing treatment. Clinical evidence indicates an increase in fear of tumour recurrence which may account for the maintenance of distress following therapy. Psychological distress is associated largely with side-effects of hair loss, weight gain and fatigue in chemotherapy patients (Sinsheimer & Holland, 1987). These data are convergent with other investigations of distress among cancer patients (e.g., Ganz *et al.,* 1989; Graydon, 1988).

Coping strategies also represent a variable that may influence the level of psychological distress experienced in response to cancer therapy. We found that patients predominantly reported using acceptance, positive reframing and active coping (Buick, 1996). As can be seen from Figure 2, coping outcome was clearly differentiated between radiation and chemotherapy patients. Chemotherapy patients were more likely to suppress competing activities, mentally disengage and use restraint than radiation patients. Radiation patients reported a greater use of acceptance. Repeated measure analysis showed that a number of coping responses changed over time. Three main patterns

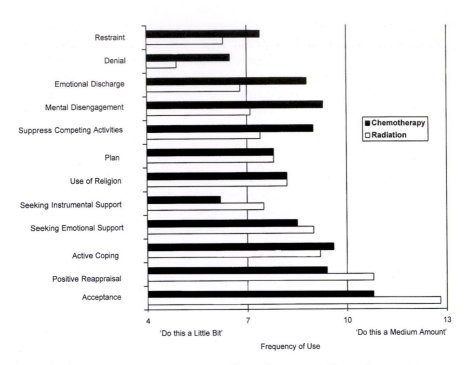

FIGURE 2   Coping Strategies Reported by Radiation and Chemotherapy Patients

of change emerged: First, a gradual decrease in use across the treatment experience indicated that positive reappraisal, seeking instrumental support, active coping, restraint, planning and suppression of competing activities were used predominantly in preparing for and during the first half of treatment. A second pattern showed the sustained use of seeking emotional support and disengaging from pre- to during treatment. The use of these coping responses declined following therapy. A third pattern of change indicated increased acceptance during treatment with gradual decline following treatment. It is also interesting to note that radiation patients had less coping flexibility than chemotherapy patients; this may reflect a greater demand on coping resources for women receiving chemotherapy as opposed to radiation.

The primary number of reported problems associated with radiation and chemotherapy treatment in cancer patients appear to involve inadequate preparation or education. Peck (1972) and Peck and Boland (1977) conducted the first systematic interviews of patients undergoing radiation. The content of the interviews suggested that patients held a pessimistic view of radiation and were unprepared for treatment. For example, very few patients knew how radiation therapy would affect them (Isler, 1971) and held many misconceptions regarding the specific nature of treatment (Peck & Boland, 1977). These results are consistent with our research assessing patients' knowledge concerning the nature and intent of radiation, prior to commencing treatment (Buick, 1996). In a sample of women receiving adjuvant radiation for primary breast cancer, 23% of patients did not know the name of the treatment: "I don't know. You just lie on the bed and they zap you". In addition, 20% of patients incorrectly stated the name of the treatment: radium treatment, radio rays, x-rays, radiology, laser beams and 'a ray thing'. Approximately one third of patients did not know the total length of their treatment, the length of the individual treatment sessions and were surprised at having further treatment after surgery. Patients predominantly expected radiation therapy to cure them, or 'destroy', 'cleanse', 'sterilise' 'whatever's left' (40%). Forty-six percent of patients were having radiotherapy because their 'doctor told them to', thus reducing the likelihood of recurrence.

Why do so many patients have inadequate information regarding treatment? A number of explanations have been postulated including patients' denial processes, lack of information from medical professionals and insufficient repetition of material. Current research has, however, overlooked the hypothesis that medical information may not be congruent with patients' perceptions or beliefs concerning the illness and its treatment. Intervention research appears to support this possibility: the results suggest that increasing patient understanding of the impending experience is associated with a more positive psychological outcome.

PSYCHOLOGICAL INTERVENTIONS FOR PATIENTS RECEIVING TREATMENT

Rainey (1985) conducted a preparatory intervention for radiation patients, examining a high information group (12 minute slide-tape programme introducing e.g., personnel, equipment, procedure) and a low information group (standard booklet). Rainey found that the high information group were better informed and had less anxiety and mood disturbance at the first and last week of treatment. The findings appear to suggest that adequate preparation for adjuvant therapy reduces distress prior to and during treatment. Forester, Kornfeld and Fleiss (1985) conducted a controlled trial in patients receiving radiation of an educational-supportive psychotherapy model. Forester *et al.* (1985) found less distress and reduced number of physical symptoms among those who received the brief weekly psychotherapy sessions. This effect was shown up to four weeks post-treatment. The results also suggest an association between the emotional and physical concomitants of treatment. In alleviating patient distress, certain physical symptoms associated with radiation may be reduced. The current body of intervention literature suggests that education increases patients' knowledge of cancer and improves psychological adjustment in the immediate short-term as well as six to 12 months post-intervention (Berglund *et al.*, 1994; Cain *et al.*, 1986).

Johnson, Lauvier and Nail (1989) investigated the effects of an informational intervention on outcomes of coping with radiation treatment of prostate cancer. The experimental intervention was delivered through tape-recorded messages containing content selected from patient descriptions of the radiotherapy experience obtained in a previous study (King *et al.*, 1985). Each message included concrete objective descriptions of a particular phase of the radiation treatment experience, e.g., onset of side effects. Johnson *et al.*'s (1989) findings support the self-regulatory theory — patient understanding of the experience emerged as an important factor with respect to: 1) mediating coping behaviour and 2) patients being able to maintain usual activities during and following radiation treatment. Increased understanding of treatment may foster problem-solving coping that results in patients being able to reduce the amount of disruption to their usual activities. The desired outcome of coping with a threatening event is to prevent disruption and discomfort from the emotional response and to minimise the negative impact on a person's life (Lazarus, 1966). In addition, cognitive schema structured by perceptual information may help to reduce the effort patients expend in organising the experience into a meaningful context. Whilst the current body of intervention literature suggests support for the processes based in self-regulation theory, additional validation is however necessary.

COGNITIVE MODELS OF CANCER

Cognitive theorists (Lazarus, 1966; Leventhal, 1970) have proposed that cognitive processes mediate response to threat. The individual's psychological structure and cognitive features of the event shape the conclusions drawn regarding the degree of threat and adequacy of coping resources. Leventhal and Diefenbach (1991) suggested that persons experiencing an illness threat employ implicit theories, that is illness schemata comprised of subjectively perceived symptoms and causal attributions, to understand the health threat and regulate health behaviour. In a study of how cancer patients coped with chemotherapy, Nerenz *et al.* (1984) noted that patients seemed to be responding to the treatment situation in terms of implicit theories about the disease and its treatment. For example, patients with malignant lymphoma appeared to determine the effectiveness of chemotherapy by monitoring the size of their palpable diseased lymph nodes. Patients who experienced a sudden disappearance of the nodes were more distressed than did those with gradual remission. The heightened distress of patients with the most rapid remission apparently reflected the fact that: 1) patients no longer had a discernible method of assessing the effectiveness of the treatment and 2) patients did not understand having to continue treatment when they were 'cured', i.e., had no tangible evidence of illness. The results suggest an implicit model of illness in which symptoms define the presence or absence of disease and mediate patients' psychological response. Leventhal and his colleagues (Leventhal & Diefenbach, 1991; Leventhal, Meyer & Nerenz, 1980; Leventhal, Nerenz & Steele, 1984) argue that disease representations such as these form implicit theories of illness that are used to guide coping and to evaluate and regulate the use of treatment. It is important to recognise that the patient's behaviour is not necessarily medically rational, but that the responses are consonant with the patient's representation of the medical problem and are, therefore, psychologically valid.

A further body of research investigating surgical interventions for breast cancer can be interpreted within the cognitive representations of illness framework. A number of investigations have suggested that patients who choose lumpectomy as opposed to mastectomy procedures hold different 'ideas' concerning breast cancer. Ashcroft,

Leinster and Slade (1985) and Margolis and Goodman (1984) found that women selecting limited resection and radiation were more concerned with insult to their body image, were more dependent on their breast for self-esteem and believed they would experience difficulty adjusting to the loss of the breast by mastectomy. In contrast, patients who selected mastectomy, predominantly perceived the breast with cancer as 'foreign' and wanted to have it removed and they were more fearful of the side effects of radiation. Interpreting these results within the Leventhal framework suggests that patients were making a decision which was congruent with their illness representation of cancer. Ashcroft *et al.* (1985) also found no difference in emotional distress between women who had chosen mastectomy or limited resection and radiation. The congruency between the illness representation and the surgical procedure may have minimised patients' emotional response to surgical intervention. Interpretation of the results in this field has predominantly centred around decision-making and sense of control paradigms. The concept of illness representations, however, extends this argument. That is, the illness representation moderates the surgical decision and the congruency between belief and action moderates patients' sense of control. Future research needs to consider the interplay among these constructs.

Illness cognitions form an interpretative framework for the generation and appraisal of emotional and coping responses. The paradigm which consistently underlies much of the work is the notion that a basic conceptual self-regulatory system, comprising assumptions, beliefs or theories regarding the disease or illness, necessitates interaction and functioning. Leventhal's model of self-regulatory behaviour (Leventhal *et al.*, 1980; Leventhal *et al.*, 1984) posits that adaptation to illness reflects the combined action of four sets of underlying factors:

1. The cognitive model of illness, that is, what the person thinks about the illness and treatment experience;
2. The emotional response to the illness and treatment;
3. The coping response directed by the illness cognitions; and
4. The person's appraisal of the coping outcome.

Nerenz *et al.*'s (1984) research with lymphoma patients indicates that illness cognitions and coping have an important role to play in adjustment to cancer therapy. However, methodological problems limit conclusions regarding the strength and exact nature of these associations. A further criticism of the illness representation research, to date, concerns the lack of work aimed at investigating the link between illness representations and coping. Implicit models of illness were developed primarily within the framework of cognition, with the aim of understanding the coping process and response. However, the current status of coping research suggests that much of this work has continued in relative detachment from that on illness representations (Skelton & Croyle, 1991). Longitudinal studies of such relationships and how these might change over time could expand the theoretical understanding of breast cancer patients' illness perceptions and coping strategies and may also benefit clinical work by identifying possible points of intervention.

In addition, research has been aimed at establishing primarily the structure and specific content of personal beliefs or illness perceptions concerning a number of illnesses, for example, diabetes (Hampson, Glasgow & Toobert, 1990; Hampson, Glasgow & Foster, 1995), osteo arthritis (Hampson, Glasgow & Zeiss, 1994), chest tuberculosis (Dalal & Singh, 1992) and coronary heart disease (De Valle & Norman, 1992). There is, however, very little work which has examined the specific content of women's illness perceptions for breast cancer. Our research is one of the first investigations to assess the cognitive and emotional representations using the self-regulatory model of behaviour. The current health psychology literature is also relatively limited in its understanding of the process of change and resistance to change in personal beliefs associated with different illnesses. This is also true for cancer. Thus, we undertook to study the process of change in illness perceptions among breast cancer patients. Furthermore, research to date has disregarded the possibility that illness cognitions are predictors of psychological adjustment to treatment. Specific attention to the cognitive basis of patients' understanding of illness and its effect, may considerably improve psychological adjustment to the treatment.

ILLNESS REPRESENTATIONS AND POST-SURGICAL THERAPY: RADIATION AND CHEMOTHERAPY

Fifty-two radiation and 26 chemotherapy patients receiving adjuvant therapy for primary breast cancer participated in a longitudinal study from pre- to three months post-treatment. The treatment groups comprised, primarily, European, middle-class women. This sample characteristic is consistent with the epidemiological figures for New Zealand, with Maori and Pacific Island women more likely to present with significantly later stage disease. The Illness Perception Questionnaire (IPQ, Weinman *et al.,* 1996), adapted for use with a breast cancer population (Buick, 1996), was used to investigate the characteristics of patients' cognitive representations of cancer and its treatment. We also designed a structured interview based on the work by Taylor, Lichtman and Wood (1984b) and Nerenz *et al.* (1984), which is designed to reflect the conceptual dimensions of the IPQ.

The Causes of Breast Cancer

Patients believed that breast cancer was caused by a combination of attributes comprising: internal beliefs centred on self and self-blame, chance, environmental hazards and genetic factors. Consistent with the results of the IPQ, content analysis of the personal theory section of the interview identified seven causal theories: myself, stress, extreme worrying, marital discord, lack of emotional expression, chance and environmental hazards (see Table 1). The category 'lack of emotional expression' gives credence to the idea of a cancer-prone personality, as described by Temoshok (Temoshok *et al.,* 1985). The wide array of causal beliefs is concordant with a number of studies reporting attributes ranging from self-blame, stress (O'Connor, Wicker & Germino, 1990; Taylor *et al.,* 1984b), having 'caught or inherited it' (O'Connor *et al.,* 1990), to environmental hazards (Timko & Janoff-Bulman, 1985). The breadth of causal beliefs may reflect the controversy surrounding the disease aetiology, of which relatively little is known. The lack of medical clarification may engender patients to search for an explanation.

Internal, self-blame attributes remained stable across the treatment experience. This constancy may represent characterological traits rather than attributes mediated by the treatment protocol. Patient responses, therefore, may tap implicit causal mechanisms for a number of illnesses, including breast cancer. This argument is concordant with Lau and Hartman's (1983) research suggesting that minor illness experiences can be extrapolated to major, life-threatening disease. In addition, self-blame attributes do not necessarily represent negative or maladaptive responses. We suggest that patients' conception of perceived control over the blame attribute

Table 1 Personal Theories as to the Cause of Breast Cancer

Hunches	Examples from Patient Interview
Myself	"My reaction to things. I obviously haven't dealt with things in a way that they aren't going to affect me. I haven't looked after myself as well as I should have".
Stress	"Stress, stress on myself. What stresses haven't I experienced is the question I've experienced a tremendous amount of stress all my life. More than most people. I think this is a physical manifestation of my stress".
Extreme Worry	"I always worrying about something, and maybe if I am like that, it might be more likely that a lump could grow".
Marital Discord	"If I hadn't married my husband I do ask myself where I would be today. I don't think you can go through all the hate I've been through and not have something wrong with you".
Lack of Emotional Expression	"I've spent so much of my life feeling angry and not being able to do anything about it. I have spent so much of my life living with this anger. I guess if has to come out someway".
Chance	"To me it's just chance. Yeah it's only chance that it happens, pure and simple, as if you were gambling".
Environmental Hazards	"We don't know what we're breathing anymore or how they process food. I think this has something to do with it".

may be an important component in determining its effect. For example, dietary attributions comprise a controllable or modifiable component. Self-blame responses may prove adaptive if the patient effects a change which results in increased feelings of control. The results from our patient interviews also support this argument. We found that patients who reported controllable self-blame attributes (i.e., "my breast cancer was caused by dietary factors", "my breast cancer was caused by getting rundown and overworked") were more likely to report engaging in modifying behaviour, e.g., change of diet, or reducing the number of hours at work. Timko and Janoff-Bulman (1985) have found that causal attributes which represent modifiable behaviour may afford patients a greater perception of invulnerability to recurrence.

Whilst internal and self-blame causal attributes for cancer appear to be stable over time, the role of chance and genetic factors appears to change; these beliefs strengthen during and following treatment. The process of change associated with patients' causal beliefs may represent an attempt to restructure illness perceptions in preparation for a period of uncertainty, when the likelihood of recurrence is a realistic expectation. Furthermore, the nature of the change in attributions suggests an attempt to establish causal dimensions of the disease not characterised by personal responsibility. This may be important for the development of patients' perceived vulnerability to recurrence following active medical intervention. Increased perceptions of chance and genetic factors places the likelihood of recurrence outside of the realm of personal responsibility — one can do little about an illness recurrence governed by 'luck of the draw', or pre-determined DNA material. Patients' causal beliefs may influence psychological adjustment to cancer in that the attributes subtract from or contribute to patients' perceived vulnerability to recurrence.

Beliefs regarding the cause of breast cancer were also clearly differentiated between radiation and chemotherapy patients (see Figure 3). Chemotherapy patients were more likely to report internal, self-blame and environmental attributes, as opposed to radiation patients who reported a greater belief in chance. The difference in pre-treatment causal attributes between groups is of importance. Why should women with primary breast cancer perceive different causes for their disease based on assignment to a particular therapy? Comparison of the causal beliefs between node positive chemotherapy and radiation patients, respectively, suggests that the notion of 'severity' plays an important role in the development of causal attributes for cancer. If histopathological markers of disease severity, e.g., axillary node involvement, accounted for differences in causal perceptions, we would expect that patients with node positive status held homogenous illness perceptions, irrespective of referral for radiation or chemotherapy. Our results did not support this hypothesis. Node positive patients assigned to chemotherapy (N = 26) as opposed to radiation only (N = 22) held discrepant causal beliefs. There was, however, no difference in causal beliefs between node positive or node negative patients referred for radiation. The results suggest that referral for chemotherapy in itself, is perceived as a marker of disease severity, impacting on patients' cognitive-interpretive framework of the illness.

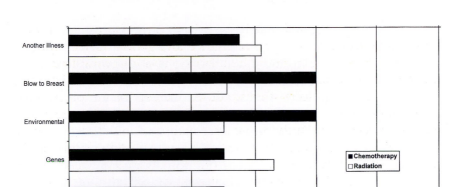

FIGURE 3   Radiation and Chemotherapy Patients' Causal Beliefs for Breast Cancer.

Patients' beliefs concerning the duration and consequences of chemotherapy also support this argument. Prior to commencing treatment, chemotherapy patients were more likely to perceive breast cancer as lasting for a long time and having a greater impact on their lives than radiation patients. Two further arguments also support the perceived severity hypothesis: First, the length of chemotherapy (6 months) when compared to radiation (4–5 weeks) may serve to reinforce patients' perceptions of severity. Second, radiation patients may compare themselves with chemotherapy patients and believe they are 'better off' — focusing on aspects of the event which denotes advantage. This argument is consistent with the notions of downward comparison (Hagopian, 1993) and secondary victimisation (Taylor, 1983).

Furthermore, we hypothesise that the procedural nature of the treatment may serve to reinforce the most salient features of the patients' illness perceptions. For example, the internalised administration (i.e., intravenous drip and ingestion of tablets) of chemotherapeutic cytotoxic agents may reinforce the internal orientation of causal attributes for cancer. Conversely, receipt of an external beam of radiation may reinforce the salient external attributes of radiation patients' illness schemata. Further research is necessary to validate this hypothesis.

Taylor *et al.* (1984b) found that attributions of responsibility to the self, environment, or chance showed no relationship with positive psychological adjustment to cancer. However, blame of another person was negatively correlated with psychological adjustment. It is interesting that attributions were unrelated to adjustment in Taylor *et al.'s* study. The authors suggested that the understanding and predicability usually created by attributions during a stressful event, were provided by cognitions other than causal attributes. Taylor *et al.'s* work raises a number of unanswered questions concerning the importance of patients' beliefs in mediating psychological adjustment. One of the issues surrounding Taylor *et al.'s* work concerns the relative importance of studying one component of the illness representation, i.e., causal attributes. Psychological adjustment to a stressful event may be derived from the overall meaning established by the interplay amongst all five components. Murray (1990) has suggested that various attribute dimensions (e.g., causal, controllability, consequences) are used to a greater or lesser degree in cognitive representations of illness. Illness representations are conceptualised, therefore, as schemata comprising clusters or groups of knowledge. Thus, we used cluster analysis procedures to separate the illness perception data set into its constituent groups or clusters. The cluster analysis technique explores the differential patterns among perceptual components comprising illness schemata. We also investigated the relationship between illness belief clusters and psychological adjustment to treatment.

Illness Belief Clusters and Psychological Adjustment to Radiation and Chemotherapy

The analyses identified two distinct clusters. As can be seen from Figure 4, the first cluster for radiation patients represented more negative illness beliefs, with the highest mean scores on the identity, internal/self-blame, duration and consequence. Patients in this cluster also scored lower on the cure/control scale, indicative of a diminished belief in the possibility of curing or controlling cancer. There was no difference between the first and second cluster on patients' beliefs concerning the role environmental hazards in causing cancer. Patients in the negative illness cluster were more likely to report psychological distress prior to commencing and up to three months post-radiation. Patients in the negative cluster were also more likely to report coping with radiation by venting of emotion, disengagement and restraint coping responses. Consequently, patients with more negative illness beliefs exhibited less coping flexibility. Patients with negative illness beliefs also reported a greater level of functional disruption, ranging from inability to work, disturbance of sleep and rest patterns and a tendency to report social withdrawal. Patterns of functional disruption were evidenced from during treatment up to three months post-radiation. Patients also reported higher severity ratings for the somatic effects of treatment.

The first cluster for chemotherapy patients was also characterised by negative illness beliefs, with the highest mean scores on the identity, internal/self-blame and consequence scales and a lower score on the cure/control dimension. There was no difference between the two illness clusters in terms of patients' beliefs regarding duration; patients' scores indicated a duration belief indicative of a greater likelihood of recurrence. Chemotherapy patients comprising the negative illness belief cluster reported a similar pattern of psychological and

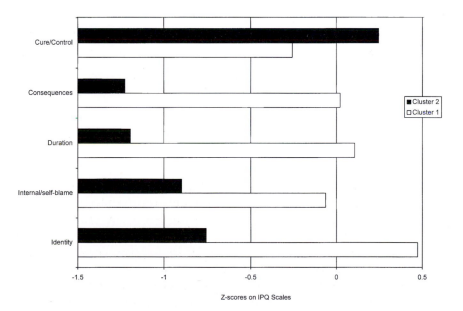

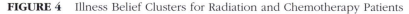

FIGURE 4 Illness Belief Clusters for Radiation and Chemotherapy Patients

behavioural responses compared to radiation patients. There was, however, a primary difference in the pattern of functional disruption associated with treatment — chemotherapy patients were more likely to continue working than radiation patients. The difference in functional outcome may reflect an attempt by chemotherapy patients to preserve lifestyle behaviours representative of their self-identity within a treatment context defined by perceptions of increased disease severity and vulnerability to recurrence.

Content analysis of patient transcripts supported the pattern of illness belief clusters. Patients who comprised the negative illness clusters were more likely to report 1) lower levels of accurate information concerning the nature and intent of treatment and 2) personal theories of causation centred on stressful life events, marital discord, extreme worrying and lack of emotional expression. It is interesting to note that patients' assignment to a more negative or positive illness belief cluster was not associated with markers of disease severity. There was no association between tumour size, metastases status, axillary node involvement, type of surgery and a more negative illness cluster. This suggests that patients' perceptions concerning disease severity and likelihood of recurrence did not reflect the actual medically-estimated risk presented by cancer. However, patients with a more negative illness belief were more likely to report a medically documented concurrent illness or problem, e.g., migraines, asthma, eczema. This finding, coupled with the results showing that patients 1) have increased attention to identity symptoms defining the label of breast cancer and 2) perceive the side effects of treatment as more severe, suggests that patients in the negative illness cluster may be more sensitive to physiological cues. This pattern of heightened physiological arousal may reflect a form of somatic introspection whereby treatment side-effects and the symptomatology associated with the concurrent medical problem exacerbate perceptions of treatment severity.

The results suggest that negative illness beliefs appear to be associated with maladaptive psychological responses. A schema composed of more moderate or positive illness perceptions evidently contrasts in its effect on psychological adjustment with a schema composed of the negative dimensions of cancer. Patients appear to use illness schemata as a framework for selecting consonant psychological and behavioural responses to the treatment as they progress through it. Our research suggests that the content of this self-regulatory system could be used as a way to identify patients at risk of poor psychological adjustment to cancer therapy. Furthermore, negative perceptions of breast cancer may interfere with patients' ability to interpret and understand the treatment experience. In turn, this may foster emotion-focused and disengagement-style coping that results in patients being unable to control the amount of disruption to their usual activities during therapy. Conversely, illness perceptions structured by appropriate or accurate information may help reduce the effort patients expend in organising the experience into a meaningful context. Illness perceptions which facilitate the development of a more positive meaning, may also directly affect adjustment to treatment by enhancing feelings of control and increased self-esteem.

The self-regulatory model of illness is also consistent with the symbolic interactionist approach which conceives of the individual deriving a self- and contextual-meaning of illness (Fife, 1990). Self-meaning concerns the perceived effect of the illness on the person's perception of self, whereas contextual-meaning addresses the perceived characteristics of the event itself. The link between these two dimensions suggests a high degree of congruence with the structure of our illness belief clusters. Patients' causal attributes may represent a derived contextual-meaning of breast cancer, i.e., the patient's perception of the self within the cancer experience. The clustering of internal, self-blame attributes with more negative, event-related perceptions of treatment is not unexpected as patients' sense of self-meaning needs to be consonant with the contextual-meaning of illness. Thompson and Janigan (1988) suggested that individuals needed a sense of coherence between their self-definitions and the events which occurred in their lives. The results from our work suggest that if this congruence exists, patients who report negative illness beliefs may hold a more negative self-definition within which the experience of cancer is defined and understood. Thus, conforming the cancer experience to pre-existing perceptions may be less overwhelming than reconstructing existing cognitions to the current situation (Marris, 1974). Whilst this parallels the self-regulatory model, the symbolic interactionist perspective extends this interplay one step further. Tangible features of the illness experience which are not consonant with the patient's perception of herself may be redefined within the parameters of the individual's self-identity. Research centred on the self-regulatory system needs to consider this interplay as it may account for the relative inflexibility of illness cognitions and hence their resistance to restructuring. Addressing negative illness clusters with psycho-education programmes may, therefore, be inadequate. The nature of self-perception may require a more indepth psychological intervention to enable patients a less negative perception of their self-identity and thus, the illness experience. Therefore if we are to concern ourselves with the clinical implications, this hypothesis suggests that approaches to care which encourage positive self-identity amongst patients may be efficacious.

ILLNESS PERCEPTIONS IN MEDICAL STAFF AND LAYPERSONS

The amount of work which has assessed the cognitive basis of stereotypes held by physically healthy people towards those with cancer is surprisingly small. Illness stereotype research falls directly within the parameters of cognitive representations. Illness stereotypes can be viewed as cognitive schemata comprising groups of attributes that organise the individual's knowledge base and understanding of ill people. These perceptions may not necessarily be accurate and thus, affective and behavioural responses directed toward ill populations based on inaccurate perceptions may result in inappropriate outcomes. Peters-Golden's (1982) work highlights the differential perceptions of cancer held by healthy women in the community and women who had been diagnosed with breast cancer, ranging from 3 weeks to 21 years. Healthy people reported that they would attempt to 'cheer up' a cancer patient. Conversely, patients reported that 'unrelenting optimism' was disturbing. In addition, healthy people believed that cancer patients did not want to discuss their illness and were concerned primarily with the cosmetic aspects associated with surgical intervention. This perception contrasted with cancer patients who reported apprehensions concerning recurrence and death.

There is also limited research investigating the cognitive basis of medical professionals' perceptions of cancer patients. Current research indicates that the discrepancy between those attitudes held by medical professionals and those held by patients may actually affect patients' subsequent health behaviour (Baumann & Leventhal,

1985; Meyer, Leventhal & Gutmann, 1985). Neuling and Winefield (1988) reported that women recovering from breast cancer surgery desired informational support exclusively from physicians. Dunkel-Schetter (1984) found that breast cancer patients perceived the lack of information from physicians to be problematic. Rose (1990) found that cancer patients (59% breast cancer) desired informational support from health professionals more than friends and family. Our research has confirmed these findings: radiation therapists' and oncology nurses' perceptions of breast cancer and its treatment are incongruous with the actual experience reported by patients. Whilst these incongruities are not favourable for patient care, they are encouraged by a medical model which does not consider the differences in illness beliefs between the practitioner and patient. Research within the discipline of health psychology has become very patient focused. One of the limitations associated with this orientation is the lack of research addressing medical education issues for health workers.

We compared the illness perceptions reported by 78 healthy matched controls from the community, 27 radiation therapists and 16 oncology nurses involved in the administration of chemotherapy, with patients receiving cancer therapy (Buick, Petrie & Probert, 1996). The focus of the study was on medical professionals' and physically healthy women's perceptions of breast cancer, rather than on any necessarily factual aspects of the disease. Subjects were instructed to rate the 'typical' psychological and behavioural response of the 'average' woman receiving treatment for breast cancer. The rationale underlying the instructions was to tap into subjects' self-concept of breast cancer. Research has shown that the self is a natural reference point when thinking about and evaluating other people's behaviour (Markus, Smith & Moreland, 1985).

We found that causal perceptions of cancer were disparate among laypersons, medical professionals and breast cancer patients (see Figure 5; Buick, Petrie & Probert, 1996). Physically healthy women and radiation therapists had stronger beliefs concerning the role of internal/self-blame and chance attributes, than patients. These results are consistent with Payne (1990) who found that stress and 'bottling up' of emotions were perceived as primary causes of breast cancer in a lay population. Our work suggests that radiation therapists, treating patients on a daily basis, conceive of breast cancer as caused by 'something the patient has done'. The results suggest that cancer patients may be 'double stigmatised', i.e., for having cancer and causing cancer. Research has shown that people are more likely to avoid cancer patients if they view the patient as contributing to the disease (Curbow, Andrews & Burke, 1986). Oncology nurses, however, showed the opposite pattern of results to radiation therapists: nurses were more likely to believe that breast cancer was caused by chance. Physically healthy women's perceptions of the length and impact of treatment were comparable to chemotherapy, but not radiation patients. Lay perceptions of breast cancer appear, therefore, to be structured by information pertaining to the chemotherapeutic as opposed to radiation therapy experience. Medical professionals' perception of the consequences of treatment and duration of cancer did not match patients' beliefs: oncology nurses underestimated, whereas radiation therapists overestimated the impact of treatment and perceived duration of the disease. It is possible that illness perceptions held by medical professionals may reflect a self-protection mechanism. Personnel treating breast cancer may develop a cognitive-interpretive framework of the patient's experience which allows for continued functioning within the cancer context, without engendering an overwhelming sense of responsibility or emotional involvement.

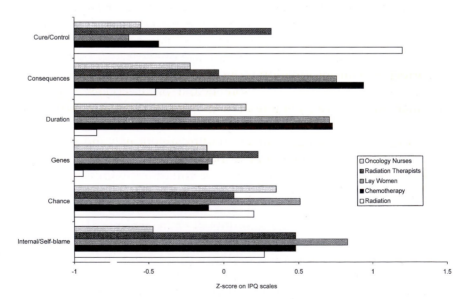

FIGURE 5   Laypersons' and Medical Professionals' Perceptions of Breast Cancer

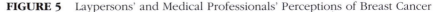

Laypersons and medical professionals also overestimate the degree of psychological distress associated with cancer therapy. Laypersons' total score for distress was two times greater than the score for either radiation or chemotherapy patients. Medical personnel also believed that patients sought instrumental and emotional support. Physically healthy women believed that patients would use denial and venting of emotion to cope with treatment. Conversely, patients reported the predominant use of positive reappraisal, acceptance and active coping. Our results are consistent with Derogatis, Abeloff and McBeth (1976) who found that physicians overestimated levels of anxiety than patients rated themselves. Katz *et al.* (1987) also found that medical students and hospital nurses perceived cancer patients as more physically and psychologically impaired than people with heart disease, AIDS and diabetes. Our work suggests that patients may experience too little or inappropriate support as medical personnel and public perceive the needs of patients incorrectly. These findings raise the question of whether medical staff have the appropriate skills to determine the psychological and behavioural needs that patients require to meet the demands of treatment.

The hypothesis from self-regulation theory posits that the effect of intervention on coping outcome is mediated by increasing patients' understanding of their experience (Johnson *et al.*, 1989). Consistent with this argument, we found that the majority of patients who comprised the negative illness clusters were more likely to report incorrect or misinformation concerning radiation therapy. Our results suggest the need for more health professionals to provide accurate information, congruent with patients' illness perceptions. The possibility remains, that receipt of information which facilitates cognitive understanding of illness and treatment may aid in restructuring patients' negative illness beliefs. Medical information or preparation procedures which are not congruent with the information content and belief structure of patients' illness perception may be encoded within the information hierarchy at a low level. The outcome of this lower ordering encoding means that it is unlikely that the information will be retrieved and acted upon within the treatment setting. Patients respond to radiation and chemotherapeutic protocols in a way that is congruent with the content of their illness schemata. In addition, patients' feelings of control and self-esteem may also be diminished through lack of information or inappropriate support by others. Appropriate information may help to restore patients' sense of control by providing them with information concerning, e.g., the cause, consequences and nature of treatment. Perceptions of control may also be enhanced by information programmes which teach patients ways of managing the treatment and its side effects. In turn, this information and support may feed into more outlook-mediated constructs, such as optimism. Patients who feel they have adequate skills to cope with treatment side effects may construe a more positive meaning from the treatment experience.

Our results suggest that biased perceptions on the part of medical staff and laypersons may compromise the quality of assistance which is offered. Educational programmes that aim at the reduction in cognitive biases through the disclosure of inappropriate perceptions should be directed at lay and medical professional communities.

PRACTICAL IMPLICATIONS AND SUMMARY

The theory of self-regulation provides a unique conceptual framework with which to understand the illness experience. Our work clearly raises the possibility that illness perceptions of cancer and its treatment could serve as clinical markers and provide some indication of the level of psychological and functional adaptation patients will be able to achieve and sustain. Future research needs to address the development of illness perception measures as clinical diagnostic tools for detection of 'at risk' patients. In addition, research needs to ascertain not only long-term relationships between illness perceptions and psychological adjustment, but also to examine the role of implicit theories of illness in the physical outcome of cancer. The notions of 'severity' and perceived invulnerability also appear to be an important adjunct to the self-regulatory model of illness. Vulnerability perceptions may exacerbate the development of beliefs concerning the consequences, controllability and causality of cancer. Given that illness belief clusters may represent measures of perceived invulnerability to cancer recurrence, it is important to determine the origins of these perceptions.

Interventions which provide accurate information concerning the nature and consequences of treatment may prepare patients for a change in reduction in psychological and functional capabilities. These accurate expectations may reduce the discrepancy between what patients believe the experience should be like and what actually occurs. The results from our work, however, suggest that there are different patterns of interplay amongst the components comprising illness perceptions. It is erroneous, therefore, to assume that all patients will respond to a psychological intervention in a uniform fashion. There is no one successful intervention strategy for all patients, but that some interventions are successful when individual's illness perceptions are considered and when the intervention and individual styles are congruent. Successful management of cancer patients will, therefore, play into and subsidise the patient's cognitive-interpretative framework, arguably through its influence on schematic compositions patients have formed of the experience. Without understanding the cognitive-interpretative framework from which patients derive meaning for and a conceptualisation of the cancer experience, interventions targeted at enhancing patients' psychological adjustment to treatment may well adopt an unintended 'hit-and-miss' approach.

The results from our work also suggest that incongruities exist between physically healthy individuals and patients diagnosed with cancer. These findings present a problem for health educators. The question then becomes one of changing stereotypes in order to increase acceptance and understanding of cancer patients. The relative stability of material encoded within cognitive schemata further suggests that an effective method may be to change the content of illness stereotypes held by physically healthy people, rather than completely eradicate the schemata. The concept of changing cognitions, however, raises a number of questions as the nature of illness cognitions is characterised by experience-based and over-learned perceptual patterns. Future research needs to establish the most effective intervention methods to effect cognitive modification. In addition, the discrepancies between medical professionals' and patients' illness representations has clear implications for the development of medical education programmes for health workers. In addition, the results from our work investigating medical professionals' and laypersons' perceptions of breast cancer, suggest that the self-regulatory model of behaviour provides a useful framework for assessing the perception and organisation of other people's illness experiences. The self-regulatory model can also be used

broadly and systematically as an interpretive framework for compre-
hending the thoughts, feelings and behaviours of physically healthy
individuals and medical personnel towards the physically ill.

REFERENCES

Andersen, B.L., Karlson, J.A., Anderson, B. & Tewfik, H.H. (1984)
Anxiety and cancer treatment: Response to stressful radiotherapy. *Health Psychology*, **3**, 535–551.

Ashcroft, J.J., Leinster, S.J. & Slade, P.A. (1985) Breast cancer-patient
choice of treatment: Preliminary communication. *Journal of
Royal Society of Medicine*, **78**, 43–46.

Baltrusch, H.J.F. & Santagostino, P. (1989) The Type C behavior
pattern: New concepts. *International Journal of Psychophysiology*, **7**, 126–127.

Baltrusch, H.J.F., Stangel, W. & Titze, I. (1991) Stress, cancer and
immunity. New developments in biopsychosocial and psy-
choneuroimmunologic research. *Acta Neurologia*, (Napoli) **13**,
315–327.

Bauman L.J. & Leventhal, H. (1985) I can tell when my blood pressure is up, can't I? *Health Psychology*, **4**, 203–218.

Bennett, I.C., McCaffrey, J.F., Baker, C.A., Burke, M.F., Lee, J.F. &
Balderson, G.A. (1990) Changing patterns in presentation of
breast cancer over the past 25 years. *Australian and New
Zealand Journal of Surgery*, **60**, 665–671.

Berglund, G., Bolund, C., Gustafsson, U.L. & Sjoden, P.O. (1994)
One-year follow-up of the 'Starting Again' group rehabilitation
programme for cancer patients. *European Journal of Cancer*,
30A, 1744–1751.

Bond, G.G. & Wellisch, D.K. (1990) Psychosocial care. In C.M. Haskell
(Ed.), *Cancer Treatment*, 3rd ed., (pp. 893–904). Philadelphia:
W.B. Saunders & Co.

Buick, D.L. (1996) *Psychological adjustment to radiation and
chemotherapy: The role of illness perceptions.* Unpublished
Doctoral Dissertation: University of Auckland School of Medicine.

Buick, D.L., Petrie, K.J. & Probert, J. (1996) *Illness beliefs, coping and
emotional distress: How do healthy women and medical staff
perceive women with breast cancer?* Paper presented at the

American Psychosomatic Society Annual Meeting, Williamsburg, USA.

Burish, T.G. & Carey, M.P. (1984) Conditioned response to chemotherapy: Etiology and treatment. In B. Fox & B. Newberry (Eds.), *Impact of psychoendocrine systems in cancer and immunity* (pp. 311–320). New York: Hogrefe.

Cain, E.N., Kohorn, E.I., Quinlan, D.M., Latimer, K. & Schwartz, P.E. (1986) Psychosocial benefits of a cancer support group. *Cancer*, **57**, 183–189.

Cheang, A. & Cooper, C.L. (1985) Psychosocial factors in breast cancer. *Stress Medicine*, **1**, 61–66.

Curbow, B., Andrews, R.M. & Burke, T.A. (1986) Perceptions of the cancer patient: Causal explanations and personal attributions. *Journal of Psychosocial Oncology*, **4**, 115–134.

Dalal, A.K. & Singh, A.K. (1992) Role of causal and recovery beliefs in the psychological adjustment to chronic disease. *Psychology and Health*, **6**, 193–203.

Derogatis, L.R., Abeloff, M.D. & McBeth, C.D. (1976) Cancer patients and their physicians in the perception of psychological symptoms. *Psychosomatics*, **17**, 197–201.

De Valle, M.N. & Norman, P. (1992) Causal attributes, health locus of control beliefs and lifestyle changes among pre-operative coronary patients. *Psychology and Health*, **7**, 201–211.

DeVita, V.T. (1985) Principles of chemotherapy. In V.T. DeVita, Jr., S. Hellman & S.A. Rosenberg (Eds.), *Cancer: principles and practice of oncology* (pp. 257–285). Philadelphia: Lippincoutt.

Dunkel-Schetter, C. (1984) Social support and cancer: Findings based on patients' interviews and their implications. *Journal of Social Issues*, **40**, 77–98.

Fife, B.L. (1994) The conceptualization of meaning in illness. *Social Science and Medicine*, **38**, 309–316.

Fisher, B., Bauer, M. & Margolese, R. (1985) Five-year result of randomised clinical trial comparing total mastectomy and segmental mastectomy with or without radiation in the treatment of primary breast cancer. *New England Journal of Medicine*, **312**, 666–673.

Forester, B.M., Kornfeld, D.S. & Fleiss, J. (1985) Psychotherapy during radiotherapy: Effects on emotional and physical distress. *American Journal of Psychiatry*, **142**, 22–27.

Frytak, S. & Moerter, C.G. (1981) Management of nausea and vomiting in the cancer patient. *Journal of the American Medical Association,* **245**, 393–396.

Ganz, P.A., Polinsky, M.L., Schag, C.A. & Heinrich, R.L. (1989) Rehabilitation of patients with primary breast cancer: Assessing the impact of adjuvant therapy. *Recent Results in Cancer Research,* **115**, 244–254.

Graydon, J.E. (1988) Factors that predict patients' functioning following treatment for cancer. *International Journal of Nursing Studies,* **25**, 117–124.

Hagopian, G.A. (1993) Cognitive strategies used in adapting to a cancer diagnosis. *Oncology Nursing Forum,* **20**, 759–763.

Hampson, S.E., Glasgow, R.E. & Foster, L.S. (1995) Personal models of diabetes among older patients: Relationship among self-management and other variables. *The Diabetes Educator,* **21**, 300–307.

Hampson, S.E., Glasgow, R.E. & Toobert, D.J. (1990) Personal models of diabetes and their relations to self-care activities. *Health Psychology,* **9**, 632–646.

Hampson, S.E., Glasgow, R.E. & Zeiss, A.M. (1994) Personal models of osteoarthritis and their relation to self-management activities and quality of life. *Journal of Behavioural Medicine,* **17**, 143–158.

Holland, J.C. & Lesko, L.M. (1990) Chemotherapy, endocrine therapy and immunotherapy. In J.C. Holland & J.H. Rowland (Eds.), *Handbook of psycho-oncology: Psychosocial care for the patient with cancer* (pp. 146–162). New York: Oxford University Press.

Isler, C. (1971). Radiation therapy 2: The nurse and the patient. *RN Magazine,* **34**, 48–51.

Johnson, J.E., Lauvier, D.R. & Nail, L.M. (1989) Process of coping with radiation therapy. *Journal of Personality and Social Psychology,* **57**, 358–364.

Katz, I., Hass, G., Parisi, N., Astone, J., McEvaddy, D. & Lucido, D.J. (1987) Lay people's and health care personnel's perceptions of cancer, AIDS, cardiac and diabetic patients. *Psychological Reports,* **60**, 615–629.

Kelsey, J.L. (1993) Breast cancer epidemiology: Summary and future directions. *Epidemiologic Reviews,* **15**, 256–263.

King, K.B., Naill, L.M. Kreamer, K., Strohl, R.D. & Johnson, J.E. (1985) Patients' descriptions of the experience of receiving radiation therapy. *Oncology Nursing Forum,* **12**, 55–61.

Knobf, M.T. (1986) Physical and psychologic distress associated with adjuvant chemotherapy in women with breast cancer. *Journal of Clinical Oncology*, **4**, 678–684.

Lagios, M.D., Westdahl, P.R., Margolin, F.R. & Rose, M.R. (1982) Duct carcinoma in situ: Relationship of extent of noninvasive disease to frequency of occult invasion, multicentricity, lymph-node metastases and short term treatment failures. *Cancer*, **50**, 1309–14.

Lau, R.R. & Hartman, K.A. (1983) Commonsense representations of common illness. *Health Psychology*, **2**, 167–185.

Lazarus, R.S. (1966) *Psychological stress and the coping process.* New York: McGraw Hill.

Leventhal, H. (1970) Findings and theory in the study of fear communications. In L. Berkowitz (Ed.), *Advances in experimental social psychology* (Vol. 5, pp. 119–186). New York: Academic.

Leventhal, H. & Diefenbach, M. (1991) The active side of illness cognitions. In J.A. Skelton & R.T. Croyle (Eds.), *Mental Representations in health and illness* (pp. 247–272). New York: Springer-Verlag.

Leventhal, H., Meyer, D. & Nerenz, D. (1980) The common sense representation of illness danger. In S. Rachman (Ed.), *Contributions to medical psychology* (Vol. 2, pp. 7–30). New York: Pergamon Press.

Leventhal, H., Nerenz, D. & Steele, D. (1984) Illness representations and coping with illness threats. In A. Baum & J. Singer (Eds.), *A handbook of psychology and health. Volume 4: Social psychological aspects of health* (pp. 219–252). New Jersey: Erlbaum.

Margolis, G.L. & Goodman, R.L. (1984) Psychological factors in women choosing radiation therapy for breast cancer. *Psychosomatics*, **25**, 464–469.

Markus, H., Smith, J. & Moreland, R.L. (1985) Role of self-concept in the perception of others. *Journal of Personality and Social Psychology*, **6**, 1494–1512.

Marris, P. (1974) *Loss and change.* New York: Random House.

Meyer, D., Leventhal, H. & Guttman, M. (1985) Commonsense models of illness; the example of hypertension. *Health Psychology*, **4**, 115–135.

Murray, M. (1990) Lay representations of illness. In P. Bennett, J. Weinman & P. Spurgeon (Eds.), *Current developments in health psychology*, (pp. 63–92). London: Harwood Academic.

Nerenz, D.R., Leventhal, H., Love, R.R. & Ringler, K.E. (1984) Psychological aspects of cancer chemotherapy. *International Review of Applied Psychology*, **33**, 521–529.

Neuling, S.J. & Winefield, H.R. (1988) Social support and recovery after surgery for breast cancer: Frequency and correlates of supportive behaviors by family, friends and surgeon. *Social Science and Medicine*, **27**, 385–392.

O'Connor, A.P., Wicker, C.A. & Germino, B.B. (1990) Understanding the patients' search for meaning. *Cancer Nursing*, **13**, 167–171.

Payne, S. (1990) Lay representations of breast cancer. *Psychology and Health*, **5**, 1–11.

Peck, A. (1972) Emotional reactions to having cancer. *American Journal of Roentgenology, Radium Therapy and Nuclear Medicine*, **114**, 591–599.

Peck, A. & Boland, J. (1977) Emotional reactions to radiation treatment. *Cancer*, **40**, 180–184.

Peters-Golden, H. (1982) Breast cancer: Varied perceptions of social support in the illness experience. *Social Science and Medicine*, **16**, 483–491.

Petrie, K.J., Buick, D.L., Weinman, J. & Booth, R. (1996) Positive effects of illness reported by Myocardial Infarction and Breast Cancer Patients. Manuscript submitted for publication.

Rainey, L.C. (1985) Effects of preparatory patient education for radiation oncology patients. *Cancer*, **39**, 744–750.

Rose, J.H. (1990) Social support and cancer: Adult patients' desire for support from family, friends and health professionals. *American Journal of Community Psychology*, **18**, 439–464.

Rotman, M., Rogow, L., DeLean, G. & Heskel, N. (1977) Supportive therapy in radiation oncology. *Cancer*, **39**, 744–750.

Sinsheimer, L.M. & Holland, J.C. (1987) Psychological issues in breast cancer. *Seminars in Oncology*, **14**, 75–82.

Skelton, J.A. & Croyle, R.T. (1991) Mental representation, health and illness: An introduction. In J.A. Skelton & R.T. Croyle (Eds.), *Mental representations in health and illness* (pp. 1–9). New York: Springer-Verlag.

Smith, L.L. & McNamara, J.J. (1977) Social work services for radiation therapy patients and their families. *Hospital and Community Psychiatry*, **28**, 752–754.

Spicer, D.V. & Pike, M.C. (1994) Epidemiology of breast cancer. In R.A. Lobo (Ed.), *Treatment of post-menopausal women: Basic and clinical aspects* (pp. 315–324). New York: Raven Press.

Taylor, S.E. (1983) Adjustment to threatening events: A theory of cognitive adaptation. *American Psychologist*, **38**, 1161–1173.

Taylor, S.E., Lichtman, R.R. & Wood, J.V. (1984a) Compliance with chemotherapy among breast cancer patients. *Journal of Personality and Social Psychology*, **3**, 553–562.

Taylor, S.E., Lichtman, R.R. & Wood, J.V. (1984b) Attributions, beliefs about control and breast cancer patients. *Health Psychology*, **46**, 489–502.

Temoshok, L. & Dreher, H. (1992) *The Type C connection: The behavioral links to cancer and your health.* New York: Random House.

Temoshok, L., Heller, B.W., Sagebeil, R.W., Blois, M.S., Sweet, D.S., DiClemente, R.J. & Gold, M.L. (1985) The relationship of psychosocial factors to prognostic indicators in cutaneous malignant melanoma. *Journal of Psychosomatic Research*, **29**, 139–153.

Thompson, S. & Janigan, A. (1988) Life schemes: a framework for understanding the search for meaning. *Journal of Social and Clinical Psychology*, **7**, 260–268.

Timko, C & Janoff-Bulman, R. (1985) Attribution, vulnerability and psychological adjustment: the case of breast cancer. *Health Psychology*, **4**, 521–544.

Vecchia, C.L., Decarli, A. & Parazzini, F. (1987) General epidemiology of breast cancer on northern Italy. *International Journal of Epidemiology*, **16**, 347–355.

Weinman, J., Petrie, K.J., Moss-Morris, R. & Horne, R. (1996) The Illness Perception Questionnaire: A new method for assessing the cognitive representation of illness. *Psychology and Health*, **11**, 431–445.

Welch, D.A. (1980) Assessment of nausea and vomiting in cancer patients undergoing external beam radiotherapy. *Cancer Nursing*, **3**, 365–371.

Yonke, G. (1967) Emotional responses to radiotherapy. *Hospital Topics*, **2**, 107–108.

14

The Role of Illness Cognitions and Coping in the Aetiology and Maintenance of the Chronic Fatigue Syndrome (CFS)

Rona Moss-Morris*

Over the past decade, a debilitating chronic illness characterised by unremitting or relapsing fatigue has been a subject of intense debate. Early reports in the 1980's labelled the illness "yuppie flu", regarding the malady as a psychosomatic reaction to the stressors of modern society (Polca, 1991). Sufferers of the illness and their advocates strongly opposed these aspersions, insisting that the cause of the illness was organic. Since 1980 a series of names for the condition have been advanced, such as chronic mononucleosis, postviral fatigue syndrome and myalgic encephalomyelitis (ME), reflecting assumptions about the possible organic nature of the illness (Steincamp, 1988). In response to the nomenclature controversy and in an attempt to define a homogeneous group of patients for research purposes, the Centre for Disease Control in Atlanta renamed the condition chronic fatigue syndrome (CFS) and published the first standardised diagnostic criteria for the illness (Holmes

---

*Preparation of this chapter was supported by a grant from the New Zealand Health Research Council.

et al., 1988). Despite this attempt at standardisation, research to date has been unable to establish a definitive aetiology and treatment for CFS. Empirical findings have been diverse and studies have found support for the role of both psychological and organic factors in the illness. To make sense of these disparate findings, cognitive behavioural models of CFS have been proposed which provide multi-causal, interactive explanations of the illness (Surawy *et al.*, 1995; Wessely *et al.*, 1991). Key factors in these models are patients' illness perceptions and coping responses, which are seen to have an important role in both the onset and perpetuation of the condition. CFS patients who participate in treatment programmes based on these paradigms report substantial reductions in their levels of fatigue and disability (Butler *et al.*, 1991; Deale *et al.*, in submission; Sharpe *et al.*, 1996). As no other form of treatment has been able to demonstrate such positive effects, it does indeed appear that cognitive behavioural factors are important in CFS.

This chapter provides a comprehensive review of the theoretical and empirical literature on illness perceptions and coping in CFS. Brief summaries of the presenting features of the illness and the aetiological debate surrounding the disorder are provided as background to the review. Current cognitive behavioural theories of CFS and the central role that illness and symptom beliefs play within these frameworks are outlined. This is followed by a review of the empirical literature on the role of symptom interpretation, illness representations, coping and cognitive distortions in both the onset and maintenance of CFS. Finally, based on this empirical evidence, suggestions are made for treatment and future research.

CHRONIC FATIGUE SYNDROME (CFS)

There are no clear pathological markers for CFS. As such, diagnosis relies on descriptive phenomenology and a range of definitions have been proposed over the last few years (Holmes *et al.*, 1988; Lloyd *et al.*, 1988; Sharpe *et al.*, 1991). In an attempt to standardise the CFS diagnosis across countries, a group of international researchers published a new consensus definition (Fukuda *et al.*, 1994). They specified that in addition to being present for at least six months, the fatigue must have a definite onset, cause substantial disruption to the individual's day-to-day activities and should not be caused by continual exertion. At least four additional key symptoms, such as muscle and joint pain, headaches, unrefreshing sleep and neuropsychological difficulties need to be reported. Medical conditions that may explain the presence of chronic fatigue, psychiatric illnesses with psychotic features and recent substance abuse problems preclude a diagnosis of CFS.

Prevalence rates of CFS have varied according to the diagnostic criteria used. The most recent statistics suggest that while 18.3% of the general population report chronic fatigue, only 1% meet central criteria for CFS and an even fewer 0.2% attribute their excessive tiredness to the CFS (Pawlikowska *et al.*, 1994). Well-educated, middle aged white women are traditionally reported as being over-represented in CFS samples (e.g. Manu, Lane & Mathews, 1993; Ramsay & Dowsett, 1992). However, community based and primary care studies have found that this over-representation reflects a gender and socioeconomic diagnostic and help-seeking bias, rather than an illness bias (Euba *et al.*, 1995; Lloyd *et al.*, 1990).

Although CFS has become an increasingly recognised diagnosis over the last decade, debate still rages over the organic versus psychological nature of the illness. Initially, those who favoured CFS as an organic disease focused their attention on CFS as a viral disorder. Despite a number of different viruses being investigated, no consistent relationship has been found between viruses and CFS (see Mawle, Reyes & Scott Schmid, 1994 for review). Further, a prospective primary care study was unable to find any evidence that viral infections predict the onset of CFS (Wessely *et al.*, 1995), although one study has found a link between glandular fever and a post viral fatigue syndrome (White *et al.*, 1995). Biological research has had greater success investigating neuroendocrine, neurobiological and immune aspects of CFS (see Bearn & Wessely, 1994 for review). Regional brain deficits, changes in neurotransmitter function and immune activation have all been reported in this population.

Nonetheless, the increasing evidence for a neurobiological basis to CFS does not necessarily confirm that it is an organic disorder. Neurobiological changes are frequently found in a number of psychiatric disorders and immune dysfunction can be related to stress (Bearn & Wessely, 1994). Premorbid psychological distress is a strong risk factor for developing chronic postviral fatigue (Wessely *et al.*, 1995) and psychiatric disorders are common in CFS patients. A number of studies have shown that they have a significantly higher frequency of depression, anxiety and somatisation disorder when compared to both the general population and medically ill patients, with up to 75% of CFS patients meeting criteria for a concurrent psychiatric disorder (e.g. Manu *et al.*, 1993; Wessely & Powell, 1989; Wood *et al.*, 1991). Some researchers have interpreted these findings to mean that CFS is a psychiatric disorder which presents in a predominantly somatic fashion (Lane, Manu & Mathews, 1991; Manu *et al.*, 1993). Others suggest that concurrent psychiatric disorder could reflect a common biological marker, an overlap in symptoms, or an understandable reaction to an often unacknowledged, disabling illness (Abbey & Garfinkel, 1991; Ray, 1991). Therefore, it would be problematic and most likely inaccurate to place CFS in a purely functional framework. Rather, the evidence to date suggests that explanations of CFS need to incorporate a broad range of factors and be flexible enough to include the possibility that a number of aetiological pathways may exist. Recent cognitive behavioural approaches to the disorder incorporate both organic and psychological features of the illness in explaining how the illness might develop and be maintained over time.

Cognitive Behavioural Models of CFS

Wessely *et al.* (1991) proposed the formative cognitive behavioural model of CFS. They suggested that an organic insult such as a virus precipitates a cycle of psychological responses, which mediate between the acute organic illness and the chronic syndrome. In other words, while organic factors precipitate the illness, cognitive behavioural factors perpetuate the condition. Wessely *et al.* (1991) explain that when resuming normal activity levels following a viral infection, it is common to experience symptoms of physical deconditioning. If people attribute these symptoms to signs of ongoing disease rather than deconditioning, they will tend to resort to rest and inactivity in an attempt to "cure" the symptoms. A cycle of avoidance and symptom experience develops, which can lead to loss of control, demoralisation and possible depression and anxiety. These psychological states can further perpetuate the illness through generating more physical symptoms.

Surawy *et al.* (1995) expanded this earlier formulation to include an explanation of predisposing factors. They suggest that predisposed people are highly achievement orientated and base their self-esteem and the respect from others on their ability to live up to certain high standards. When such people are faced with precipitating factors which affect their ability to perform, such as a combination of excessive stress and an acute illness, their initial reaction is to press on and keep coping. This behaviour leads to exhaustion. In making sense of the situation a physical attribution for the exhaustion is made, which protects their self-esteem by avoiding the suggestion that their inability to cope is a sign of personal weakness. Physical attributions result in people focusing on the somatic rather than emotional aspects of their illness. Symptoms which could be physiological concomitants of chronic psychological distress or inactivity such as fatigue, poor concentration and muscle pain, are interpreted as signs of an ongoing disease. This somatic interpretive bias leads to a perpetuating cycle of avoidance of activity in an attempt to reduce symptoms. However, reduced activity conflicts with achievement orientation and may result in bursts of activity in an attempt to meet expectations. These periodic bursts of activity inevitably exacerbate symptoms and result in failure, which further reinforces the belief that they have a serious illness. As time goes by, efforts to meet previous standards of achievement are abandoned and patients become increasingly preoccupied with their symptoms and illness. This results in chronic disability and the belief that one has an ongoing incurable illness.

These models account for the high incidence of psychiatric disorder in CFS without ruling out organic factors in the illness. However, neither psychiatric disorder nor viral illness by themselves are sufficient conditions for the development of CFS. Rather, the necessary factor is the patient's bias for attributing symptoms to disease rather than other factors. Similar to Leventhal's self-regulatory model of illness representations (Leventhal, Nerenz & Steele, 1984), these illness beliefs are seen to direct ways of coping, such as avoiding activity, which in turn influences outcome or disability. In fact, cognitive behavioural models of CFS suggest that illness representations play an even more critical role in this disorder than in other medical conditions, in that they not only determine outcome, but also contribute to the onset of the condition. Additional support for this view comes from studies which have used cognitive behavioural therapy (CBT) with CFS patients.

Cognitive Behavioural Therapy for CFS

Five CBT trials with CFS patients have been completed. Of these, two reported that CBT was no more effective than standard medical care, immunological treatment (Lloyd, Hickie & Wakefield, 1993) or no treatment (Friedberg & Krupp, 1994), while three others found that CBT was significantly more effective than relaxation therapy (Deale *et al.*, in submission), standard medical care (Sharpe *et al.*, 1996) and no treatment (Butler *et al.*,1991). The conflicting results most likely reflect the different approaches used in the individual trials. The successful trials could be distinguished from the non-successful ones in that they were based on the models of CFS summarised above and combined a gradual return to activity with gentle challenging of patients' existing illness beliefs. Patients were presented with the idea that precipitating and perpetuating factors of their illness might be different. They were taught that symptoms do not necessarily signal ongoing disease and that avoiding activity to reduce symptoms causes further symptoms. Activity levels and rest times were monitored according to predetermined goals set by the patients, rather than on how well or badly they were feeling at the time. Sharpe *et al.*'s (1996) study measured patients' illness perpetuating beliefs and avoidance of activity before and after treatment. These variables were substantially reduced following CBT, suggesting that altering illness beliefs and increasing activity were important treatment mechanisms.

CFS patients in these successful CBT trials reported substantial and continued improvement in their general functioning, levels of fatigue and depression up to a year post-treatment, although few reported complete resolution of symptoms (Butler *et al.*, 1991; Deale *et al.*, in submission; Sharpe *et al.*, 1996). A four year follow-up of the first successful CBT trial showed that patients who initially responded to treatment sustained their level of functional improvement, while those who initially refused or did not benefit from treatment were still substantially disabled by their CFS (Bonner *et al.*, 1994).

One of the unsuccessful CBT trials also included graded activity as part of the treatment, but failed to address illness or symptom beliefs (Lloyd *et al.*, 1993). In fact, as they combined their CBT trial with an immunological trial, the concurrent administration of immunoglobin injections may even have confirmed patients' beliefs about the essentially physical nature of the illness (Sharpe, 1995). It has also been suggested that the number of CBT sessions included in this trial were too few to bring about significant change (Chalder, Deale & Wessely, 1995; Sharpe, 1995). The rationale behind Friedberg and Krupp's (1994) CBT trial was distinctly different from the successful trials. Rather than challenging existing illness beliefs and increasing activity, patients were encouraged to accept their symptoms, to tolerate illness limitations and to restructure their lifestyle in keeping with the confines imposed by the illness. Although this programme had some effect on depressive symptoms, there were no significant changes in stress symptoms or fatigue severity. Overall it appears that for CBT to be effective, beliefs about the illness must be addressed.

Despite positive findings, CBT to date has largely been based on theoretical frameworks drawn from clinical observation and the underlying mechanisms involved have not been empirically confirmed. While the successful trials have shown substantial improvements, few patients report a complete recovery and a small percentage do not improve. Empirical confirmation of how cognitive and behavioural factors contribute to CFS should provide more definite guidelines for future CBT programmes.

THE SELF-REGULATORY MODEL OF ILLNESS REPRESENTATIONS APPLIED TO CFS

Over the last few years we have conducted a series of studies using the self-regulatory model of illness representations (Leventhal, *et al.* 1984) to guide our empirical investigation of cognitive and behavioural factors in CFS. This work has focused on gaining a clearer picture of the nature of CFS patients' illness representations and how these representations influence both coping and outcome. Before discussing the findings on patients' misperceptions of their illness as a whole, I have summarised the results from a body of research on symptom misrepresentations in CFS. The representation of symptoms is key to the self-regulatory model, which suggests that the experience of symptoms and subsequent interpretation of these symptoms form the illness identity around which other illness beliefs develop. When people experience symptoms they will attempt to label them. Conversely, people who have an illness label will search for symptom information consistent with this label. A wide range of diverse symptoms are integral to the label of CFS, which make people exceptionally vulnerable to interpreting bodily sensations, emotional and neuropsychological responses as part of their illness.

Subjective Symptom Reports Versus Objective Measurements

Research aimed at objectifying CFS patients' symptoms, inadvertently perhaps, provided the initial insight that cognitive factors were contributing to patients' experience of symptoms. A primary complaint of CFS sufferers is muscle fatigue and physical exhaustion. Physiological studies, however, have found that these subjective complaints bear little relationship to objective laboratory tests of muscle strength or cardiovascular response (Lloyd, Hales & Gandevia, 1988; McCluskey & Riley, 1992). Muscle abnormalities were consistent with deconditioning rather than pathology. CFS patients' perceptions of their peak exercise workload were significantly greater than those of healthy controls and other medical patients, although objective measures showed no differences in heart rate responses and respiratory exchange ratios between the groups.

At least 18 studies have investigated another key CFS complaint, neuropsychological symptoms. A recent review of this research found that whereas there was some evidence of mild neuropsychological impairment, the most consistent finding was that there was no relationship between objective performance on standardised tests and subjective reports of cognitive difficulty (Moss-Morris *et al.*, 1996). Subjective reports were, however, consistently correlated with higher levels of psychopathology and somatic complaints. CFS patients also reported higher levels of mental fatigue in response to the testing situation than both healthy and psychiatric controls. This was in contrast to their objective performance which appeared to be unaffected by up to three hours of testing.

In general, CFS patients' experience of physical exertion, cognitive difficulty and both mental and muscle fatigue, appears to be more convincingly related to disturbances in subjective perceptions than actual abnormalities. The factors causing these misperceptions still need to be explored. One possibility, consistent with cognitive behavioural formulations of the illness, is that CFS patients have an attention bias for somatic related information and a tendency to misinterpret normal bodily sensations and cognitive failures as signs of disease. The following section demonstrates that CFS patients have a particularly negative view of their illness. This negative illness schema may encourage priority processing of symptom relevant information, leading to the misperception of the significance of these symptoms.

The Nature of the Illness Representation

We have used the Illness Perception Questionnaire (IPQ, Weinman *et al.*, 1996) to ascertain if CFS patients have characteristic cognitive representations of their illness. Consistently high scores on the identity, consequences and time-line scales, suggests that CFS patients believe their illness has a wide range of symptoms, a profound impact on their lives and is likely to last a long time (Moss-Morris, Petrie & Weinman, 1996; Moss-Morris & Petrie, 1996a).

These negative illness beliefs do not appear to be just a consequence of having a chronic physical illness. When compared to patients with rheumatoid arthritis, diabetes and chronic back pain on the IPQ, CFS patients had significantly higher illness identity and consequences scores (Weinman *et al.*, 1996). The CFS group were also more likely to attribute their illness to a virus or pollution and significantly less likely to attribute the illness to their own behaviour.

In a recent study we compared illness beliefs in CFS and depressed patients (Moss-Morris & Petrie, 1996a). The similarities between these two conditions and the fact that depressed patients are known to evaluate events in an overly negative fashion (e.g. Beck, Rush, Shaw & Emery, 1979), made it particularly interesting to ascertain whether CFS patients' negative views of their illness could distinguish them from depressed patients. This study comprised a total of 53 patients meeting research criteria for CFS (Fukuda *et al.*, 1994), 14 of whom also had a current DSM-III-R diagnosis of depression. Twenty patients with a current primary DSM-III-R diagnosis of either major depression or dysthymia were included as a comparison group. The groups were matched in aggregate for age, education and gender.

The IPQ was adapted to be relevant to both CFS and depressed patients. The 12 item illness identity scale was lengthened to 28 symptoms, which included core symptoms of both depression

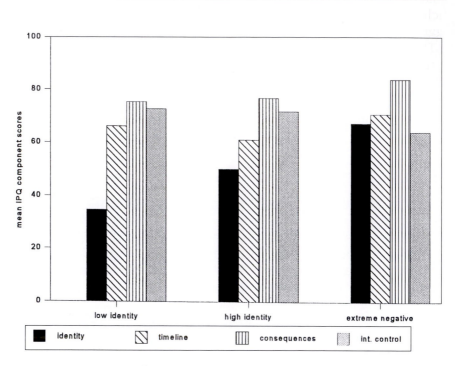

FIGURE 1   Illness Perception Questionnaire (IPQ) clusters

and CFS. The causal items were dropped from the questionnaire and a separate 19 item attributional scale was used. We also decided to analyse the IPQ data in a different way. Previously we had compared groups on individual dimensions of the illness representation. However, illness representations are conceptualised as schemata containing groups of beliefs. As such, we performed a cluster analysis on the IPQ data to investigate how varying ratings on the individual subscales clustered together. Figure 1 shows the three distinct clusters of beliefs which emerged from this analysis. The first two clusters could only be distinguished by the second having a higher illness identity score, while the third represented the most negative beliefs, with the highest mean scores on the identity, time-line and consequences scales and the lowest score on internal control/curability.

At the second stage of the analysis we looked at how the patient groups were distributed across the IPQ clusters. Figure 2 shows the primary depressed patients fell evenly into the first two clusters, with none of them falling into the extreme negative cluster. Very

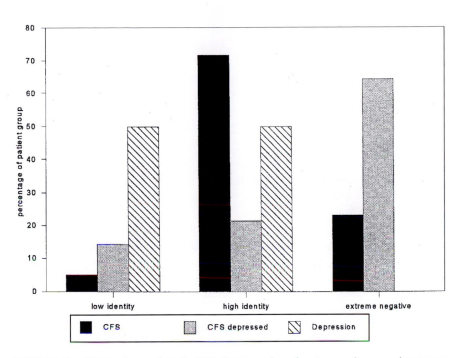

FIGURE 2 Comparison of CFS, CFS depressed and primary depressed groups across IPQ clusters

few CFS and CFS depressed patients fell into the low identity cluster. The CFS group were largely represented in the high identity cluster, whereas the majority of the CFS depressed patients fell into the extreme negative cluster. Overall, primary depressed patients appear to view their illness in a less negative fashion than CFS patients, with CFS depressed patients having the most negative view of their illness. The extent to which patients attribute symptoms to their CFS seems to be particularly notable. The mean number of symptoms endorsed by the CFS group on the 28 item identity scale was 25.2. They were no less likely to endorse psychological symptoms as part of their illness than depressed patients, but significantly more likely to endorse the physical symptoms.

Although they see psychological symptoms as part of their illness, CFS patients do not generally believe these symptoms are caused by psychological factors. We also asked patients in this study to assign a percentage to which they considered 19 different causes contributed to their illness (Moss-Morris & Petrie, 1996a).

Beliefs about cause clearly differentiated between the two groups (see Figure 3). On average, the CFS group attributed 70% of their illness to physical causes, compared to 15% in the depressed group. The most popular physical attribution for the CFS group was a virus, followed by alternative factors such as pollution and candida. Recent stressful events and overwork were the most endorsed psychosocial factors. The depressed group most strongly endorsed recent stressful events, followed by self attributions, such as my "mental attitude" or "emotional state". Interviews with CFS patients have frequently revealed an interactive model of causal factors where stress is seen as causing immune system depletion which results in viral infection (Ware, 1993). However, it is clear from our results that the psychological factors are perceived to play a much less significant role in causing the illness.

Drawing from attributional theories of depression (Abramson, Seligman & Teasdale, 1978) we also asked patients to rate the major cause of their illness on four dimensions; locus (how much the

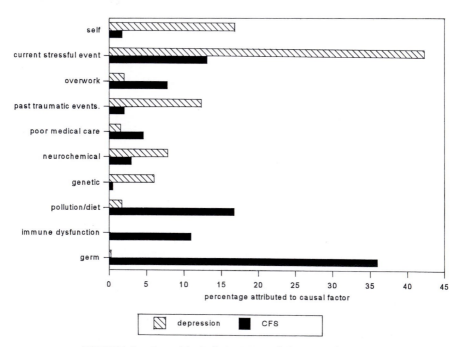

FIGURE 3   Causal beliefs in CFS and depressed groups

cause relates to something about themselves), global (how much the cause influences other areas of their lives), stable (how likely the cause is to be ongoing), and control (how controllable is the cause). Depressed patients characteristically make internal, stable, global and uncontrollable attributions for negative events (see Sweeney, Anderson & Bailey, 1986 for review). Such attributions appear to lead to feelings of personal failure and helplessness. Previous research has concluded that the major differentiating factor between CFS and depressed patients is external versus internal attributions for their illness (Powell, Dolan & Wessely, 1990). These authors suggested that an external attributional style protected CFS patients' self esteem, but possibly promoted a sense of helplessness and lack of responsibility for health. External attributions that are seen to be ongoing, uncontrollable and to affect a number of aspects of one's life would be particularly detrimental to feeling helpless in the face of one's illness.

As with the IPQ data, we performed a cluster analysis on the four attributional dimensions. Three clusters emerged. Figure 4 shows the first two were characterised by low scores on the locus dimension, representing beliefs that the cause was due to external circumstances. These two clusters differed, however, on the other three dimensions. The first cluster reflected beliefs that the cause was also global, stable and uncontrollable, while the second reflected that the cause was unstable, specific and controllable. The final cluster represented the typical depressive attributional style; internal, stable, global and uncontrollable. The majority of the depressed group fell within this final cluster, while almost 80% of the CFS groups fell within the two external clusters (see Figure 5). CFS depressed patients were over-represented in the external, stable, global cluster. The locus dimension appears to be the major distinguishing attributional feature between CFS and primary depression. The stable, global and uncontrollable dimensions appear to be largely a feature of both depressed groups.

Not only are illness representations distinct in CFS, but they remain remarkably stable over time. The six month test-retest correlations for illness identity, consequences and control/cure were all greater than .70, while time-line had a significant correlation of .54 (Moss-Morris & Petrie, 1996b). These correlations were substantially higher than those obtained from a myocardial infarction group at 3 and 6 months follow-up (Weinman *et al.*, 1996).

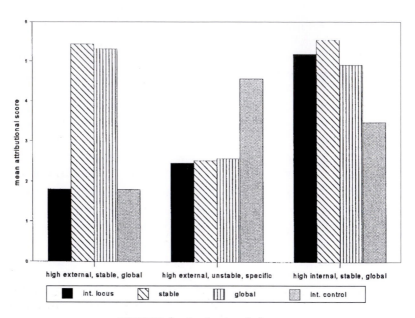

FIGURE 4 Attributional clusters

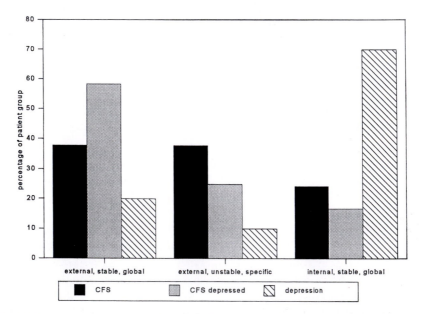

FIGURE 5 Comparison of CFS, CFS depressed and primary depressed groups across attributional clusters

In summary, CFS patients appear to have very definite unchanging views about their illness. Their illness representation is characterised by an illness identity incorporating a broad range of symptoms. Attributions about the illness are typically external and physical, and beliefs about the chronicity and consequences of the illness are generally negative. Comparisons with other medical and psychiatric chronic illness groups reveal that these negative beliefs and lack of personal responsibility for their illness are not solely a consequence of having a chronic disabling condition. CFS patients with concurrent depression have the most pessimistic illness beliefs and make more helpless illness attributions.

Illness Representations and Adjustment to CFS

If illness representations play a role in maintaining CFS, it is critical that they demonstrate a relationship with disability in this disorder. Analysis of both clusters of the IPQ and individual dimensions suggests that this is indeed the case. Perhaps of particular importance for the concept of illness representations, was the finding that although there were no differences in both the self-reported disability or sickness related unemployment between depressed and CFS patients, there were differences between the three IPQ clusters presented in Figure 2 (Moss-Morris & Petrie, 1996a). The extreme negative beliefs cluster had significantly higher self-reported disability scores than both the other two clusters. In addition, 78% of patients in this cluster were unemployed due to sickness, compared to 52% in the high illness identity cluster and only 15% in the low identity cluster. Illness representations appear to be a better predictor of disability than nosological grouping. Regression analyses indicated that illness identity and serious consequences were the main predictors of concurrent disability and also predicted both self reported disability and sickness related unemployment six months later (Moss-Morris *et al.*, 1996; Moss-Morris & Petrie, 1996b).

Whereas physical attributions are clearly distinguishing features of the illness, we have been unable to demonstrate a relationship between specific causal beliefs and disability. In two separate studies we have measured a range of specific illness attributions, the number of attributions made, the ratio of physical to psychological attributions and the degree to which CFS patients rated the cause of their illness as external, stable, global and uncontrollable (Moss-Morris *et al.*, 1996; Moss-Morris & Petrie, 1996b). None of these measures was positively associated with disability. Also to our surprise and contrary to Powell *et al.*'s (1990) prediction that external attributions protected self esteem, we were unable to find a relationship between causal attributions and self esteem measured by Rosenberg's (1965) self esteem scale. However, when comparing the attributional clusters derived from the CFS and depressed samples (see Figure 4) on outcome measures, the internal cluster had significantly higher distress and depression scores. Investigation of the cluster differences on individual items of the Beck Depression Scale (1978), revealed that most of the variance was accounted for by items that measured feelings of sadness, guilt, failure and personal weakness, providing some support for the protective role of external attributions. We also found that within a CFS sample, patients' emotional attributions such as stress were negatively associated with psychological well-being, but positively associated with vitality (Moss-Morris *et al.*, 1996). As such, emotional attributions while associated with the affective components of distress, may protect against the physical manifestations.

Findings from other studies suggest that labelling of symptoms may be a more important predictor of the onset of CFS and ongoing disability than specific causal attributions. Although one longitudinal study did find that viral attributions were related to disability over a two year period (Sharpe *et al.*, 1992), consistent with our results, two prospective primary care studies found no relationship between specific viral attributions and the development of CFS (Cope *et al.*, 1994; Wessely *et al.*, 1995). However, Cope *et al.* (1994) found that a preference for attributing common symptoms to physical factors, rather than to psychological or environmental factors, was the most important risk factor for developing CFS after a viral infection. Wilson *et al.* (1994) reported that the more firmly a large cohort of CFS sufferers attributed their symptoms to a disease process, the more likely they were to remain functionally impaired three years later. Interestingly, both these studies measured immune dysfunction in conjunction with these cognitive variables and concluded that immunological variables predicted neither the onset nor ongoing disability in CFS.

Results from cross-sectional, longitudinal and prospective studies have therefore confirmed that illness and symptom beliefs contribute to both the onset and perpetuation of CFS. The relationship between illness beliefs and disability is largely accounted for by illness identity, serious consequences and a bias for interpreting symptoms as physical in nature. The specific causal beliefs held by CFS patients appear to be less important in relation to disability, but attributing the illness to external factors may protect against feelings of depression and failure.

Illness Representations, Coping and Adjustment

The previous section has discussed the effects that illness representations have on determining outcome and disability in CFS. Drawing from Leventhal *et al.*'s (1984) self-regulatory model, we would also expect illness representations to guide the way in which patients cope with their illness. Certainly, CFS patients' illness beliefs appear to be related to coping in a logical fashion. Illness identity, serious consequences and time-line were positively associated with disengagement strategies, venting emotions and focusing on symptoms, but negatively associated with limiting coping strategies such as reducing stress and exercise (Moss-Morris *et al.*, 1996; Moss-Morris & Petrie, 1996b). Disengagement strategies such as avoiding thinking about or dealing with the problem and coping by venting emotions are consistently related to poor adaptation to chronic illnesses (Petrie & Moss-Morris, in press). As such, more negative illness beliefs appear to be related to the maladaptive coping strategies. On the other hand, patients who believed they had some control over the illness were less likely to use disengagement strategies and more likely to use strategies such as positively reinterpreting the situation, actively trying to deal with the illness and limiting activity and stress. One way CFS patients feel in control of their illness is by limiting activity. In fact, most patients believe that rest and reduced activity is helpful in controlling symptoms, while maintaining activity is unhelpful (Ray, Jefferies & Weir, 1995). These beliefs are reflected in patients' choice of coping strategies. Patients who believed that resting was helpful were more likely to accommodate to the illness by limiting activity and stress (Ray *et al.*, 1995). Therefore, in understanding the choice of coping strategies, one has to take into account both illness beliefs and patients' expectations of what is likely to be helpful in dealing with the illness.

Also in support of the self-regulatory model are studies which have found that coping strategies influence adaptation to CFS

(Antoni *et al.*, 1994; Moss-Morris *et al.*, 1996; Ray *et al.*, 1993; Ray *et al.*, 1995; Sharpe *et al.*, 1992). Disengagement strategies and focusing on symptoms have shown consistent relationships to both disability and psychological distress, while maintaining activity, distracting from symptoms and seeking emotional support have been negatively associated with functional impairment (Antoni *et al.*, 1994; Moss-Morris *et al.*, 1996; Ray *et al.*, 1993; 1995). Limiting activity and stress has a particularly interesting relationship to adjustment in CFS. Both longitudinal and cross-sectional results have shown that limiting strategies result in higher levels of dysfunction (Moss-Morris & Petrie, 1996b; Ray *et al.*, 1993; 1995; Sharpe *et al.*, 1992). Work seems to be particularly affected. Limiting strategies predicted fewer working hours per week, a decreased likelihood of increasing work hours and higher levels of self reported disruption to work six months later (Moss-Morris & Petrie, 1996b). In contrast, these same strategies were strongly related to feelings of positive well-being. At first glance these findings appear contradictory: surely a decreased capacity to work and participate in day-to-day activities would lead to feelings of demoralisation and distress? However, as discussed above, limiting strategies were negatively associated with pessimistic illness beliefs and positively related to internal control. Limiting strategies may provide CFS patients with a sense of control over the illness and a feeling that they are actively doing something to deal with the problem. Decreasing activity and stress levels could also help to temper symptoms and reduce the distress of illness unpredictability (Ray *et al.*, 1995). Further, believing they need to accommodate to the illness may provide people with a legitimate reason to remove themselves from situations they had previously found stressful.

Two of the coping strategies which have been consistently linked to disability also seem to distinguish CFS patients from others. Blakely *et al.* (1991) compared coping in CFS patients, chronic pain patients and healthy controls. The CFS group were significantly more likely than the others to use disengagement strategies in dealing with stressful situations. When compared to depressed patients in the way they coped with their illness, the major strategy to differentiate between the groups was limiting coping (Moss-Morris & Petrie, 1996a). Both CFS and CFS depressed patients used more limiting strategies than primary depressed patients, with the CFS non-depressed group scoring highest on this scale.

In general, the findings suggest that two disparate pathways of illness perceptions, coping and disability may exist. CFS patients who hold excessively negative beliefs tend to give up or withdraw from dealing with the illness. Rather than actively choosing to limit their activity, their negative illness beliefs and stable, external attributions may lead to feelings of helplessness and loss of control, resulting in a passive withdrawal from activity and heightened negative affect. Patients with excessively negative illness beliefs and external stable attributions are more likely to have concurrent depression, so it may be that negative affect contributes to both the formation of the negative illness schemata and the maintenance of the illness cycle. On the other side is the group of patients with less pessimistic illness beliefs, who nevertheless experience a number of symptoms which they strongly attribute to signs of a physical disease. These patients believe that rest is the effective way of dealing with their symptoms and as a result choose to limit their exposure to stress and activity. They feel more in control of their illness, are psychologically better adjusted to their condition, but are still unduly disabled.

COGNITIVE MODELS OF PSYCHOPATHOLOGY APPLIED TO CFS

Up until this point, I have focused on work which is directly relevant to the self-regulatory model of illness perceptions. This model is essentially a health psychology framework, developed to facilitate our understanding of how patients with medical conditions adjust to their illnesses. At the beginning of this chapter I made reference to the fact that CFS is difficult to understand within either a purely medical or psychiatric model. As such, it may also be useful to draw from cognitive models of psychopathology to facilitate our understanding of underlying mechanisms in CFS.

Ingram (1990) proposed a model of psychopathology which differentiated between three underlying cognitive mechanisms; schema, operations and products. In the case of depression, the central pathogenic schemata include a negative view of the self, the world and the future. Cognitive operations such as self focused attention and absorption, ensure that information consistent with these central schemata is given priority processing. Products of this processing system include distortions in thinking such as selective abstraction (focusing on the negative aspects of an experience), overgeneralising (assuming that the negative consequences of one experience applies to similar experiences in the future) and catastrophising (expecting the worst possible outcome to occur). In turn, these negative thoughts or distortions help to maintain the central schemata.

There is some evidence that catastrophic thinking and dysfunctional attitudes in CFS contribute to the experience of disability. In one study we asked CFS patients what they thought would be the consequence of pushing themselves beyond their present physical state (Petrie, Moss-Morris & Weinman, 1995). One third of the patients had highly exaggerated expectations, such as having a total collapse or even dying. People who had catastrophic expectations about their illness were significantly more disabled and fatigued than non-catastrophisers. Antoni *et al.* (1994) found that classic depressive cognitions such as distortions in thinking and negative self statements were related to disability in both CFS depressed and non depressed groups. However, as there was no primary depressed group in this study it is difficult to ascertain how unique these cognitions were to CFS patients. It is possible that these depressive cognitions would be related to disability in any group of chronically ill patients and thus are merely a reflection of the relationship between negative affect and disability.

Based on our earlier findings on illness representations in CFS, we hypothesised that whereas depressed patients' schema are dominated by negative self perceptions, CFS patients' view of themselves is dominated by perceptions of themselves as seriously ill people. These illness schema lead to somatic rather than self absorption, and to distortions in thinking specific to somatic rather than interpersonal events. To test these hypotheses we compared four groups; CFS patients with and without depression, primary depressed patients, and healthy controls who had no history of either depression or CFS, on measures of cognitive distortion, self focusing, self esteem and self rated health (Moss-Morris & Petrie, 1996a). Our measure of cognitive distortions was adapted from the Cognitive Error Questionnaire (CEQ, Lefebvre, 1981). We divided this questionnaire into two subscales; the Somatic CEQ which measured distortions specific to the experience of everyday symptoms, such as muscle aches and fatigue, and the General CEQ which measured distortion related to a range of everyday interpersonal events.

Table 1 Means and standard deviations of cognitive variable for CFS, CFS depressed, primary depressed and healthy control groups.

	CFS n = 39	CFS depressed n = 14	Primary depressed n = 20	Healthy controls n = 38
Somatic CEQ	28.33 (9.7)*	31.64 (6.4)*	32.72 (11.2)*	20.13 (5.8)
General CEQ	22.15 (8.9)	26.17 (7.9)	35.15 (11.9)*+	21.74 (6.6)
Self esteem	31.24 (4.7)	27.71 (5.3)*	24.86 (5.7)*#	33.11 (4.1)
Self focusing	31.02 (7.0)	33.77 (6.5)	35.97 (6.3)*#	31.48 (6.3)
Self rated health	4.05 (.79)*	4.00 (.96)*	3.15 (1.1)*+	1.76 (.68)

*significantly different from controls p < .0001
#significantly different from CFS patients p < .05
+significantly different from both CFS groups p < .0001

Both scales incorporated errors of catatrophising, selective abstraction and overgeneralisation.

Multivariate analysis controlling for demographic factors showed that the four groups were significantly different on all the cognitive measures (see Table 1). The results generally supported the hypotheses, with the depressed groups having lower self esteem and being more self focused, and the CFS groups rating themselves as least healthy. All three patient groups scored significantly higher on the Somatic CEQ when compared to healthy controls. However, there was no difference between both the CFS groups and healthy controls on the General CEQ, with the depressed group scoring significantly higher on this subscale than all three other groups. The depressed patients also had equivalent scores on both CEQ subscales, while the CFS groups had substantially higher scores on the Somatic subscale.

We also investigated the relationships between cognitive distortion and both illness perceptions and outcome in CFS (Moss-Morris & Petrie, 1996b). The Somatic CEQ was associated with the pessimistic illness beliefs, serious consequences and chronic time-line. As such, a negative illness schema may produce distortions in thinking such as viewing the outcome of symptoms as catastrophic, selectively attending to symptoms and expecting symptoms to reoccur in similar or related situations. In turn, these distortions in thinking may help to maintain the negative illness schema. The General CEQ was unrelated to these illness beliefs, but was highly correlated with self esteem, suggesting that cognitive distortions related to interpersonal events may be both generated by a negative self schema and help to preserve this negative self image.

The CEQ scores remained extremely stable over a six month period, but were only weakly able to predict outcome in CFS. Our cross-sectional data suggested that while the General CEQ was related to psychological distress, the Somatic CEQ was related to unemployment and physical disability, although these relationships were substantially weaker six months later. The weak main effects may be because somatic distortions impact on disability through interaction with negative illness beliefs. Regression equations showed that the interaction between serious consequences and the somatic CEQ measured at time one had a significant predictive effect on disability six months later.

The results from our studies based on models of psychopathology, provide further evidence that CFS and depression from a cognitive point of view, are distinct conditions. Neither depressed nor non-depressed CFS patients show the generalised distortions in thinking characteristic of depressed patients. Their errors in thinking are specific to somatic events. CFS patients, unless they are depressed, have good self esteem and are no more self focused than healthy controls.

Practical Implications and Conclusions

By empirically testing concepts from models of both health psychology and psychopathology, we have been able to demonstrate that CFS patients have unique underlying cognitions and coping styles which appear to contribute to their disability. CFS patients have a dominant view or schema of their illness comprised of a strong illness identity, external attributions for their condition and pessimistic beliefs about the consequences and time-line of their illness. Patients who develop chronic fatigue post-virally have demonstrated a propensity to label a wide range of everyday symptoms as physical in nature (Cope *et al.*, 1994). This propensity may contribute to the formation of CFS patients' illness schema, particularly their strong illness identity. Pessimistic illness beliefs are associated with a tendency to make negative inferences about the consequences of symptoms. This suggests that negative illness schema direct the processing of information and result in thought processes that help to maintain the negative illness beliefs. CFS patients also have characteristic ways of coping with their illness.

These include disengaging from dealing with the illness or actively limiting activity and stress.

The relationships identified between these illness cognitions, coping and disability provide some guidelines for interventions, many of which have already been incorporated within existing successful CBT programmes (Butler *et al.*, 1991; Sharpe *et al.*, 1996; Deale *et al.*, in submission). Perhaps one of the most important distinctions to bear in mind during treatment is between specific causal beliefs and symptom attributions. Although CFS patients usually hold definite views about the specific causes of their illness, these beliefs are generally unrelated to ongoing disability. As such, intervening to change existing causal beliefs appears unnecessary and could only serve to alienate patients and confirm that they are misunderstood. However, teaching patients to re-label and reinterpret their symptoms where appropriate, could be the key to both altering pessimistic illness beliefs and improving functioning and levels of fatigue. Current CBT programmes emphasize that symptoms experienced during the initial stages of resuming activity are signs of deconditioning rather than ongoing disease. In other words, patients are provided with an alternative explanation for their symptoms. Similarly, alternative explanations could also be found for some of the psychological and neuropsychological symptoms reported by CFS patients. For instance, being distressed can sometimes be a natural reaction to an external event rather than purely being related to the illness, while being unable to remember something simple can be a sign of stress or preoccupation with other issues. This re-labelling process also assists in altering somatic distortions, as reasonable rather than catastrophic explanations are given for symptoms. Combining this cognitive re-structuring with graded activity gives patients an opportunity to test out new beliefs in a controlled environment. Graded activity also provides an alternative to both limiting and disengagement coping strategies. Our data suggested that limiting activity gave patients a sense of control over their illness and a feeling of well-being. Carefully graded activity where patients are encouraged to set their own realistic goals ensures that a sense of internal control is maintained. For patients who tend to disengage from dealing with their illness, graded activity provides a concrete and non threatening way of coping. Finally, as concurrent depression in CFS is associated with the most extreme negative illness beliefs, helpless attributions and lower self esteem, where appropriate, treatment may also need to be geared towards dealing with the depression.

In conclusion, empirical work on illness perceptions and coping strategies provides convincing support for the cognitive behavioural models and treatment of CFS. However, research to date has relied exclusively on self-report instruments to measure cognitive constructs. This approach is vulnerable to response bias and the findings only reflect conscious cognitive processes and do not give a clear picture of the dynamic processes involved. There is now a wealth of laboratory studies which have investigated the information processing biases of patients with depression and anxiety (see Mathews & McCleod, 1994 for review). Similar designs adapted for CFS populations will provide a more accurate account of how underlying cognitions influence the processing of information in this group. Further, the relationship between cognitive and/or behavioural constructs and biological variables warrants further attention. Cognitive behavioural models of CFS emphasise the importance of the interactions between these factors. However, studies on CFS still tend to reflect the Cartesian duality of medicine, focusing either on psychological or biological measures.

REFERENCES

Abbey, S.E. & Garfinkel, P.E. (1991) Chronic fatigue syndrome and depression: Cause, effect, or covariate. *Reviews of Infectious Diseases*, **13**, Suppl 1, S73–S83.

Abramson, L.Y., Seligman, M.E.P. & Teasdale, J. (1978) Learned helplessness in humans: Critique and reformulation. *Journal of Abnormal Psychology*, **87**, 49–74.

Antoni, M.H., Brickman, A., Lutgendorf, S., Klimas, N., Imia-Fins, A., Ironson, G., Quillian, R., Jose Miguez, M., van Riel, F., Morgan, R., Patarca, R. & Fletcher, M.A. (1994) Psychosocial correlates of illness burden in chronic fatigue syndrome. *Clinical Infectious Diseases*, **18**, Suppl 2, S73–S78.

Bearn, J. & Wessely, S. (1994) Neurobiological aspects of the chronic fatigue syndrome. *European Journal of Clinical Investigation*, **24**, 79–90.

Beck, A.T. (1978) *Depression Inventory*. Center for Cognitive Therapy: Philadelphia.

Beck, A.T., Rush, A.J., Shaw, B.F. & Emery, G. (1979) *Cognitive therapy of depression.* New York: Guilford Press.

Blakely, A.A., Howard, R.C., Sosich, R.M., Murdoch, J.C., Menkes, D.B. & Spears, G.F.S. (1991) Psychiatric symptoms, personality and ways of coping in chronic fatigue syndrome. *Psychological Medicine*, **21**, 347–362.

Bonner, D., Ron, M., Chalder, T., Butler, S. & Wessely, S. (1994) Chronic fatigue syndrome: A follow up study. *Journal of Neurology, Neurosurgery and Psychiatry*, **57**, 617–621.

Butler, S., Chalder, T., Ron, M. & Wessely, S. (1991) Cognitive behaviour therapy in chronic fatigue syndrome. *Journal of Neurology, Neurosurgery and Psychiatry*, **54**, 153–158.

Chalder, T., Deale, A. & Wessely, S. (1995) Cognitive behavior therapy for chronic fatigue syndrome (letter to the editor). *The American Journal of Medicine*, **98**, 419–420.

Cope, H., David, A., Pelosi, A. & Mann, A. (1994) Predictors of chronic "postviral" fatigue. *Lancet*, **344**, 864–368.

Deale, A., Chalder, T., Marks, I. & Wessely, S. (in submission) Cognitive behavior therapy for chronic fatigue syndrome: A randomized controlled study.

Euba, R., Chalder, T., Deale, A. & Wessely, S. (1995) A comparison of the characteristics of chronic fatigue syndrome in primary and tertiary care. *British Journal of Psychiatry*, **167**, 1–6.

Friedberg, F. & Krupp, L.B. (1994) A comparison of cognitive behavioral treatment for chronic fatigue syndrome and primary depression. *Clinical Infectious Diseases*, **18**, Suppl 1, S105–S110.

Fukuda, K., Straus S.E., Hickie, I., Sharpe, M.C., Dobbins, J.G. & Komaroff, A. (1994). The chronic fatigue syndrome: A comprehensive approach to its definition and study. *Annals of Internal Medicine*, **121**, 953–959.

Holmes, G.P., Kaplan, J.E., Gantz, N.M., Komaroff, A.L., Schonberger, L.B., Straus, S.E., Jones, J.F., Dubois, R.E., Cunningham-Rundles, C., Pahwa, J., Tosato, G., Zegans, L.S., Purtilo, D.T., Brown, N., Schooley, R.T. & Brus, I. (1988) Chronic fatigue syndrome: A working case definition. *Annals of Internal Medicine*, **108**, 387–389.

Ingram, R.E. (1990) Self-focused attention in clinical disorders: Review and a conceptual model. *Psychological Bulletin*, **107**, 156–157.

Lane, T.J., Manu, P. & Mathews, D. (1991). Depression and somatiz-ation in the chronic fatigue syndrome. *The American Journal of Medicine*, **91**, 335–343.

Lefebvre, M.F. (1981). Cognitive distortion and cognitive errors in depressed psychiatric and low back pain patients. *Journal of Consulting and Clinical Psychology*, **49**, 517–525.

Leventhal, H., Nerenz, D.R. & Steele, D.S. (1984) Illness representa-tions and coping with health threats. In A. Baum & J.E. Singer (Eds.), *Handbook of psychology and health: Vol IV* (pp. 221–252). New York: Erlbaum.

Lloyd, A.R., Hales, J. & Gandevia, S.C. (1988) Muscle strength, endurance and recovery in the post-infection fatigue syndrome. *Journal of Neurology, Neurosurgery and Psychiatry*, **51**, 1316–1322.

Lloyd, A.R., Hickie, I., Boughton, B.R., Spencer, O. & Wakefield, D. (1990) Prevalence of chronic fatigue in an Australian popula-tion. *The Medical Journal of Australia*, **153**, 522–528.

Lloyd, A.R. Hickie, C. & Wakefield, D. (1993) Immunologic and psychologic therapy for patients with chronic fatigue syndrome: A double-blind, placebo-controlled trial. *The American Journal of Medicine*, **94**, 197–203.

Lloyd, A.R., Wakefield, D., Boughton, C. & Dwyer, J. (1988) What is myalgic encephalomyelitis. *Lancet*, **1**, 1286–1287.

Manu, P., Lane, T.J. & Mathews, D.A. (1993) Chronic fatigue and chronic fatigue syndrome: Clinical epidemiology and aetiologi-cal classification. *Ciba Foundation Symposium*, **173**, 23–42.

Mathews, A. & MacLeod, C. (1994) Cognitive approaches to emotion and emotional disorders. *Annual Review of Psychology*, **45**, 25–50.

Mawle, A.C. Reyes, M. & Scott Schmid, D.C. (1994) Is chronic fatigue syndrome an infectious disease? *Infectious Agents and Disease*, **2**, 333–341.

McCluskey, D. & Riley, M. (1992) Exercise testing in patients with chronic fatigue syndrome. In B.M. Hyde, J. Goldstein & P. Levine (Eds.), *The clinical and scientific basis of myalgic encephalomyelitis/chronic fatigue syndrome* (pp. 364–371). Ottawa: Nightingale Research Foundation.

Moss-Morris, R. & Petrie, K.J. (1996a) Discriminating between chronic fatigue syndrome and depression: A cognitive analysis.

Paper presented at the Fourth International Congress of Behavioral Medicine, Washington D.C., USA.

Moss-Morris, R. & Petrie, K.J. (1996b) Cognitive mechanisms in the maintenance of disability in chronic fatigue syndrome. Paper presented at the American Psychosomatic Society Annual Meeting, Williamsburg, USA.

Moss-Morris, R., Petrie, K.J., Large, R.G. & Kydd, R.R. (1996) Neuropsychological deficits in chronic fatigue syndrome: *Artifact or reality? Journal of Neurology, Neurosurgery & Psychiatry*, **60**, 00–00.

Moss-Morris, R., Petrie, K.J. & Weinman, J. (1996) Functioning in chronic fatigue syndrome: Do illness perceptions play a regulatory role? *British Journal of Health Psychology*, **1**, 15–25.

Pawlikowska, T., Chalder, T., Hirsch, S.R., Wallace, P., Wright, D.J.M. & Wessely, S.C. (1994) Population based study of fatigue and psychological distress. *British Medical Journal*, **308**, 763–308.

Petrie, K.J., Moss-Morris, R. & Weinman, J. (1995) Catastrophic beliefs and their implications in the chronic fatigue syndrome. *Journal of Psychosomatic Research*, **39**, 31–37.

Petrie, K.J. & Moss-Morris, R.E. (in press) Coping with chronic illness. In A. Baum, C. McManus, S. Newman, J. Weinman & R. West (Eds.). *Cambridge handbook of psychology, health and medicine*. Cambridge University Press.

Polca, J. (1991) On the track of an elusive disease. *Science*, **254**, 1726–1728.

Powell, R., Dolan, R. & Wessely, S. (1990) Attributions and self-esteem in depression and chronic fatigue syndromes. *Journal of Psychosomatic Research*, **34**, 665–673.

Ramsay, A.M. & Dowsett, B. (1992) Myalgic encephalomyelitis, then and now, an epidemiological introduction. In B.M. Hyde, J. Goldstein & P. Levine (Eds.), *The clinical and scientific basis of myalgic encephalomyelitis/chronic fatigue syndrome* (pp. 81–84). Ottawa: Nightingale Research Foundation.

Ray, C. (1991) Chronic fatigue syndrome and depression: Conceptual and methodological ambiguities. *Psychological Medicine*, **21**, 1–9.

Ray, C., Jefferies, S. & Weir, W.R.C. (1995) Coping and chronic fatigue syndrome: Illness responses and their relationship with fatigue, functional impairment and emotional status. *Psychological Medicine*, **25**, 937–945.

Ray, C., Weir, W.R.C., Stewart, D., Miller, P. & Hyde, G. (1993) Ways of coping with chronic fatigue syndrome: Development of an illness management questionnaire. *Social Science and Medicine*, **37**, 385–391.

Rosenberg, M. (1965) *Society and the adolescent self-image*. Princeton, NJ: Princeton University Press.

Sharpe, M. (1995) Cognitive behavior therapy for chronic fatigue syndrome (letter to the editor). *The American Journal of Medicine*, **98**, 420.

Sharpe, M.C., Archard, L.C., Bantavala, J.E., Borysiewicz, L.K., Clare, A.W., David, A., Edwards, R.H.T., Hawton, K.E.H., Lambert, H.P., Lane, R.J.M., McDonald, E.M., Mowbray, J.F., Pearson, D.J., Peto, T.E.A., Preedy, V.R., Smith, A.P., Smith, D.G., Taylor, D.J., Tyrell, D.A., Wessely, S. & White, P.D. (1991). A report — Chronic fatigue syndrome: guidelines for research. *Journal of the Royal Society of Medicine*, **84**, 118–121.

Sharpe, M., Hawton, K., Seagroatt, V. & Pasvol, G. (1992) Follow up of patients presenting with fatigue to an infectious diseases clinic. *British Medical Journal*, **305**, 147–152.

Sharpe, M., Hawton, K., Simkin, S., Surawy, C., Hackman, A., Klimes, I., Peto., T., Warrel., D. & Seagroatt, V. (1996) Cognitive behaviour therapy for chronic fatigue syndrome: A randomized controlled study. *British Medical Journal*, **312**, 22–26.

Steincamp, J. (1988) *Overload: Beating M.E.* New Zealand: Cape Catley Ltd.

Surawy, C., Hackmann, A., Hawton, K. & Sharpe, M. (1995) Chronic fatigue syndrome: A cognitive approach. *Behavior Research and Therapy*, **33**, 535–544.

Sweeney, P.D., Anderson, K. & Bailey, S. (1986) Attributional style in depression: A meta-analytic review. *Journal of Personality and Social Psychology*, **50**, 974–991.

Ware, N.C. (1993) Society, mind and body in chronic fatigue syndrome: An anthropological view. *Ciba Foundation Symposium*, **173**, 62–82.

Weinman, J. Petrie, K.J., Moss-Morris, R. & Horne, R. (1996) The Illness Perception Questionnaire: A new method for assessing the cognitive representations of illness. *Psychology and Health*, **11**, 431–445.

Wessely, S., Butler, S., Chalder, T. & David, A. (1991) The cognitive behavioural management of the post-viral fatigue syndrome. In R. Jenkins & J. Mowbrey (Eds.), *Postviral fatigue syndrome* (pp. 305–334). Chichester: John Wiley & Sons.

Wessely, S., Chalder, T., Hirsch, S.R., Pawlikowska, T., Wallace, P. & Wright, D.J.M. (1995) Postinfectious fatigue: Prospective cohort study in primary care. *The Lancet*, **345**, 1333–1338.

Wessely, S. & Powell, R. (1989) Fatigue syndromes: a comparison of chronic "postviral" fatigue with neuromuscular function. *Journal of Neurology, Neurosurgery and Psychiatry*, **52**, 940–948.

White, P.D., Grover, S.A., Kangro, H.O., Thomas, J.M., Amess, J. & Clare, A.W. (1995). The validity and reliability of the fatigue syndrome that follows glandular fever. *Psychological Medicine*, **25**, 917–924.

Wilson, A., Hickie, I., Lloyd, A., Hadzi-Pavlovic, D., Boughton, C., Dwyer, J. & Wakefield, D. (1994) Longitudinal study of outcome of chronic fatigue syndrome. *British Medical Journal*, **308**, 756–759.

Wood, G.C., Bentall, R.P., Göpfert, M. & Edwards. R.H.T. (1991) A comparative psychiatric assessment of patients with chronic fatigue syndrome and muscle disease. *Psychological Medicine*, **21**, 619–628.

15

Illness Representations and Recovery from Myocardial Infarction

Keith J. Petrie & John A. Weinman*

Diseases of the heart are a leading cause of death in many Western countries. Approximately 1.5 million Americans suffer a myocardial infarction (MI) each year and 500,000 of these are fatal. Costs of the condition in terms of direct medical care services and indirect costs through loss of earnings and social security or insurance payments are considerable (Ades, Huang & Weaver, 1992; Picard *et al.*, 1989). Advances in medical technology and treatment for myocardial infarction mean that fewer patients die in the acute stage of the illness. However, these gains contrast with the small progress achieved in understanding and improving the rehabilitation phase following MI. The problems that MI patients face in changing their lifestyle, health care behaviour and returning to productive work can be more debilitating than the physical effects of the MI itself. Many patients, for instance, do not return to work following MI although they are physically capable of doing so. With greater numbers of patients surviving MI, understanding the processes that direct the recovery phase of the illness has gained in importance as an area for research.

*Preparation of this chapter was supported by a grant from the New Zealand Health Research Council.

MI brings with it a number of immediate psychological effects that have implications for longer term behaviour change. The initial period after the MI is typically marked by intense emotional and social disturbance for the patient and their immediate family. The MI patient can experience high levels of anxiety and depression during this period as they become aware of the full impact of the illness. This can produce psychological difficulties, intense fears about a further MI and for many patients, low expectations of regaining health and vigour.

Previous research has pointed to patients' beliefs and perceptions of their illness being critically important in the recovery phase of MI. Maeland and Havik (1987) found patients' in-hospital expectations of their future work capacity to be a strong predictor of eventual return to work. Byrne (1982) has also shown MI patients holding negative models of their illness to be less likely to return to work and to have lower levels of functioning regardless of the severity of their MI. Some have noted that MI patients often develop quite idiosyncratic ideas about their illness and recovery that are rarely disclosed or discussed in medical consultations. Logan (1986), in a study of patient drawings in cardiac patients, noted that some patients had clearly erroneous models of what damage had occurred to their heart following MI. In one example, he discusses a patient who believed that the large vessel supplying the blood to his heart had become almost completely blocked following his MI. A full explanation to counter this misconception resulted in an improvement in his angina symptoms and mood.

An extreme form of negative health perceptions is seen in "cardiac invalidism" (Riegel, 1993). Here patients adopt an extremely passive, dependant and helpless role in the belief that any form of overly vigorous activity will bring on another MI. A hypersensitivity to bodily symptoms means that normal sensations may be misconstrued to indicate over-exertion or an impending fatal MI. This pattern often results in the overuse of medical services mainly for reassurance about symptoms. Cardiac invalidism is often supported by the patient's spouse who becomes overprotective and may permanently take on many of the household tasks previously undertaken by the patient. This form of adaptation is difficult to change and can become a self-fulfilling negative spiral; deconditioning accompanies decreases in fitness with the result that any exertion is likely to be more acutely felt by the patient and interpreted as further confirmatory evidence for limiting activity.

Much of the available data in the MI area points to the fact that psychological variables assume primary importance over medical ones in influencing recovery following MI (e.g. Diederiks *et al.*, 1991; Garrity, 1975) and that both patient's and spouse's perceptions about the illness are critical in rehabilitation and the return of social and occupational functioning (Garrity, 1975). However, to date, this work on psychological factors and recovery from MI has not been based on any clear theoretical framework and has tended to focus predominately on psychopathology. Risk factors such as the Type-A behaviour pattern and hostility have received a great deal of attention (Case *et al.*, 1985; Shekelle, Gale & Norusis, 1985) as has the role of depression (Frasure-Smith, Lesperance & Talajic, 1993; Levine *et al.*, 1996) and social isolation (Appels, 1990) in research examining the influence of psychological factors on outcome from MI.

We believe the self-regulatory model of Leventhal and his colleagues (Leventhal, Meyer & Nerenz, 1980) has a useful application in understanding patients' behaviour following MI. This model provides a framework for understanding which illness perceptions may be important at various stages of the recovery process and may eventually offer a guide to the development of more effective interventions in the rehabilitation phase of the illness. Implicit in the illness perception approach is the view that the patient is an active participant in the treatment and recovery process. This approach fits with our own view of the MI patient. Rather than being a passive depository of information from medical and nursing staff, he/she is actively constructing a working model of how the MI came about, how long it will last and what consequences the illness will have for their lives in the future. Potential educational and rehabilitation programmes are evaluated by the patient from this standpoint and accepted or discarded depending on how they fit into the working cognitive model of their illness.

In this chapter we outline the application of the illness perception approach to MI recovery. Initially, we consider how an illness perception approach may provide a more in-depth understanding of the acute phase of MI, in particular how it relates to treatment delay. We then examine how the causal attributions that the patient and spouse make are related to subsequent positive changes in health habits and behaviour. The role of illness perceptions in predicting attendance at cardiac rehabilitation programmes and return to work is also discussed. In the latter part of the chapter we look at the relationship of illness perceptions to emotion and coping as part of the self-regulatory model. We complete this chapter with an attempt to pull these various parts together to form a model of how illness perceptions operate following a MI.

The data on which this chapter is based has been drawn from the *Heart attack recovery project* — a research project based in Auckland, New Zealand. The study followed 143 first time heart attack patients aged 65 years or under for 12 months following their admission to hospital. Subjects in the study completed assessments in hospital and at 3, 6 and 12 months after their admission. Spouses also completed questionnaires about their perceptions of their partner's illness. This study used a new instrument called the Illness Perception Questionnaire (IPQ) (Weinman *et al.*, 1996) to measure the illness perception components of identity, time line, control/cure and consequences. This new measure provides an efficient way of comprehensively assessing the patient's perceptions of their illness, which was previously only possible through semi-structured interviews.

MAKING SENSE OF EARLY MI SYMPTOMS

The onset of a heart attack provides an excellent model of how patients make sense of symptoms and rapidly build implicit cognitive models about what may be causing their physical distress. Unlike many other serious illnesses, the onset of myocardial infarction is typically sudden. Individuals go from feeling well to feeling sick very rapidly. Often the illness is signalled by pain in the chest or left arm, as well as nausea and sweating. The recognition of these symptoms as a possible MI or serious illness often occurs only after the person has mentally discarded other potential causes for their symptoms; *"This must be indigestion from tonight's meal — I will take some antacid tablets"* or *"Perhaps I strained my muscles while I was working today"*. By generating possible causes and starting the treatment appropriate to these lay models, the individual has commenced a psychological process to satisfactorily explain and manage their pain and symptoms. This process may conclude with the person seeking medical assistance for their symptoms, but in many cases of MI, death occurs prior to the individual seeking such help.

The cognitive process of excluding potential diagnoses is explained cogently by Leventhal's self-regulation model which highlights the critical role of appraisal in this process. In a manner very analogous to scientific inquiry, personal hypotheses about acute symptoms are adopted or discarded on the basis of how usefully they provide a coherent explanation and direct successful coping strategies. Successful strategies are, in patient terms, ones that provide relief from symptoms and pain as well as being consistent with the patient's model of the illness. In the case of MI, initial strategies to manage symptoms based on personal models of indigestion or muscle strain are typically unsuccessful at causing a reduction in pain and are usually soon discarded. Short-term strategies instituted by the patient seeking to understand and manage their early symptoms may ultimately delay the seeking of medical care and worsen long-term prognosis. Most fatalities from MI occur within one hour of the onset of symptoms and more than 50% of patients in this category die without ever reaching hospital.

The recent advent of thrombolytic therapy for treating the acute stage of MI has focused more attention on understanding and reducing patient delay between the onset of symptoms and the initiation of treatment. Clinical trials have demonstrated that thrombolysis therapy has a far more beneficial effect the earlier it is instituted following the onset of symptoms. Early thrombolytic therapy can limit the amount of damage from the MI and alter the course of the illness (ISIS-2 Collaborative Group, 1988). A recent study showed a 45% mortality reduction in a group treated by thrombolysis within one hour of the onset of symptoms compared to a group not treated by thrombolysis (GSSI, 1986). The effectiveness of early thrombolytic treatment has encouraged more research into the factors influencing delay. Mass media campaigns have also been developed to provide information about early symptoms of myocardial infarction and to highlight the importance of quick action in response to chest pain. In the United States, the National Heart, Lung and Blood Institute recently developed a *National Heart Attack Alert Program* to increase community awareness of the symptoms of acute myocardial infarction as a means of reducing treatment delay for MI.

The period of delay from the onset of symptoms to arrival at hospital varies widely between countries and between urban and rural areas. However, a consistent finding is that regardless of location, the patient's decision time is the main component of total treatment delay (Dracup *et al.*, 1995). In our Auckland sample, the median period of delay was 2 hours 30 minutes. A large multi-site Italian study of 5,301 patients found a median time of 3 hours 50 minutes (GISSI, 1995), while a similar US study of 212,990 patients from 904 hospitals found an average delay of 2 hours. In this study, older patients, women and those who arrived at hospital during the daytime hours had significantly greater delay times (Maynard *et al.*, 1995). Other research has found patients with a history of angina or heart failure to take longer to recognise the early symptoms of the MI as a serious health threat (Meischke, Eisenberg & Larsen, 1993; Schroeder, Lamb & Hu, 1978).

The adoption by patients of a more serious illness model — *"Maybe I am having a heart attack"*, or even the contemplation of this as a possibility — *"I should call a doctor about my symptoms"*, is strongly influenced by a number of factors in MI patients. The strength of the pain experienced is influential in increasing motivation for a satisfactory explanation. Pain also acts as a strong cue to the person about the dangerous nature of the condition (GISSI, 1995). We have found previous personal experience with heart disease through a family history of the disease seems to facilitate the adoption of a more serious illness model and to reduce delay from the onset of symptoms to arrival at hospital (Petrie, Weinman & Sharpe, 1996). Interestingly, Cameron (1996) in this volume has also identified a family history of cancer as being associated with vulnerability beliefs and an increased availability of cancer illness representations. Previous studies with other illnesses have also found that personal experience with an illness leads to an over-estimation of its frequency (Jemmott, Ditto & Croyle, 1988). It seems likely that this process also influences the perception of the likelihood of MI and facilitates earlier treatment.

We also found the identity component of the patient's illness perception had an impact on treatment delay. Illness identity represents the symptoms that individuals perceive as being associated with their heart condition. These symptoms may in some cases differ from those seen as part of the condition from a strictly medical point of view. For example, about one third of MI patients in our sample identified dizziness and sore eyes as symptoms caused by their heart condition. We found while there was no difference between patients who delayed versus those that didn't on the number of physical symptoms they associated with their condition, those patients who reached hospital earlier were more likely to associate breathlessness as being part of their illness (Petrie,

Weinman & Sharpe, 1996). Previous research has been largely unsuccessful in identifying differences in symptoms between patients who delay and those that reach care early. However, it may be that the critical factor in this relationship is not the symptoms per se, but the patient's cognitive model of what particular symptoms signal a myocardial infarction that is critical. One of the difficulties of encouraging early action in this area is that for some patients the symptom onset is slow rather than sudden and may subside and reoccur over time, thus adding difficulties in the interpretation of symptoms (Dracup *et al.*, 1995).

Another important factor influencing the interpretation of early symptoms of a heart attack is the influence of significant others. This is particularly so in individuals whose normal coping style is to seek out others for advice and support. Others provide a way of checking out personal ideas about symptoms and are an important source for advice about appropriate action. We have found treatment delay in MI patients to be significantly shorter in those who coped with their MI by seeking out the advice of others about what to do. While previous research has pointed out the fact that most patients do typically discuss their symptoms with those around them, it may be the speed with which this occurs that may be critical in the delay process.

The early identification of myocardial infarction symptoms represents a real life and death example of the Leventhal self-regulatory model in action. The cognitive processes involved in recognition of MI symptoms as representing a serious threat to health are influenced by previous knowledge about the symptoms of heart disease, either through a family history or personal experience. The early seeking out of advice and support from others seems to facilitate the identification of symptoms as potentially threatening and thus reduce treatment delay. Interventions designed to alter lay models about what symptoms indicate myocardial infarction are likely to have significant influence on delay times.

CAUSAL ATTRIBUTIONS

For most people, a heart attack is a very frightening experience. When individuals are confronted with an unexpected negative event such as a physical assault, accident, or serious illness, there is a powerful inclination to find a cause for the event (Bulman & Wortman, 1977). Knowing the cause of an illness or other traumatic incident helps make the experience less anxiety provoking and the future more predictable. Once a diagnosis of myocardial infarction has been made, most patients spontaneously develop ideas about the cause of their illness. The process of finding a cause or causes for the MI helps patients make sense of their illness experience and provides a framework to guide their future actions to cope with the disease.

Many patients have clearly developed ideas about the cause of heart attacks based on first-hand knowledge of people they have known who have had myocardial infarctions or from information taken from the mass media. The popular media image of a heart attack victim is a harried male executive who has brought the illness on through constant overwork and relentless job stress. Usually the victim is seen as not having enough time off for relaxation and their health may be already compromised by smoking, being overweight and paying scant regard to a healthy lifestyle or diet. In fact, people's ideas about why someone is susceptible to a heart attack is much more clearly defined in our culture than for other common illnesses such as diabetes, arthritis, or cancer. The availability of these causal models makes the MI patient's attributional search considerably easier than for other illnesses.

Our sample of MI patients were asked to rate a list of 24 possible causes of their illness based on a five-point scale for how likely each one was to have caused their illness. This list was generated from recent studies of attributions following MI (Affleck *et al.*, 1987; De Valle & Norman, 1992). Figure 1 shows the 12 most common attributions for patients in our study. Stress was the cause most patients identify as being the reason for their MI. Further stress items such as "the type of work I do" and "overwork" also appear in the top 12 rated causes. Other common causal attributions relate to an unhealthy lifestyle; "eating fatty foods", "lack of exercise", "smoking", "being overweight" and "a poor diet". Stress has been found to be the most common perceived cause of heart attacks in a number of studies in both the United States (Affleck *et al.*, 1987; Rudy, 1980) and the United Kingdom (De Valle & Norman, 1992).

The search for causes of illness is not limited to patients, but is also common in others close to the patient (Taylor, Lichtman & Wood, 1984). Causal attributions can also provide the spouse with a

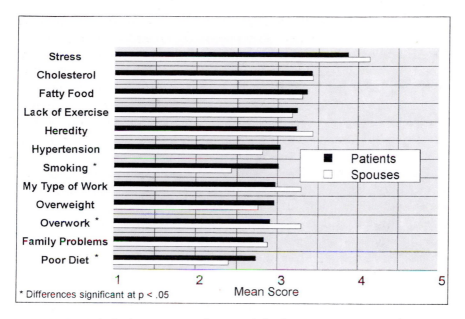

FIGURE 1   Beliefs about causes of myocardial infarction in patients and spouses

greater sense of control in a situation which many find very stressful. Studies have found a large percentage of spouses to show increased rates of psychological distress and symptoms of anxiety during the time their partner is in hospital (Bedsworth & Molen, 1982) and up to one year after their partner's MI (Mayou, Foster & Williamson, 1978; Skelton & Dominian, 1973).

In our study we also had spouses rate the cause of their partner's heart attack on the same scale. The spouses' ratings are also presented in Figure 1 and show a high degree of concordance with patients about the relative importance of various causes. However, some differences did exist between patients and spouses; patients rated smoking and a poor diet as significantly more important than spouses, while spouses rated overwork on the part of their partner higher than patients. These differences may represent a self protective bias on the part of the spouse, many of whom may also smoke and presumably eat a similar diet.

One important aspect of causal attributions is the ways in which they can influence perceived control and involvement in future behaviour. Thus we were interested in seeing whether patients' and spouses' attributions predict later changes in health behaviour after the patient leaves hospital. Previous research has produced inconsistent findings on the relationship between causal attributions and health behaviour change, with some studies finding an association (Bar-On, 1987; De Valle & Norman, 1992) and others finding no relationship (Croog & Richards, 1977; Rudy, 1980). A possible explanation for this inconsistency is that previous work on attributions and illness have largely categorised causal attributions under four headings; self, others, chance, or the environment (Turnquist, Harvey & Andersen, 1988). These categories, however, may be more reflective of the attributions and research concerns of psychologists rather than those of patients. For a more extensive discussion of this and related issues, see the chapter by Marteau in Section 2 of this book.

Most patients make considerable changes in their diet and exercise patterns in the six months following their MI. Relevant data from our MI sample are shown in Figure 2. We found that patients make significant changes in their diet following their MI by eating less red meat, fried food and food high in salt or sugar. Patients also increased their consumption of bran or high fibre food, fruit, and ate breakfast more often. The frequency with which patients engaged in strenuous exercise also increased and smoking rates dropped markedly.

Factor analysis of patients' most common causal attributions resulted in three interpretable attributional factors for MI patients. The first factor, labelled *lifestyle*, had high loadings on "eating fatty foods", "lack of exercise", "being overweight", "high levels of cholesterol" and "smoking". The second factor we labelled *stress*, loaded highly on "overwork", "stress" and "my type of work". The third factor, called *heredity*, loaded high on "heredity" and "high blood pressure". A further factor analysis of the spouses' causal attributions also resulted in three similar factors. Two factors, *lifestyle* and *stress*, were closely related to the patient factors and were significantly correlated. The third spouse factor was labelled *family distress* and loaded highly on "depression", "arguing with people", as well as "family problems and worries".

Examining the relationship between attributions and changes in health behaviour six months following MI, we found the belief by patients that the MI was caused by a faulty lifestyle was significantly related to overall improvements in diet and to an increase in the frequency of strenuous exercise (Petrie *et al.*, 1996). Attributions

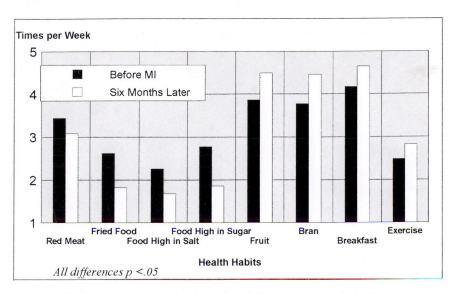

FIGURE 2 Changes in health habits following myocardial infarction

related to stress or to heredity were unrelated to later changes in health behaviour. We found a similar pattern in the data for spouses. In spouses, the attribution of the MI to lifestyle was also significantly correlated with an increase in their partner's frequency of strenuous exercise and to positive dietary changes.

These data suggest that causal attributions are very common following MI and show a high degree of agreement between patient and spouse. There appears to be widespread cultural belief that stress is the major cause of heart attacks and this causal attribution would seem important to modify if changes are required in dietary and health behaviour. Patient beliefs about heart attacks seem to group into three main causes; stress, lifestyle and heredity factors which are different from the way causal attributions have been previously grouped and analysed by researchers. It seems from our data that causal attributions are important determinants of later changes in health behaviour. They provide important guideposts for patients and their spouses by directing coping towards controlling a future myocardial infarction. Patient and spousal beliefs that the MI was caused by a faulty lifestyle were precursors to making changes in the types of foods eaten at home and participation in regular exercise. However, the belief that the MI was caused by stress, which is the most common attribution made by patients, had no relationship with later lifestyle changes.

CARDIAC REHABILITATION PROGRAMME ATTENDANCE AND RETURN TO WORK

After the acute phase of myocardial infarction, patients are typically directed into a cardiac rehabilitation programme. Rehabilitation programmes are aimed at helping the patient adjust to their illness, modifying the risk factors for a future MI, limiting or reversing the extent of cardiac disease, as well as improving return to social and occupational functioning. Most rehabilitation programmes include graduated exercise training, education about cardiac disease and guidelines for lifestyle change. Cardiac rehabilitation programmes are now also widely used with patients who have undergone coronary artery bypass surgery, coronary angioplasty and also for patients with stable angina pectoris.

The effectiveness of cardiac rehabilitation programmes has been reviewed recently. This analysis showed benefits for patients in terms of exercise tolerance, a reduction in smoking, improvement in psychological well-being, a reduction in the cardiovascular symptoms of angina and heart failure and a reduction in mortality (Wenger *et al.*, 1996). The extent of benefit in terms of reduced mortality from cardiac rehabilitation programmes is, however, difficult to quantify when put in the context of recent improvements in cardiac medication such as ACE inhibitor therapy and the fact that randomized controlled studies have often used highly selected samples.

Despite the likely benefits of cardiac rehabilitation for MI patients, a significant proportion of patients fail to attend any rehabilitation sessions or drop out prematurely (Goble *et al.*, 1991). In our study of first time MI patients we found 31% of patients failed to turn up to cardiac rehabilitation (Petrie *et al.*, 1996). Previous research is suggestive of the fact that patients choosing not to attend rehabilitation may have different views of their illness than patients who do attend. A recent study found that patients who were judged by staff to view their illness less seriously were less likely to attend cardiac rehabilitation (Ades *et al.*, 1992), and others have argued that a rehabilitation programme cannot be successfully started with myocardial infarction patients unless they have developed compatible personal models of their illness (Garrity, 1975).

We tested this by examining differences in illness perceptions between MI patients who attended rehabilitation and those who did not. We found illness perceptions measured by the IPQ shortly after admission to hospital were associated with later rehabilitation attendance. Although patients who attended rehabilitation programmes did not differ in terms of the medical seriousness of their MI or their age, they did have a significantly stronger belief that their illness could be controlled or cured (Petrie *et al.*, 1996). This suggests that the decision to participate in rehabilitation is strongly influenced by the patient's beliefs about their illness and, in particular, the perceived efficacy of rehabilitation in changing the course of their heart condition.

A significant number of MI patients fail to return to work even although they are medically capable of doing so. Past research has identified that cardiac rehabilitation seems to have a minimal impact on the patient's decision to return to work (Wenger *et al.*, 1996). Patients with a poorer education, a more unstable job history, higher levels of psychological distress and greater levels of family instability have been noted as being at risk for not returning to work after MI (Oldridge, 1991). Previous research however, has not systematically examined how patients' beliefs about their illness relate to the speed with which they return to work. We looked at this aspect in the *Heart attack recovery project.* The median time in our study for patients previously in full time employment to return to work was six weeks. We found that rehabilitation attendance was unrelated to the speed of return to work. However, those MI patients who returned to work within six weeks were characterised by a perception that their illness held less serious consequences and would last a shorter time. The patient's belief about the future consequences of their illness also predicted disability outside work. We found the perception that the illness held grave consequences also predicted future disability in the patient's social interaction, work around the home and recreation (Petrie *et al.*, 1996). These results suggest that more importance should be taken of patients' illness beliefs when planning rehabilitation and other interventions designed to improve function and return to work after MI. Patients may benefit from assessment of their personal ideas about their heart attack and perhaps an intervention designed to alter misconceptions and overly negative or catastrophic views of their illness and recovery. Previous work suggests that catastrophic thinking may be associated with greater levels of dysfunction in chronic illness (Petrie, Moss-Morris & Weinman, 1995). A difficulty in identifying patients' beliefs about their illness is that these are rarely volunteered by patients in medical consultations for the fear of being thought as stupid or misinformed by the doctor. The patient may also be reluctant to express ideas that put them in conflict with the doctor on whom the patient is reliant on for ongoing care. Moreover, patients are rarely asked for their ideas or views about their illness in medical consultation. The outcome of this process is that patients' illness beliefs remain essentially private.

THE DEVELOPMENT AND STABILITY OF ILLNESS PERCEPTIONS

With any chronic health problem, patients' representations of their illness may develop over a period of time, particularly if their problem is one that does not readily fit with an existing personal model. Leventhal, Nerenz and Steele (1984) found that many of their patients initially conceptualise their illness in acute terms, on the basis of their perceptions of its identity and time-line. Thus, the initial expectation with most conditions is that the illness will go away either because that is its natural time-course, or because treatment will be effective. The early symptoms of MI may well activate acute non-cardiac representations and this may be one reason for the delays in seeking help which we have discussed earlier in the chapter. However, it is important to note that cardiac representations can also be generated in response to the non-cardiac symptoms associated with general or abdominal pains. This reflects the strength of heart disease prototypes in which Leventhal *et al.* (1984) call "the generalised pool of illness information current in the culture", as well as the potential salience of heart disease to the individual (e.g. one's father or brother had a heart attack).

Once any disease has been diagnosed or confirmed, then this information will generally have a direct influence on the patient's representation, but there are often considerable discrepancies between doctors' and patients' perceptions (e.g., Lacroix, 1991). The onset of MI is sudden and means that it is possible to examine and compare patients' representations from the onset of the illness. We have found in our data that within a few days of experiencing their first MI, patients report clear beliefs about the identity, cause, cure/control, consequences and time line of their illness. While many of these beliefs are shared across the sample (e.g., the pattern of causal attributions — as discussed earlier), there is con-

siderable variation in the extent to which patients assess the severity of their heart attack or see it as amenable to cure or control.
Thus, at the onset of a MI, patients do seem to have ready access to
prototypic or shared representations with some common ideas
about causal factors but with large individual variation in other
illness perceptions, which are instrumental in influencing subsequent behaviour and adaptation.

Previous work on illness perceptions in other illness groups has
not used prospective studies or repeated designs and there is very
little information available about the way illness perceptions change
over time. Self-regulatory process changes will occur in response to
new symptoms and information, or as the result of negative coping
appraisals. In contrast, other approaches to the study of illness, such
as attribution theory, indicate that causal attributions can remain
quite stable and influential over long time periods (Turnquist,
Harvey & Andersen, 1988). MI offers an excellent opportunity to
examine this issue since it is possible to track illness perceptions
from the time of onset of illness. In our study we have assessed
patients' perceptions of their MI on four occasions, shortly after the
onset, then at 3, 6 and 12 months afterwards.

The different dimensions of illness perceptions were compared
over the four time periods, using a repeated measures one-way
ANOVA. The results show that, although there is considerable variance in illness perceptions at each point in time, two dimensions
show evidence of stability and two show a significant change over
time. Patients' perceived control or amenability to cure of their MI
showed a significant decrease over the 12 months from onset and
their perceptions of time-line showed a highly significant increase
over the same time period. Although perceived consequences of MI
showed a small but consistent decline, this was not significant and
the identity scores showed an initial reduction, but returned to
baseline levels at 12 months.

The apparent stability of the identity and consequences dimensions
may reflect the fact that, for many patients, there are relatively few
further symptoms and that prototypic perceptions of heart disease are
readily available. Prohaska *et al.* (1985) and Bishop (1987) have
demonstrated that lay beliefs of heart disease are well defined and
hence these are not only readily accessed shortly after MI onset but
remain largely unchanged during the following year. The increasing
time-line perceptions may reflect what Leventhal *et al.* (1984)

describe as the change from an acute to a more chronic view of the disease over time and a similar pattern of cognitive change may be reflected in the reducing beliefs in the possibility of cure and control.

It is possible that part of this apparent consistency in patients' representations of their MI may reflect the methodology we have used. By asking patients to complete the same questionnaire at regular intervals may induce a need to be consistent and hence this may mask real variation. Systematic studies of the way in which questionnaire information is processed and the demand characteristics which are involved also show that respondents may actively strive to produce consistent responses (see Sheeran & Orbell, 1996).

Clearly, it will be necessary to establish the extent to which the relative stability of certain illness representations following MI are a function of the assessment procedure. If, as we suggest, there are good reasons for stability in these patients, then the implications of this are important for patient rehabilitation and recovery. It indicates the need to identify patient cognitions at an early stage in order to identify barriers to rehabilitation and recovery.

ILLNESS PERCEPTIONS AND RECOVERY

In this chapter we have aimed to demonstrate how the illness perception approach may be applied to develop a clearer understanding of the patient's experience following myocardial infarction. Examining the way individuals conceptualise their symptoms and illness, from the development of initial symptoms through to the rehabilitation phase, offers a new way of understanding the impact of a heart attack and many of the problematic behaviours that may accompany the condition. Delays in seeking treatment for cardiac symptoms can have a major influence on the outcome of the disease. While previous research has focused in an atheoretical way on the demographic and clinical factors associated with delay, illness perceptions offer the opportunity to understanding treatment delay as a dynamic process. Moreover, intervention programmes aimed at reducing delay should have measurable effects on the availability of a myocardial infarction representation.

Throughout the course of their illness we see the individual as an active participant who is always seeking a rapprochement between their illness model and their everyday experience. What is perhaps remarkable with MI is the speed with which clear cognitive models of illness are developed and how some change over time as the individual is confronted with the reality of the condition. In our study, the data indicate that on the whole, initial optimism about the time course and control or curability of the disease changed towards a more chronic illness model. However, there was considerable variation within the group and against this general shift there were some individuals whose ideas changed in the opposing direction. The relationship of changes in illness perceptions to overall emotional adjustment is an area that is in need of further investigation.

Patients' beliefs about whether their heart attack was caused by stress, genetic factors, or poor health habits act as a clear starting point for individuals when deciding to make changes in their personal health behaviours. For many, a heart attack is seen as a clear warning of the consequences of smoking, a poor diet and a sedentary lifestyle. However, many other patients do not make these associations and may see personal stress or family problems as the main reason for their illness. From this standpoint, changes to health behaviours make little sense. This process does not exclusively belong to the patient. Beliefs about the cause of the illness in the patient's family can, as we have seen, also influence these lifestyle changes. Spouses and family members can be effective agents for change in this area by offering prompts, encouragements and positive reinforcements for new behaviour.

Cardiac rehabilitation programmes have been shown to make a positive impact on many patients following MI. However, a considerable number of patients either do not attend or drop out from courses prematurely. We have found that the patient's view of their illness is an important factor in both rehabilitation attendance and in how quickly patients return to work following their MI. Our results suggest that highly negative or catastrophic thinking about illness is an important area for future intervention programmes. If such thinking can be identified early in the recovery process and interventions developed to foster realistic models and expectations, then improvements in the rates of functioning can be anticipated. These findings might also partially explain recent relating post-MI depression to clinical outcome (e.g., Lesperance, Frasure-Smith & Talajic, 1966), since similar negative cognitive distortions may be associated with depression and these can serve to interfere with rehabilitation and recovery. An important challenge for the future is to develop techniques that access private views of illness in situations where patients may feel reluctant to discuss these freely.

Another is to develop effective interventions for changing individuals' catastrophic and negative cognitions about their illness. Progress in these areas is likely to improve the adjustment and recovery of function in patients following myocardial infarction.

REFERENCES

Ades, P.A., Huang, D. & Weaver, S.O. (1992) Cardiac rehabilitation participation predicts lower rehospitalization costs. *American Heart Journal*, **123**, 916–921.

Affleck, G., Tennen, H., Croog, S. & Levine, S. (1987) Causal attributions, perceived benefits control and recovery from a heart attack. *Journal of Social and Clinical Psychology*, **53**, 339–355.

Appels, A. (1990) Mental precursors of myocardial infarction. *British Journal of Psychiatry*, **156**, 465–471.

Bar-On, D. (1987) Causal attributions and the rehabilitation of myocardial infarction victims. *Journal of Social and Clinical Psychology*, **5**, 114–122.

Bedsworth, J.A. & Molen, M.T. (1982) Psychological stress in spouses of patients with myocardial infarction. *Heart and Lung*, **11**, 450–456.

Bishop, G.D. (1987) Lay conceptions of physical symptoms. *Journal of Applied Social Psychology*, **17**, 127–146.

Bulman, J.R. & Wortman, C.B. (1977) Attributions of blame and coping in the "real world": Severe accident victims react to their lot. *Journal of Personality and Social Psychology*, **35**, 351–363.

Byrne, D.G. (1982) Psychological responses to illness and outcome after survived myocardial infarction: A long-term follow-up. *Journal of Psychosomatic Research*, **26**, 105–112.

Cameron, L. (1997) Screening for cancer: illness perceptions and illness worry. In K.J. Petrie & J. Weinman (Eds.), *Perceptions of illness and health: Current research and applications*. London: Harwood Academic.

Case, R.B., Heller, S.S., Case, N.B. & Moss, A.J. (1985) Type A behaviour and survival after acute myocardial infarction. *New England Journal of Medicine*, **312**, 737–741.

Croog, S.H. & Richards, N.P. (1977) Health beliefs and smoking patterns in heart patients and their wives: a longitudinal study. *American Journal of Public Health*, **67**, 921–930.

De Valle, M. & Norman, P. (1992) Causal attributions, health locus of control beliefs and lifestyle changes among pre-operative coronary patients. *Psychology and Health*, **7**, 201–211.

Diederiks, J.P., Bar, F.W., Hoppener, P. & Vonken, H. (1991) Predictors of return to former leisure and social activities in MI patients. *Journal of Psychosomatic Research*, **35**, 687–696.

Dracup, K., Moser, D.K., Eisenberg, M., Meischke, H., Alonzo, A.A. & Braslow, A. (1995) Causes of delay in seeking treatment for heart attack symptoms. *Social Science and Medicine*, **40**, 379–392.

Frasure-Smith, N., Lesperance, F. & Talajic, M. (1993) Depression following myocardial infarction. *Journal of the American Medical Association*, **270**, 1819–1825.

Garrity, T.F. (1975) Morbidity, mortality and rehabilitation. In W.D. Gentry & R.B. Williams (Eds.), *Psychological aspects of myocardial infarction and coronary care*. St Louis, Missouri: Mosby.

GISSI. (1986). Effectiveness of intravenous thrombolytic treatment in acute myocardial infarction. *Lancet*, **1**, 397–401.

GISSI. (1995) Epidemiology of avoidable delay in the care of patients with acute myocardial infarction in Italy. *Archives of Internal Medicine*, **155**, 1481–1488.

Goble, A.J., Hare, D.L., Macdonald, P.S., Oliver, R.G., Reid, M.A. & Worcester, M.C. (1991) Effect of early programmes of high and low intensity exercise on physical performance after a transmural acute myocardial infarction. *British Heart Journal*, **65**, 126–131.

Jemmott, J.B., Ditto, P.H. & Croyle, R.T. (1988) Commonsense epidemiology: Self-based judgements from laypersons and physicians. *Health Psychology*, **7**, 55–73.

ISIS-2 Collaborative Group. (1988) Randomized trial of intravenous streptokinase, oral aspirin, both, or neither among 17, 187 cases of suspected acute myocardial infarction: ISIS-2. *Lancet*, **2**, 349–360.

Lacroix, J.M. (1991) Assessing illness schemata in patient populations. In J.A. Skelton & R.T. Croyle (Eds.), *Mental representation in health and illness* (pp. 193–220). New York: Springer-Verlag.

Lesperance, F., Frasure-Smith, N. & Talajic, M. (1996) Major depression before and after MI: its nature and consequences. *Psychosomatic Medicine*, **58**, 99–110.

Leventhal, H., Meyer, D. & Nerenz, D. (1980) The common sense representation of illness danger. In S. Rachman (Ed.), *Contributions to medical psychology* (pp. 7–30). New York: Pergamon Press.

Leventhal, H., Nerenz, D. & Steele, D. (1984) Illness representations and coping with health threats. In A. Baum & J. Singer (Eds.), *A Handbook of psychology and health* (Vol. 4, pp. 219–252). Hillsdale, NJ: Lawrence Erlbaum Associates.

Levine, J.B., Covino, N.A., Slack, W.V., Safran, C., Safran, D.B., Boro, J.E., *et al.* (1996) Psychological predictors of subsequent medical care among patients with hospitalized with cardiac disease. *Journal of Cardiopulmonary Rehabilitation*, **16**, 109–116.

Logan, R.L. (1986) Patient drawings as aids to the identification and management of causes of distress and atypical symptoms of cardiac patients. *New Zealand Medical Journal*, **99**, 368–371.

Maeland, J.G. & Havik, O.E. (1987) Psychological predictors for return to work after a myocardial infarction. *Journal of Psychosomatic Research*, **31**, 471–481.

Maynard, C., Weaver, W.D., Lambrew, C., Bowlby, L.J., Rogers, W.J. & Rubison, M. (1995) Factors influencing the time to administration of thrombolytic therapy with recombinant tissue plasminogen activator (data from the national registry of myocardial infarction). *American Journal of Cardiology*, **76**, 548–552.

Mayou, R., Foster, A. & Williamson, B. (1978) The psychological and social effects of myocardial infarction on wives. *British Medical Journal*, **18**, 699–701.

Meischke, H., Eisenberg, M.S. & Larsen, M.P. (1993) Prehospital delay interval for patients who use emergency medical services: The effect of heart related medical conditions and demographic variables. *Annals of Emergency Medicine*, **22**, 1597–1601.

Oldridge, N.B. (1991) Compliance with cardiac rehabilitation services. *Journal of Cardiopulmonary Rehabilitation*, **11**, 115–127.

Petrie, K.J., Moss-Morris, R. & Weinman, J. (1995) The impact of catastrophic beliefs on functioning in Chronic Fatigue Syndrome. *Journal of Psychosomatic Research*, **39**, 31–37.

Petrie, K.J., Weinman, J. & Sharpe, N. (1996) Illness perceptions and treatment delay after myocardial infarction. Manuscript in preparation.

Petrie, K.J., Weinman, J., Sharpe, N. & Buckley, J. (1996) Role of patients' view of their illness in predicting return to work and functioning after myocardial infarction: longitudinal study. *British Medical Journal*, **312**, 1191–1194.

Petrie, K.J., Weinman, J., Sharpe, N. & Walker, S. (1996) Causal attributions and health behaviour change following myocardial infarction. Manuscript submitted for publication.

Picard, M.H., Dennis, C., Schwartz, R.G., Ahn, D.K., Kraemer, H.C., *et al.* (1989) Cost-benefit analysis of early return to work after uncomplicated acute myocardial infarction. *American Journal of Cardiology*, **63**, 1308–1314.

Prohaska, T.R., Leventhal, E.A., Leventhal, H. & Keller, M.L. (1985) Health practices and illness cognition in young, middle aged and elderly adults. *Journal of Gerontology*, **40**, 569–578.

Riegel, B.J. (1993) Contributions to cardiac invalidism after acute myocardial infarction. *Coronary Artery Disease*, **4**, 215–220.

Rudy, E.B. (1980) Patients' and spouses' causal explanations of a myocardial infarction. *Nursing Research*, **29**, 352–356.

Schroeder, J.S., Lamb, I.H. & Hu, M. (1978) The prehospital course of patients with chest pain: analysis of the prodromal, symptomatic, decision-making, transportation and emergency room periods. *American Journal of Medicine*, **64**, 742–747.

Sheeran, P. & Orbell, S. (1996) How confidently can we infer health beliefs from questionnaire responses? *Psychology and Health*, **11**, 273–290.

Shekelle, R.B., Gale, M. & Norusis, M. (1985) Type A score (Jenkins Activity Survey) and risk of recurrent coronary heart disease in the aspirin myocardial infarction study. *American Journal of Cardiology*, **56**, 221–225.

Skelton, M. & Dominian, J. (1973) Psychological stress in wives of patients with myocardial infarction. *British Medical Journal*, **14**, 101–103.

Taylor, S.E., Lichtman, R.R. & Wood, J.V. (1984) Attributions, beliefs about control and adjustment to breast cancer. *Journal of Personality and Social Psychology*, **46**, 489–502.

Turnquist, D.C., Harvey, J.H. & Andersen, B.L. (1988) Attributions and adjustment to life-threatening illness. *British Journal of Clinical Psychology*, **27**, 55–65.

Wenger, H.K., Froelicher, E.S. *et al.* (1996) *National practice guideline: cardiac rehabilitation* Maryland: US Department of Health and Human Services.

Weinman, J., Petrie, K.J., Moss-Morris, R. & Horne, R. (1996) The illness perception questionnaire: A new method for assessing the cognitive representation of illness. *Psychology and Health*, **11**, 431–445.

16

Virtual Narratives: Illness Representations in Online Support Groups

Kathryn P. Davison & James W. Pennebaker*

Illness representations are a central concern for health psychologists because patients' lay models direct attitudes, health behaviours and recovery processes. The bulk of empirical groundwork to date has been laid in identifying components of these constructions — symptoms, causes, consequences, etc. — and their health impact. A more elusive and clinically essential challenge is to understand the construction process, that is, how illness representations are formed, modified and maintained. Leventhal (1983), Bishop (1991) and others have noted that the dynamic nature of representations must be examined within the larger contextual system of the patient.

Although intrapsychic in nature, illness representations are *socially* generated. Patients develop attitudes and expectations by talking with others, hearing their stories and comparing them with their own experience. Although the ideas surrounding many illnesses are first formed within the family or among peers, once individuals are diagnosed with a serious and chronic disease, the ways

*Preparation of this chapter was made possible by grants from the National Science Foundation (SBR9411674) and the National Institute of Health (MH52391) to the second author.

they comprehend their illness is by talking with experts, reading and searching out others who have also been diagnosed with the same disease. Many of us as children remember our grandparents talking at length with their friends about their common (or unique) symptoms, illnesses and disabilities. As we get older, many of us can better appreciate the social and informational value of socially sharing illness perceptions.

If illness representations are, to a great degree, socially constructed, where and how do people talk about disease? To what degree do people with different diseases differ in the ways they talk about and socially compare their diseases with others? These questions lie at the heart of our paper. Rather than focus on the illness representations directly, we are more concerned with the social and linguistic dynamics associated with talking about chronic illness.

One reason social and health psychologists have not studied the ways in which people naturally discuss their diseases with similar others is that most discussions are informal rather than routine. If a woman is diagnosed with breast cancer, for example, friends who may have had similar experiences may talk individually with her. Only in recent years have support groups emerged wherein groups of people with the same disease are encouraged to convene to discuss common issues and problems (Jacobs & Goodman, 1989). Although support groups are growing in popularity for some diseases, many people with diseases are unable to attend support meetings because of the limitations of the disease or other considerations such as distance, time, etc.

Within the last five years, a quiet revolution has been taking place within the support group movement. In addition to the traditional group meetings of people with diseases, individuals have been turning to the computer world of Internet. With a modem and basic software, thousands of people with a variety of diseases are able to locate discussion or support groups arranged by diseases. Without leaving home, people are able to read comments and letters from others and to respond in a public forum. Because the interactions are public and exchanges take place within hours or, in some cases, seconds, the support groups take on many of the qualities of face-to-face interactions. The advent of the Internet, particularly of online support groups, offers a unique opportunity to gain insights about the development and maintenance of illness models. Moreover, the willingness and motivation of patients to participate in such groups constitutes psychologically valuable information. What kinds of information do patients seek from each other? What can we infer about their coping styles from their writing behaviour? Who talks and what does their language tell us about their life and concerns? Information about supportive behaviours colours in the social context of illness perceptions.

In this chapter we present the reasoning and results of our initial inquiries in this area, a study of virtual support groups for six disease conditions: heart disease, breast cancer, prostate cancer, arthritis, diabetes and chronic fatigue syndrome (CFS). Our discussion falls broadly into four sections. We begin by providing the reader with an overview of the virtual community in general and online support groups in particular, the source of our samples. We then compare the relative tendencies of patients to participate in these support groups. The second section focuses on the distinguishing linguistic characteristics of the support groups. How do the features of language usage reflect the expressive style of the patients and their beliefs about their illness? We discuss our approach to the study of language in health processes and social dynamics. The third section contains qualitative judgments about the kind of collective voice that emerges from these patient groups and the fourth section concludes with implications and future directions.

THE ADVENT OF THE INTERNET

The "Internet" refers to a collection of over 20,000 linked computer networks whose original impetus came largely from government, military, research and academic centres, due to their heavy trafficking in records and information (Ferguson, 1996). The "Net", as it is most commonly known, constitutes a completely new kind of infrastructure system, something quite like a virtual highway system — one can "travel" to many different "locations" by indicating a specific address. Some locations, known as "web pages", are like billboards along the highway in which commercial and promotional information are featured. Other locations are linked in turn to extensive complications of information, entertainment, social exchange, or referral.

The Internet is no longer the preview of academics and computer hacks. It now concludes millions of private individuals as well. It has been estimated that Internet access is growing at the rate of 20% per month and already one in nine American households has access to the Net (Ferguson, 1996). This stupendous growth rate is at least partly due to the development of commercial online servers, businesses designed to promote online participation. The commercial servers, such as America Online (AOL), Compuserve, Prodigy and Microsoft News Network (MSN) offer user-friendly access interfaces that make search and navigation much simpler for the novice. A "newbie", someone new to the online community, can use a search service to locate areas of interest and point and click their way across the net. Each of the commercial servers is like a private subset of the internet: they feature their own collection of information and exchange and they each offer access to the wider realms of the Net. One can subscribe to AOL and search the same information on the Net as a Compuserve client, but AOL subscribers do not have access to the features and groups of Compuserve.

From a social psychological standpoint, the most intriguing aspect of the online community is the *interactive* component: chat rooms, newsgroups and mailing lists. Chat rooms are virtual sites where those who are "in" the room can interact via keyboard conversation. Mailing lists are composed of individual subscribers and a coordinator (the listserver) who send and receive letters (known as "posts") to each other as a group. A subscriber to a mailing list receives in his or her e-mail box all of the posts made by the group members each day. Newsgroups (known as bulletin boards or message boards on the commercial servers) are like mailing lists, in that groups of people are considered subscribers; but instead of posts collecting in each subscriber's mailbox, the "news" is featured at a particular site for all concerned to read. In fact, some support groups are configured so that subscribers can elect to participate in either a mail or news format.

Online services offer patients and their families access to other patients, to supporting foundations, to warehouses of journal articles and technical papers and to doctors willing to offer friendly advice. Vendors of every imaginable treatment and dietary supplement vie for the attention and business of patient groups. In fact, health management issues have contributed strongly to the growth of the online community: a recent US poll conducted by the Louis Harris agency indicated that subscribers of online services rated information about health and disease as their top concern. In the health arena, then, the Internet offers a medium of education and exchange actively sought after by consumers.

It is important at this point to bear in mind there are subtle but marked differences between commercial online support groups and Internet support groups which reflect their historical and organisational orientation: Internet support groups are purely patient-driven, the result of committed patients and agreeable system operators. Support groups on the commercial servers are the product of commercially motivated and programmatic marketing strategies. For instance, America Online may contract with a particular business to design and implement the health aspects of their community and so the result is a "menu" of support group types that the supplier perceives as valued by the customer. Furthermore, as described above, groups on the Internet are accessible to all online subscribers, while groups featured by the commercial servers are accessible only to their own customers.

EXPRESSIONS OF SUPPORT: GROUPS, POSTS AND WORDS

Illness representations themselves play a role in predicting the relative rates of information- and support-seeking behaviours by different patients and their families. For example, Bishop (1987) classified health problems according to a multidimensional scaling system (MDS), essentially a 2×2 system: life-threatening (or not) and contagious (or not). Contagious illnesses (e.g., flu, chicken pox or cold) carry such powerful organic causal attributions and are largely acute, so mutual support is not a goal for those sufferers and their families.

Non-contagious illnesses, on the other hand, are characterised by more ambiguous causal models and time-lines. Under these circumstances, we reasoned, patients would be motivated to seek information and support from those who have undergone similar treatments. We chose for these research purposes six non-contagious conditions that represent both life-threatening (breast cancer, prostate cancer, diabetes and heart disease) and non-life-threatening (arthritis and CFS) health problems. Within the life-threatening category, we selected breast and prostate cancers because their incidence rates are equivalent, each one affects almost exclusively members of just one sex and both involve intimate anatomy. Diabetes and heart disease were selected because they represent tremendous costs to society due to their high prevalence and contributions to disability and mortality.

The Sampled Support Groups

For purposes of this project, only newsgroups and mailing lists were sampled. They offer a more well-defined and continuous identity than do chat rooms, resulting in each post (written contribution from a subscriber) functioning as a small narrative. Support groups were sampled from both Internet and commercial servers, in this case, America Online (AOL).

Internet selection criteria

The Net features well over 30,000 newsgroups and dozens of new ones are generated daily. In order to determine which groups to monitor in a systematic way, a master list of all newsgroups (nation-wide and/or international only, not regional) was compiled and keyword searches were performed for each disease category. Keywords used were: prostate, cancer, breast, heart, cardio*, fatigue, CFS, diabetes and arthritis.

From the results of those searches, all groups that were deemed to be mutual support groups, as opposed to forums for lobbyists, doctors, researchers, or other experts, were identified. In the cases in which more than one support group was available, the group that exhibited the highest rate of exchange was chosen. Most support groups for both physical and mental illness begin with the prefix "alt.support." For example, the arthritis support group is "alt.support.arthritis." The notable exception in the case of our sample is the most active support group for breast cancer, which is "breast-cancer@morgan.ucs.mun.ca."

AOL selection criteria

Group identification and selection on AOL was much more straight-forward, reflecting the user-friendly aims of its developers. AOL's "Health Channel" features a list of numerous health concerns and diagnostic categories. Selection of a particular diagnostic category results in a menu of selections regarding that condition, one of which is always "bulletin boards". Clicking on the bulletin board icon takes the user to the newsgroup set up for that condition. Message boards were available for all of the subject conditions with the exception of CFS, which may be due to its relative newness as a health concern.

Posting Frequencies

For a period of two weeks, every post made in the selected groups was collected and saved as a separate text file. A total of 3062 posts were collected from the Net and 831 from AOL. For the purposes of the analyses, posts of 10 words or less were deleted, leaving a total of 3,703. Each post was treated as a "case", so by the end of the two-week period it was possible to have a sense of the relative frequency with which individuals contributed from each group. For instance, prostate cancer and breast cancer occur at the same rate in the U.S. and mortality rates for the two conditions are about the same. As can be seen in Figure 1, rates of participation were strikingly different. Even more striking was relative sparseness of support group activity on the part of heart patients or their families. Heart disease, which is responsible for more deaths each year than the

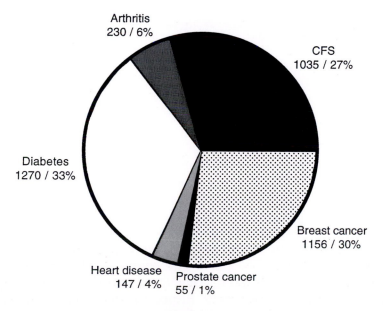

FIGURE 1

four other leading causes combined, is unique in the lack of supportive exchange by its constituency. By contrast, sufferers of CFS participate at quite high rates. More posts were made by CFS sufferers in the two-week sampling period than by all of the AOL support groups combined. We suspect that the ambiguity of disease prototype and lack of organic basis combine to stimulate a feverish search for a collective model. The components of illness perceptions — cause, cure, consequences, time-line, symptoms, label, etc., are all subjects for comparison and discussions.

Less surprising was the volume of contributions made by arthritis and diabetes patients. Diabetics are faced with the burden of constant monitoring of blood glucose levels. Consequences of non-monitoring are serious and methods of monitoring are various. Stories, comparisons of approaches and dietary strategies are valuable aspects of their combined coping modes.

Contributor Features: Type and Length

To assess support group behaviours it is necessary to identify the role of experts and family members in the group process. If contributions to a support group come entirely from health care professionals and relatives of the patient, patients' absences indicate their lack of motivation to participate. Therefore, posts were categorised according to contributor type: 1) personal, written by the patient; 2) friend or family member; or 3) expert or sales representative. As can be seen in Figure 2, in most cases the contributions were made by the patients themselves. Notable exceptions were the heart disease and prostate cancer patients. In a similar vein, prostate cancer and heart patient support groups featured higher percentages of posts by family and friends than did the other groups.

Coupled with information about types of contributors, the lengths of the post enhances the outline of the kind of disclosure occurring in the group. Some posts are quite brief, in which a patient seeks the name of a particular medication or monitor, or wants to know if someone has information about a rare aspect of a broad disorder category. Others are quite long, in which a patient may begin by asking for help in addressing a symptom and then engages in a journalistic monologue about their situation: the emotional impact of their condition, the reactions of family members, the attitude conveyed by their doctor and sometimes their relation-

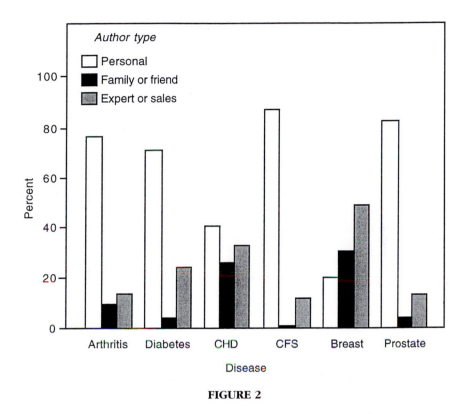

FIGURE 2

ship to the group. Table 1 contains a summary of the mean word counts of each of the condition groups. Arthritis, heart disease and prostate cancer patients wrote fewer words than did breast cancer, chronic fatigue and diabetes patients. While the differences are interesting, these indices are somewhat superficial and need to be considered together with more in-depth information about their language usage and styles of expression.

Finally, it is instructive to see the degree to which people writing about their own disease are males or females. An independent rater read each post and coded whether it was written by a male, female, or could not be evaluated. Assessment of sex was based on objective criteria (e.g., person either identified him or herself by sex or made reference to having a husband or wife). Of the 2,880 posts that were written by the person with the disease (as opposed to family member or expert), 1,543, or 54%, could be identified as male or female. Of the posts that could be identified, 84% were written by women. As would be expected, the rate differed by disease. The percentage of posts written by females was as follows: arthritis = 63%, breast cancer = 95%, diabetes = 51%, heart disease = 48%, prostate cancer = 0% and chronic fatigue = 91%.

LANGUAGE FEATURES BY DISEASE

As suggested by the number of posts and the number of words per post, people with different diseases approach online support groups in different ways. A cursory reading of the posts suggest that some newsgroups are more emotional and personal than others. Others are more concerned with objective data surrounding their disease. How can we best capture these differences in the ways people write? This is a problem that we have repeatedly faced over the last several years in studying the most relevant dimensions of emotional disclosure within the laboratory (e.g., Pennebaker, 1993). Within social and health psychology, two strategies to studying speech or writing samples have emerged: judges' ratings and computerised text analyses.

Rating Dimensions of Text

Judges' ratings of text have a long and rich tradition within psychology. In our own work where we have had people write about traumatic experiences, we have employed 3–5 independent judges to determine the degree to which each person's separate writing sample expressed negative emotion, positive emotion, indicated causal thinking, showed insight and self-reflection. In addition to being time-intensive, inter-judge reliabilities are only modest, ranging from mean correlations to .2 to .5 (Cronbach alphas depend on the number of judges and with 5 judges, boost the reliabilities up to the .6 to .9 range). Interestingly, when judges are required to rate particularly upsetting emotional writing or speech samples, the samples themselves evolve into projective tests, reducing their judged reliability. We have systematically found that the more self-relevant the topic of the text, the more skewed that judges' ratings are compared to those who have not experienced issues central to the specific text.

The phrase by phrase approach has been used by Gottschalk and Gleser (1969). Their method, which is heavily psychoanalytic in orientation, requires trained raters to evaluate each clause of a sentence. Stiles (1992) has developed a method of communication analysis called Verbal Response Modes (VRM) which also requires rating on a phrase-by-phrase basis. Similarly, Hughes, Uhlmann and Pennebaker (1994), in a study on the relationship between autonomic activity and writing about emotionally upsetting experiences, found that phrases that judges rated as expressing emotions or certain cognitive dimensions correlated with concurrent electrodermal activity. Phrase analyses, like overall text analyses, suffer from the subjective biases of human judges. Indeed, if the goal is to assess the general flavour of a text, measures of word usage are strongly related to average judged phrase assessments. For example, the data from the Hughes *et al.* (1994) experiment correlated phrases judged to be emotional (both positive and negative), cognitive (self-reflective and causal in thinking style) and self-referential with actual word counts based on predetermined word lists tapping these same dimensions. Results indicated that overall, judges' ratings of phrases and single word counts were significantly correlated for dimensions of negative emotionality, $r = (22) = .64$, positive emotionality, $r (22) = .66$, cognitive mechanisms, $r (22) = .61$ and self references, $r (22) = .91$ (Francis, 1993).

Based on a limited sample, individual word counts served as a stand-in for judges' ratings of phrases. Yet a word count is also linked to judges' ratings of the overall emotionality (positive and negative) of a writing sample and its use of cognitive mechanisms (insight and causation) and identity references. Pennebaker and Francis (in press), for example, required three judges to rate written emotional essays of 37 students who wrote about "their deepest thoughts and feelings about coming to college" for three consecutive days, 15 minutes per day. Judges' overall ratings of the essays were then compared with word counts of dimensions relevant to the overall ratings. Judges' ratings and word counts were significantly related to each other for the central dimensions of overall negative emotionality ($r = .56$), positive emotionality (.38), insight (.59) and causation (.35). Indeed, the mean interjudge correlation is virtually always lower than the correlation between word count and the average of all judges' ratings. The point, then, is that word counts can reliably serve as a proxy for overall ratings.

Establishment of a Computer-Based Text Analysis Procedure: LIWC

To bypass the problems of judges and the rating process, we have developed a text analysis computer program, LIWC (Linguistic Inquiry and Word Count). The program analyses text files on a word-by-word basis. A text file can be a single person's post on a computer bulletin board, the contents of an interaction among two or more people, samples of spoken language in particular settings, or any type of verbal sample that exists within a computer text file. Each word within the file is compared against an extended list of words divided into 61 dimensions, or dictionary scales.

On the broadest level, four general text dimensions are tapped: emotions, cognitive mechanisms, content domains and language composition (see Francis, 1993, for a description of the program). Selection of scales was guided both by results from judges' ratings of written essays in the first author's work on disclosure and by current trends in health and social psychology. Scales, for example, were created to tap basic dimensions of positive and negative emotions (e.g., Watson & Pennebaker, 1989), including anger and hostility/paranoia (Barefoot, 1992), anxiety and depression (e.g., Friedman & Booth-Kewley, 1987) and optimism (Scheier & Carver, 1987). A variety of cognitive mechanisms were also measured, including words that measured causal reasoning — although not specific styles of attribution (Peterson, Seligman & Vaillant, 1988), use of insight or self-reflection (e.g., Pennebaker, 1993) and use of a thinking style called "undoing" where people try to undo events that have already occurred (Davis *et al.*, 1995; see also the domain of self-discrepancy discussed by Higgins, Vookles & Tykocinski, 1992). Words reflecting various dimensions of identity were also measured, including singular self references (I, me) and plural self-references (we, our). In addition to these global dimensions, a wide variety of linguistic categories were also constructed.

The sums of each of the scales are converted to percentage of total words. For example, across the 2,880 personal posts from both the Net and AOL, 1.5% of the words are negative emotion words and 2.8% are positive emotion words. Interestingly, these percentages are much closer to essays by college students and adults writing about traumatic experiences as part of laboratory experiments than to control essays dealing with trivial topics (negative emotions for trauma writers = 2.0%, for control topics = 0.6%; positive emotions for trauma writers = 3.1%, for control topics = 1.2%).

A cautionary note must be included about LIWC. Language is highly contextual. A word count program usually fails to code irony, sarcasm and metaphors properly. A word that is negative in one context ("what he did made me *mad*") can be positive in another ("I'm *mad* about the cute guy in my class"). Nevertheless, a system such as LIWC is probabilistic in the analyses of computer posts. Although there will be some misclassifications of specific words, the reliability and validity findings indicate that the LIWC strategy serves as an efficient marker of overall text dimensions within a given essay.

Difference in Language Use by Disease Status

Each of the posts written by the people with the diseases themselves (as opposed to family or friends, or experts, such as physicians, or merchandisers) were separately analysed by the LIWC program. Only those posts with at least 30 words were used. The

Table 1   Text Analysis Results by Internet Disease Group

	Arthritis	Diabetes	CHD	CFS	Prostate Cancer	Breast Cancer	F-Ratio
Negative emotion	1.87a	1.62a	1.69ab	1.78a	1.08ab	1.24b	9.68
Positive emotion	2.44ab	2.31a	1.77a	2.65b	1.79abc	3.04c	10.90
Insight	2.62abc	2.29a	2.41abc	2.81b	2.94abc	2.57c	5.88
Cause	1.34ab	1.32a	0.95bc	1.02c	1.45abc	0.91c	9.88
Self-reference	6.39a	5.18b	6.96ac	7.16c	4.79ab	6.52a	26.64
Present tense	10.60a	9.41b	9.37bc	9.34b	8.05bc	8.68c	8.11
Negations	1.39a	2.04b	1.74abc	1.77c	1.54abc	1.69c	6.22
Articles	5.28a	6.04b	5.42ab	5.99b	7.05bc	5.70ac	3.25
Word count	103a	133c	114ac	141c	103abc	163b	7.67
% Big words	18.1a	17.2a	18.0a	15.8b	18.8ab	15.7b	10.66
N	127	736	48	732	10	810	

All F-ratios are statistically significant at $p < .01$ (5, 2462 df). Means with different subscripts differ at $p < .05$. Word count refers to mean number of words per post. % Big words refers to the mean percentage of all words within the posts that are greater than 6 letters. All other means are percentages based on total words per post.

percentage of words for each of the major linguistic categories were subjected to a series of oneway analyses of variance (ANOVAs) with disease status serving as the independent variable. Post-hoc comparisons between groups were computed based on least-squares solutions. As depicted in Table 1, the groups differed significantly along all of the major language dimensions.

Emotion Words

Negative and positive emotion words are based on extensive dictionaries that capture the use of 541 negative and 328 positive words and word stems. Previous studies have found that use of emotion words is highly correlated with judges' ratings of the writers' true emotions. Further, a recent meta-analytic approach examining emotion word use and longterm health based on six previous writing studies indicated that a moderate use of negative emotion words and a high use of positive emotion words were most predictive of longterm health (Pennebaker & Francis, in press). Inspection of the negative and positive emotion word use categories from the internet and AOL posts reveals an intriguing set of patterns. Negative emotion words were used most frequently by the users of the arthritis, diabetes and CFS bulletin boards and the least by the breast and prostate cancer board users. Conversely, those posting on the breast cancer boards had by far the highest percentage of positive emotion word use.

Cognitive Words

In previous studies, individuals' expanding usage of two cognitive categories — insight and causal words — has been correlated with longterm health. That is, the more that people use these terms over the course of their writing within the disclosure studies, the more their health improves. The insight category refers to words that tap self-reflection or higher level thinking. Examples of the 116 words making up this category include realise, understand, consider and think. Causal words are those that attempt to tap causal thinking or overt inference-making. Examples of the 52 words in this dictionary include because, reason, effect and infer.

As can be seen in the table, diabetes use the fewest insight-related words, whereas the CFS, arthritis and breast cancer writers use significantly more of these words. Causal words, on the other hand, are used with the greatest frequency by arthritis and diabetes groups and least by CFS and breast cancer groups. Compared to students writing about traumatic experiences, the means of all the user groups are lower for insight words (users mean = 2.55, disclosure studies mean = 3.26), but comparable for causal words (users = 1.01, disclosure studies = 1.12). The general pattern, then, suggests that all of the groups are searching for meaning and/or are engaged in cognitive effort is somewhat different ways. Whereas the diabetics are using causal language, the breast cancer and CFS users are relying more on insight and self-reflection. Interestingly, the arthritis users tend to use both styles.

Language Composition Variables

The remaining variables in Table 1 tap some standard linguistic categories that have been used previously by psychologists. The use of self-references, for example, is a central feature of Wiener and Mehrabian's (1968) verbal non-immediacy concept. When people use words such as I, my and mine, they are embracing the topic more than if they avoid these terms, "My disease" is certainly more personalised than "that disease". In addition, use of self-reference has also been linked to incidence and mortality from heart disease as well as hostility levels (Barefoot, 1992). Interestingly, CFS and heart disease patients use by far the highest rates of self-references, with diabetics and prostate cancer bulletin board users distancing themselves the most. It should be noted that the overall levels of self-reference use is far below that used by college students writing about personal traumas (bulletin board users = 6.30, disclosure studies mean = 11.30).

Verb tense, too, has been considered to be a marker of verbal non-immediacy. Whereas present tense suggests that individuals are focusing on problems and issues as they are occurring, use of past tense may be a distancing technique to move the topic away from the writers' current psychological space. Whereas arthritis users are most likely to use present tense, the two cancer groups rely on present tense at the lowest rates and, indeed, use past tense verbs at the highest rates.

Negations include words such as no, not, never, can't and don't. According to McClelland (1979), use of negations serve as a verbal form of inhibition. Further, high rates of negations reflect attempts to block basic drives for power. Indeed, McClelland found that negation usage was linked to high blood pressure. In the present study, negations were indeed used most frequently by diabetics, CFS and heart disease uses. Interestingly, the overall rates of negations were quite low in the present samples (mean = 1.80) compared to students writing about emotional traumas (mean = 2.35).

In everyday language, over 4% of all the words we use are articles: a, an, the. In an intriguing paper, Bucci (1995) suggests that article usage is a powerful indicator of concrete thinking. That is, when people are speaking about conceptual, personal and/or emotional topics, nouns are more likely to be named or identified by a pronoun such as "my car" as opposed to "a car". In the present study, prostate cancer, diabetes and CFS user groups used significantly more articles than arthritis and breast cancer groups. Consistent with the self-reference results, all of the user groups employed more articles in their postings (mean = 5.87) than participants in disclosure studies writing about traumas (mean = 4.82).

Finally, Table 1 includes the percentage of words used with six or more letters. This measure simply taps the degree to which writers employ large words — often considered a distancing or intellectualisation technique. As can be seen, breast cancer and CFS users tend to use relatively fewer large words in their writing. Overall, however, the illness user groups tend to use far more words with six or more letters (15.8%) than do students writing about traumas (13.6%).

Profiles of Disease Groups and Their Representations

While the LIWC program offers a systematic way of examining and comparing linguistic patterns, it would be a disservice not to flesh out the character of the exchanges that are skeletally framed by the LIWC findings. Even a casual reading of the groups uncovers markedly different styles of expression which characterise the condition groups. Arthritis patients are clear and serene communicators. Spammers (salespeople promoting untested "miracle" cures) are ignored. Polite requests are made. Helpful hints are requested and extended. Sentences have a consistent length and flow. Painful symptoms are conveyed without drama. Diabetes patients, by contrast, carry a much more strident tone. Their exchanges indicate an extensive understanding of their disorder, sensitivity to criticism or disagreement and occasionally outright hostile tones, towards each other and certainly towards spammers. "Between the lines" is an undercurrent of emotional volatility.

Breast cancer patients are the most engaging of the sampled groups. Their essays contain a degree of warmth and individuation that is unique. They have a nurturing quality towards each other that is quite touching and sometimes even cloying. Consistent with others' observations and despite the well-known torture of the predominant treatment course, they express virtually no negative emotion. Hardships and emotional duress are endured with a loving and patient attitude and much encouragement of others. Their style of expression is strikingly consistent with classic observations in the literature about the coping style of cancer patients in general (e.g., Greer, Morris & Pettingale, 1979; Temoshok & Dreher, 1992).

Individuals suffering from CFS are perplexing. On the one hand, their plight is obviously a serious one, causing much misery and obvious disability. On the other hand, there is a character to their exchanges that can only be described as affected: not snobbish or false, but reactive. More than any others, CFS patients' essays featured discussions of suffering overwhelmingly punctuated with repetitive exclamation points, parenthetical giggles and catastrophic conclusions. How is it that individuals who are too tired to function or to make their children's lunches can write hundreds of words and spend hours at the computer reading the posts by others and comparing symptoms of exhaustion? Skelton (1991) found that when a patient's condition lacks an identifiable organic basis and affects more than one aspect of their functioning (e.g., home, work, relationships), their credibility among health care workers is drastically reduced. One can only speculate that this group's suffering evokes little sympathy in the doctor's office.

Moreover, of all the groups, they have the most rigidly defined boundaries about illness prototypes. This seems ironic in view of its status as a diagnosis of exclusion. Contributors' posts indicate that they are familiar with the latest research and discussions of chronic fatigue: authors who include in their writings suspected psychological factors or psychosocial treatment strategies are viewed as anathema, practically subhuman in their callous and ignorant statements. One sufferer who asked if anyone else had been helped by cognitive-behavioural therapy never received a reply. Another poster who wrote in about her cognitive symptoms ("brain fog") received dozens of comparative comments within a day's time: anecdotes about lost keys, poor typing skills and impaired memory. A potential danger of group support is an unwillingness to tolerate multiple conceptualisations and coping strategies. Such intolerance reduces the kind of information available to group members, distilling and distorting, in turn, the collective illness schema.

Contained in the nearly 4,000 contributions are efforts to gather information, to establish (consensual) disease-specific norms about time-line and consequences, to engage in appropriate monitoring behaviours and to gauge the best identifiable course of action under the circumstances. Patients offer each other good information, on the whole, about short term gains and long term losses, such as stories about their experiences with hazardous side effects of medicines. Diabetics, for instance, offered numerous accounts of negative reactions to different kinds of insulin products and warned each other of the dangers of hypoglycemic reactions. There are also accounts of short term sacrifices and long term gains, such as dietary changes and other lifestyle modifications that are difficult to implement. One arthritic man wrote that removing salt from his diet had assuaged his symptoms. Asymptomatic arthritis is not something that would particularly thrill scientists, but for the patient it is the most prized health outcome and it costs other patients little to try his technique.

Lay models of illness evidenced on the Net are hardly lay models. It is easy to tell that a significant portion of the patients who participate in support groups are collecting information from a scientific perspective as well. They are educated about the methods and measures of key indices relevant to their conditions: blood glucose in the case of diabetics, the Prostate Specific Antigen (PSA) in the case of prostate cancer patients, estrogen positive status or not in the case of breast cancer patients and Rheumatoid Factor in the case of arthritis patients. Patients who have tried alternative approaches to treatment report successes and failures to the others: they are their own laboratories. In the chronic fatigue sample, for instance, some found that Evening Primrose Oil was helpful, others did not. Another patient reported that acupuncture had been helpful and yet another reported that the needles sent her into agonies.

Another interesting feature is what is not tolerated in the groups: support groups are supposed to be non-commercial forums in which patients can exchange information. Non-members who contribute and mention any product or treatment favourably are treated with scorn at best, more often with outrage and carry the quirky appellation of "spammers". Interestingly, a patient who reports about the effects of a product or treatment is not chastised as long as it is prefaced with "Just my experience".

In sum, the models reflected in these support groups represent a different viewpoint, a kind of ongoing, recursive and collective cost-benefit analysis in which their own definitions of living integrity are factored more strongly and uniquely into the health goal equation. Participants want to know how they can avoid aggravating their condition unnecessarily. They exchange information about the suspected role of stress and how to avoid it, dietary concerns, alternative approaches, iatrogenic risks and other habits suspected of driving symptoms. What emerges is a consensual model with some flexibility to allow for individual differences.

CONCLUSIONS AND SUGGESTIONS

This sample represents our first study of support group behaviours and like most exploratory work, raises more questions than answers. Before we discuss implications, it is helpful to review the aims of the study and the unique features of our sample in order to bear in mind what is, and what is not, available in the data as it stands. We know that patients turn to people in their social world to gain information about symptom interpretation and disease management before they consult a doctor (Sanders, 1982). People think and talk and define their lives by personal and social relationships. Models of illness are socially derived (Mechanic, 1972; Sanders, 1982). This reasoning is central to illness representation theory as a social construct (Anderson, 1983) and is consistent with social learning (e.g., Bandura, 1982).

The patients in our sample, by definition, are not passive types looking for a doctor who assumes control, but are active copers, seeking information and support from their peers. Medicine, in its attempts to be objective and removed from the messy contextual considerations of everyday life, has also removed itself from the experiential meaning structure and hence has a hard time gaining a foothold. The patients, then, have eagerly adopted the use of computer support groups to fill the gap left by traditional western medicine. These support groups on the Net are informative sources for naturalistic observation of social processes. The computerised support system constitutes a weak cue, allowing the group to define itself and its concerns.

Using computer-based support groups as reflections of natural social processes is both artificial and, at the same time, a reflection of the real world. The sample is self-selected and so generalisability may be limited. However, the Internet community is growing at such a pace that soon it should not represent such a potential selection bias. Self-selection, however, is inherent in the study of existing mutual support groups. Some kinds of data usually available to researchers is missing: age, race, severity of condition, educational status, physical attractiveness and sometimes even sex. Measurement issues are numerous.

What *is* available is a verbal profile, one that conveys a more complete and natural picture of patient concerns than questionnaires or office visits can uncover. A kind of de-individuation occurs, in which those who might be tempted can make caustic remarks and not suffer the usual social repercussions; and on a more benign note, personal disclosure that might not occur face to face is more easily voiced. Unlike other social gatherings, extroverts cannot dominate the "conversation" because all members are free to post whatever is on their mind. "Listening" time is not dominated by one individual: the participant always has the option of skimming, or totally ignoring, posts that do not appeal to them without offending the "speaker". Thus, group members have maximal flexibility in expressing themselves.

It is important to understand that many studies about illness cognition have been conducted using healthy samples; by contrast, illness perceptions involve what Skelton and Croyle (1991) have termed "hot cognitions". Individuals who have received and lived with a diagnosis have outgrown folk models and become resident experts in their condition. The cultural and experiential contribution is quite potent. There is literally a world of difference between the illness models of a 20-year-old college student, a middle-aged Haitian with hypertension and a 15-year diabetic who surfs the Net, not only in model structure, but in personal appreciation for what the concept really involves.

Bearing that in mind, what observations can we make about the function of social support within the patient's experience of illness and its contribution to their understanding? It is particularly important is that different types of illnesses spur searches for different kinds of information. Breast cancer patients, whose illness springs seemingly out of nowhere, seem to feel the need to make sense out of their illness and to help each other along in the process. They are more reflective overall of the way cancer has changed their outlook on life, their priorities. CFS patients are desperately engaged in a search for biomedical legitimacy. Implicit in their approach is the assumption that psychological factors reduce legitimacy and hence the authenticity of their suffering. Conversely, the conspicuous absence of CHD support behaviours stands as an implicit cognition that they have little of use to learn from other patients and a reticence to discuss their health problems in light of their larger life context. Future work will need to address these questions to assess the validity of our interpretation.

Obviously, patients are not the only ones with illness representations. Doctors, within the context of the health care delivery setting, carry implicit assumptions about disease — that they offer the best solution, that their job is to point out the problem, not to rehabilitate the patient. The health care delivery system treats disease and is geared toward acute treatment strategies. Indeed, Arthur Kleinman (1995) notes: "Biomedicine presses the practitioner to construct disease, disordered biological processes, as the object of study and treatment. There is hardly any place in this narrowly focused therapeutic vision for the patient's experience of suffering." It is no wonder that patients talk to other laypeople about their illness and are reticent to see the doctor — they already know what the doctor has to say. Doctors know how to categorise disease, but are less equipped to help the patient go on living to the best of their ability. Moreover, unless the particular doctor has experienced that disease, their credibility is low. The lay model distinction knife cuts both ways — the doctor is not an expert in the experience of illness, but in the identification of it (for a more thorough discussion of these issues, see Kleinman, 1995).

Could the credibility gap and hence the treatment obstacles, be overcome by having a peer professional around to answer patients' questions and offer support? Even access to the Internet in the physician's office could help bridge the gap between the patient's world and the doctor's? Behavioural medicine studies have indicated that group interventions in the course of chronic illness result in long-term health care utilisation reductions, more than offsetting the cost of such programs (Friedman, Sobel, Myers & Caudill, 1995). Setting up local online groups could facilitate communication among local support groups and enhance their effectiveness. The Internet as an exchange forum, plus the voluntary and in some cases paid participation of doctors on the support groups, may soon serve to demystify the doctor-patient exchange. Moreover, patients who are better informed about what kinds of symptoms are normal, which are alarming, are less anxious, make fewer unnecessary calls to doctors' offices. Moreover, patients' requests for information and support are frequently responded to by multiple participants.

The present project points to a new mode of communication worthy of study. We have also introduced a unique way by which to analyse the language of the ancient internet world. The rich communication patterns we have seen in patients' daily discussions with each other offers a glimpse at the growth and maintenance of illness representations as well as the very heart of social and emotional support. Through closer examination of this evolving process, we should be able to better construct communication processes both in the physician's office and in the natural world of the person suffering from chronic disease.

REFERENCES

Anderson, J. (1983) *The architecture of cognition.* Cambridge, MA: Harvard University Press.

Bandura, A. (1982) Self-efficacy mechanism in human agency. *American Psycholigst,* **37**, 122–147.

Barefoot, J.C. (1992) Developments in the measurement of hostility. In H. Friedman (Ed.), *Hostility, coping and health* (pp. 13–32). Washington, DC: APA Books.

Bishop, G.D. (1987) Lay conceptions of physical symptoms. *Journal of Applied Social Psychology,* **17**, 127–146.

Bishop, G.D. (1991) Lay disease representations and responses to victims of disease. *Basic and Applied Social Psychology,* **12**, 115–132.

Bucci, W. (1995) The power of narrative: a multiple code account. In J.W. Pennebaker (Ed.), *Emotion, disclosure and health* (pp. 93–122). Washington DC: American Psychological Association.

Davis, C.G., Lehman, D.R., Wortman, C.B. & Silver, R.C. (1995) The undoing of traumatic life events. *Personality and Social Psychology Bulletin*, **21**, 109–124.

Ferguson, T. (1996) *Health online*. Reading, Massachusetts: Addison-Wesley.

Francis, M.E. (1993) *Analysis of the language and process dimensions found in personal disclosure: The LIWC approach*. Unpublished doctoral dissertation. Dallas, TX.

Friedman, H.S. & Booth-Kewley, S. (1987) The "disease prone" personality: A meta-analytic view of the construct. *American Psychologist*, **42**, 539–555.

Friedman, R., Sobel, D., Myers, P. & Caudill, M. (1995) Behavioral medicine, clinical health psychology, and cost offset. *Health Psychology*, **14**, 509–518.

Gottschalk, L.A. & Gleser, G.C. (1969) *The measurement of psychological states through the content analysis of verbal behavior*. Berkeley: University of California Press.

Greer, S., Morris, T. & Pettingale, K.W. (1979) Psychological response to breast cancer: Effect on outcome. *Lancet*, **2**, 785–787.

Higgins, E.T., Vookles, J. & Tykocinski, O. (1992) Self and health: How "patterns" of self-beliefs predict types of emotional and physical problems. *Social Cognition*, **10**, 125–150.

Hughes, C.F., Uhlmann, C. & Pennebaker, J.W. (1994) The body's response to processing emotional trauma: linking verbal text with autonomic activity. *Journal of Personality*, **62**, 565–585.

Jacobs, M.K. & Goodman, G. (1989) Psychology and self-help groups: predictions on a partnership. *American Psychologist*, **44**, 536–545.

Kleinman, A. (1995) *Writing at the margins*. Berkeley, CA: University of California Press.

Leventhal, H. (1983) Behavioral medicine: Psychology in health care. In D. Mechanic (Ed.), *Handbook of health, health care and the health professions* (pp. 709–743). New York: Free Press.

McClelland, D. (1979) Inhibited power motivation and high blood pressure in men. *Journal of Abnormal Psychology*, **88**, 182–190.

Mechanic, D. (1972) Social psychological factors affecting the presentation of bodily complaints. *New England Journal of Medicine*, **286**, 1132–1139.

Pennebaker, J.W. (1993) Putting stress into words: Health, linguistic and therapeutic implications. *Behaviour Research and Therapy*, **31**, 539–548.

Pennebaker, J.W. & Francis, M.E. (in press). Cognitive, emotional and language processes in disclosure. *Cognition and emotion.*

Peterson, C., Seligman, M.E.P. & Vaillant, G.E. (1988) Pessimistic explanatory style as a risk factor for physical illness: A thirty-five-year longitudinal study. *Journal of Personality and Social Psychology*, **55**, 23–32.

Sanders, G.S. (1982) Social comparison and perceptions of health and illness. In G. Sanders & J. Suls (Eds.), *Social psychology of health and illness* (pp. 129–157). Hillsdale, NJ: Lawrence, Erlbaum Associates.

Scheier, M.F. & Carver, C.S. (1987) Dispositional optimism and physical well-being: The influence of generalized outcome expectancies on health. *Journal of Personality*, **55**, 169–210.

Skelton, J.A. (1991) Laypersons' judgements of patient credibility and the study of illness representations. In J.A. Skelton & R.T. Croyle (Eds.), *Mental representations in health and illness* (pp. 108–131). New York: Springer-Verlag.

Skelton, J.A. & Croyle, R.T. (1991) Mental representation, health and illness. In J.A. Skelton & R.T. Croyle (Eds.), *Mental representations in health and illness* (pp. 1–6). New York: Springer-Verlag.

Stiles, W.B. (1992) *Describing talk: A taxonomy of verbal response modes.* Newbury Park, CA: Sage.

Temoshok, L. & Dreher, H. (1992) *The Type C connection: The behavioral links to cancer and your health.* New York: Random House.

Watson, D. & Pennebaker, J.W. (1989) Health complaints, stress and distress: Exploring the central role of negative affectivity. *Psychological Review*, **96**, 234–254.

Wiener, M. & Mehrabian, A. (1968) *Language within language: Immediacy, a channel in verbal communication.* New York: Appleton-Century-Crofts.

Index